Damages noted - stain
June 1, 2015 - Sp.

Clinical Masking Procedures

William S. Yacullo

Governors State University
College of Health Professions

Allyn and Bacon
Boston • London • Toronto • Sydney • Tokyo • Singapore

Series Editor: Kris Farnsworth
Editorial Assistant: Christine M. Shaw
Editorial-Production Administrator: Joe Sweeney
Editorial-Production Service: Walsh Associates
Composition Buyer: Linda Cox
Manufacturing Buyer: Aloka Rathnam
Cover Administrator: Suzanne Harbison

Library of Congress Cataloging-in-Publication Data

Yacullo, William Saverio.
    Clinical masking procedures / William S. Yacullo.
        p.   cm.
    Includes bibliographical references and index.
    ISBN 0-205-17352-7
    1. Auditory masking.   I. Title
RF294.5.M37Y33   1995
617.8′075—dc20   95-35670
                                                                            CIP

Printed in the United States of America

10 9 8 7 6 5 4 3 2 1   00 99 98 97 96 95

Contents

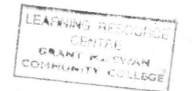

A Note to the Reader

There is considerable variability across clinics in the report form that is used for recording the results of the basic audiologic evaluation (i.e., pure-tone audiometry, speech audiometry, and acoustic immittance measurements). This book will use the audiologic assessment worksheet presented at the end of this introductory section. It includes a pure-tone audiogram, a key for audiometric symbols, commonly used audiometric abbreviations, and a table for reporting the results of speech audiometry.

Although pure-tone air- and bone-conduction thresholds can be recorded either in tabular or graphic form, graphic representation appears to be the standard way in which pure-tone audiometric results are typically reported (ASHA, 1990). ASHA (1990) has published new guidelines for audiometric symbols and procedures for graphic representation of frequency-specific audiometric findings, superseding those published by ASHA in 1974. The pure-tone audiogram and audiometric symbols used in this book are those recommended by ASHA (1990).

Contralateral masking is sometimes required when obtaining pure-tone bone-conduction and air-conduction thresholds. Different symbols are used to represent pure-tone thresholds obtained with and without contralateral masking. It should be noted that unmasked bone-conduction thresholds can be represented in two ways: *specified* and *unspecified*. First, a different bone-conduction symbol can be used depending upon whether the vibrator is placed at the right (i.e., <) or left (i.e., >) mastoid process. In other words, location of the bone vibrator is specified. *These symbols only indicate mastoid placement and not the source of the response.* Second, unmasked bone-conduction thresholds can be plotted in a way that does not suggest that the response is originating from either ear: Location of the vibrator and origin of the response are unspecified. ASHA recommends the use of an upside down "V" (i.e., ∧) for unspecified bone-conduction thresholds. You will encounter both types of unmasked bone conduction symbols in clinical practice.

When masked pure-tone thresholds are obtained, it is traditional to record the maximum masking level used at each frequency. The audiologic assessment worksheet includes a table that can be used for reporting effective masking levels in the nontest (i.e., masked) ear during air- and bone-conduction pure-tone audiometry.

The results of speech audiometry are typically presented in tabular form. The speech audiometry table used throughout this book includes space for reporting the pure-tone average (PTA), speech recognition threshold (SRT), speech detection threshold (SDT), most comfortable loudness (MCL), and loudness discomfort level (LDL); all measures traditionally are reported in dB Hearing Level (HL). The results of suprathreshold speech recognition testing are reported typically in terms of test used, sensation level (SL), and percent (%) correct achieved. Space is also provided for reporting effective masking levels used in the nontest ear during speech audiometric measures.

It is assumed that the reader is already knowledgeable of the concepts, administration, and interpretation of the basic audiologic evaluation. The following textbooks provide excellent reviews of the topic:

Kaplan, H., Gladstone, V.S., & Lloyd, L.L. (1993). *Audiometric interpretation: A manual of basic audiometry* (2nd ed.). Needham Heights, MA: Allyn & Bacon.

Katz, J. (Ed.). (1994). *Handbook of clinical audiology* (4th ed.). Baltimore: Williams & Wilkins.

Konkle, D.F., & Rintelmann, W.F. (Eds.). (1983). *Principles of speech audiometry.* Baltimore: University Park Press.

Rintelmann, W.F. (Ed.). (1991). *Hearing assessment* (2nd ed.). Needham Heights, MA: Allyn & Bacon.

Silman, S., & Silverman, C.A. (1991). *Auditory diagnosis: Principles and applications.* San Diego: Academic Press.

The American Speech-Language-Hearing Association has published many guidelines regarding procedures for audiologic assessment. Review of the following ASHA guidelines is recommended.

American Speech and Hearing Association. (1978). Guidelines for manual pure-tone audiometry. *ASHA, 20,* 297–301.

American Speech-Language-Hearing Association. (1988). Guidelines for determining threshold level for speech. *ASHA, 30,* 85–89.

American Speech-Language-Hearing Association. (1990). Guidelines for audiometric symbols. *ASHA, 32,* Supplement 2, 25–30.

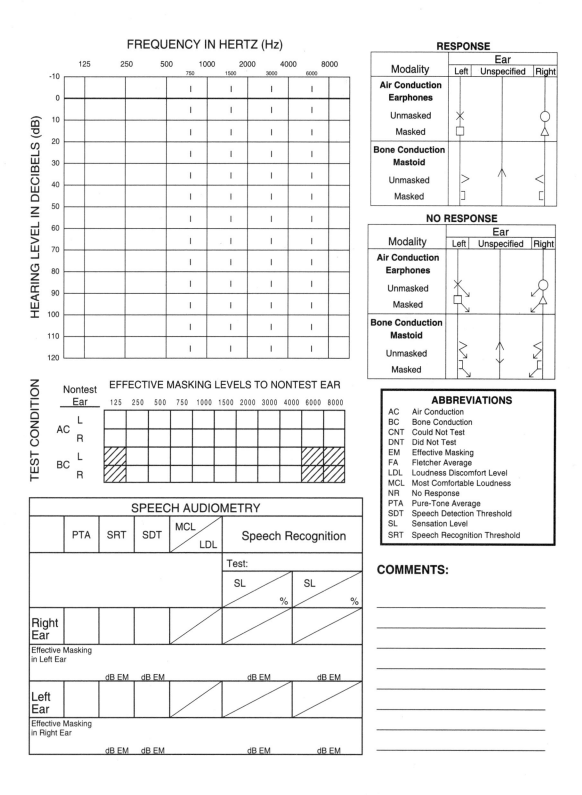

The audiologic assessment worksheet used throughout this book. The audiogram and audiometric symbols are those recommended by the American Speech-Language-Hearing Association (1990) for use during unmasked and masked pure-tone audiometry.

1
The Need for Masking

One of the major objectives of the basic audiological evaluation is to assess the auditory function of each ear independently of the other. There are some situations during both air-conduction and bone-conduction testing when this may not occur. Although a pure-tone or speech stimulus is being presented through a transducer to the test ear, the nontest ear can contribute partially or totally to the observed response. Whenever it is suspected that this is occurring during the evaluation of the test ear, a masking stimulus must be applied to the nontest ear to eliminate its participation.

There are situations during both air-conduction and bone-conduction testing when the nontest ear can contribute to a response from the test ear. Let us first consider the need for masking during air-conduction testing.

Air-Conduction Testing

Figure 1-1 illustrates how a signal presented to the test ear can reach the nontest (i.e., opposite) cochlea. Conventional supra-aural earphones (e.g., TDH-39, 49, or 50 transducers encased in MX-41/AR or Telephonics Model 51 cushions) have been placed on both ears. A pure-tone signal is presented to the test ear. If the intensity at the test earphone is sufficiently high, the nontest ear can be stimulated. This can occur in two ways. First, the air-conduction transducer can vibrate sufficiently to cause deformations of the bones of the skull. Recall that the supra-aural earphones have been coupled to the side of the skull. The outcome is stimulation of the nontest cochlea through *bone conduction*. The supra-aural earphone can function as a bone vibrator at very high intensities.

Second, sound can leak from under the test earphone, travel around the head to the nontest ear, overcome the attenuation provided by the nontest earphone, and finally reach the nontest cochlea through the normal *air-conduction* route. Thus, sound presented to the test ear can reach the nontest cochlea through both bone-conduction and air-conduction pathways.

A brief discussion of the term *attenuation* is in order. Very simply, attenuation refers to reduction of energy. *Interaural attenuation* (IA) refers to the reduction of sound energy "between ears," that is, from the test ear to the nontest ear. More specifically, it is the difference in decibels between the level of the signal at the test ear and the level at the opposite cochlea:

$$\text{Interaural attenuation} = \text{dB level}_{\text{test ear}} - \text{dB level}_{\text{nontest cochlea}}$$

Consider the two hypothetical examples presented in Figure 1-2.

1

FIGURE 1–1   Schematic diagram illustrating how sound presented to the test ear through a conventional supra-aural earphone can stimulate the nontest cochlea. There are both air-conduction and bone-conduction pathways between the signal presented at the test ear and reaching the nontest cochlea.

Adapted from G. A. Studebaker, "Clinical masking," 1979. In W. F. Rintelmann (Ed.), *Hearing assessment* (pp. 51-100). Baltimore, MD: University Park Press. Reprinted by permission.

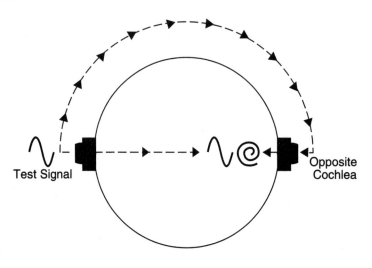

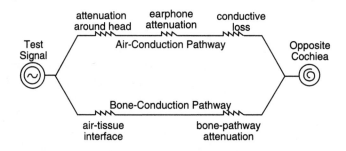

Example 1: A pure-tone signal of 90 dB HL (Hearing Level) is being presented to the test ear (Figure 1-2*A*). If 40 dB HL is reaching the nontest cochlea, then a portion of the test signal is being attenuated before it reaches the opposite ear. Because the test signal has been attenuated 50 dB before it reaches the opposite cochlea, interaural attenuation is considered to be 50 dB.

$$IA = dB \ level_{test \ ear} - dB \ level_{nontest \ cochlea}$$
$$= 90 \ dB \ HL - 40 \ dB \ HL$$
$$= 50 \ dB$$

Example 2: A pure-tone signal of 90 dB HL is being presented to the test ear (Figure 1-2*B*). If only 15 dB HL is reaching the nontest cochlea, then interaural attenuation is 75 dB.

FIGURE 1–2   Interaural attenuation (IA) is the difference between the level of the signal at the test ear and the level at the opposite cochlea. A pure-tone signal of 90 dB HL is being presented to the test ear through conventional supra-aural earphones. *Case A:* If 40 dB HL is reaching the nontest cochlea, then interaural attenuation is equal to 50 dB. *Case B:* If only 15 dB HL is reaching the nontest cochlea, then interaural attenuation is equal to 75 dB.

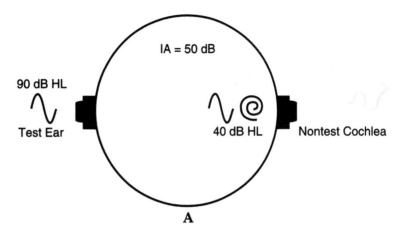

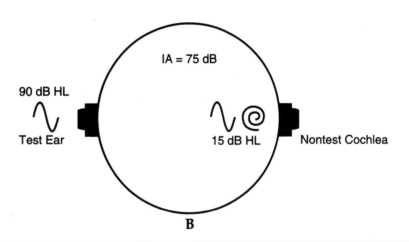

$$IA = dB\ level_{test\ ear} - dB\ level_{nontest\ cochlea}$$
$$= 90\ dB\ HL - 15\ dB\ HL$$
$$= 75\ dB$$

Ideally, large interaural attenuation is desirable during audiological testing. In fact, if interaural attenuation exceeded the equipment limits of the audiometer (e.g., 120 dB HL), masking would never be required. Unfortunately, this is not the case.

Interaural attenuation during earphone testing depends on three factors: individual subject, frequency spectrum of the test signal, and transducer type. Generally, interaural attenuation increases as the contact area of the transducer with the listener's head decreases (Zwislocki, 1953). More specifically, interaural attenuation is greater for supra-aural than circumaural earphones. Conversely, interaural attenuation is greatest for insert receivers (Killion, Wilber, & Gudmundsen, 1985; Sklare & Denenberg, 1987), partly because of their smaller contact area with the skull. Our discussion will concentrate on supra-aural earphones because they are the most frequently used clinically. The principles of clinical masking when using insert earphones are discussed in Chapter 8.

Although there are different approaches to measurement of interaural attenuation for air-conducted sound (e.g., "masking" method, method of "best beats," "compensation" method; see Zwislocki, 1953, for further discussion), the most direct approach involves measurement of *transcranial thresholds* (Berrett, 1973). Specifically, interaural attenuation (IA) is measured by obtaining unmasked air-conduction thresholds in individuals with unilateral, profound sensorineural hearing impairment and then calculating the difference between the normal and impaired ears:

$$IA = \text{Unmasked AC threshold}_{\text{impaired ear}} - \text{AC threshold}_{\text{normal ear}}$$

For example, if an *unmasked* air-conduction threshold is obtained at 65 dB HL in the impaired ear (i.e., the ear with a profound, sensorineural hearing loss) and at 5 dB HL in the normal ear, then interaural attenuation is calculated as 60 dB:

$$IA = 65 \text{ dB HL} - 5 \text{ dB HL}$$
$$= 60 \text{ dB}$$

There is the assumption that air- and bone-conduction thresholds are equal (i.e., no air-bone gaps) in the ear with normal hearing.

Table 1-1 presents interaural attenuation values for pure-tone air-conducted signals using traditional supra-aural earphones. Interaural attenuation values vary across frequency and subject, ranging from about 40 to 80 dB. Because of this very great range, Studebaker (1967a) recommends that the smallest interaural attenuation value reported (i.e., 40 dB) should be used when making decisions about the need for masking during audiological testing. This recommendation is supported by others (e.g., ASHA, 1978; Martin, 1994; Sanders, 1991). Use of a conservative interaural attenuation value of 40 dB will take into account all individuals, although it will result in the unnecessary use of masking in some instances. According to a recent survey of audiological practices in the United States, the majority of audiologists use a value of 40 dB when making a decision about the need for masking during air-conduction testing (Martin, Armstrong, & Champlin, 1994). In summary, a conservative estimate of interaural attenuation for pure-tone air-conducted sound using supra-aural earphones is 40 dB.

It should be noted that the majority of audiologists in the United States also typically use a value of 40 dB as an estimate of interaural attenuation for air-conducted speech (Martin et al., 1994) However, there are important additional variables that should be considered when selecting a value of interaural attenuation for speech. These factors will be addressed in greater detail in Chapter 4.

Bone-Conduction Testing

There are two possible locations for placement of the bone vibrator during pure-tone threshold testing—the mastoid process and the frontal bone (i.e., forehead). Although there is some evidence that forehead placement yields more reliable and valid thresholds than mastoid placement (see Dirks, 1994, for

TABLE 1–1 Range of interaural attenuation values (in dB) for pure-tone air-conducted signals using conventional supra-aural earphones.

Study	Transducer	Number of Subjects	Frequency (Hz)										
			125	250	500	750	1000	1500	2000	3000	4000	6000	8000
Berrett (1973)	TDH-39	N = 8	—	48–54	52–61	—	57–66	—	62–64	—	—	—	—
Chaiklin (1967)	TDH-39	N = 5	32–45	44–58	54–65	62–71	57–66	45–76	55–72	56–72	61–85	56–76	51–69
Coles & Priede (1970)	Not reported	N = 20	—	50–80	45–80	—	40–85	—	45–75	—	50–85	—	—
Killion, Wilber, & Gudmundsen (1985)	TDH-39	N = 6	—	45–65	52–65	53–65	52–65	47–65	50–68	50–68	52–74	—	—
Sklare & Denenberg (1987)	TDH-49P	N = 7	—	45–60	45–75	55–75	60–65	50–65	45–70	45–70	60–75	50–80	—
Snyder (1973)	TDH-39	N = 256	—	35–70	45–75	—	40–75	—	40–80	—	40–85	—	40–80

FIGURE 1–3   Schematic diagram illustrating how a signal presented through a bone vibrator placed at the mastoid process of the test ear can reach the nontest cochlea.

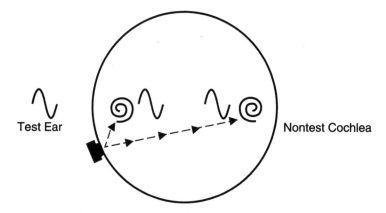

a review), the majority (97 percent) of audiologists in the United States use a mastoid placement (Martin et al., 1994). Figure 1-3 illustrates how a signal presented through a bone vibrator placed at the mastoid process of the test ear can reach the nontest cochlea. Although the bone vibrator is placed on the side of the test ear, it cannot be assumed that an observed response is in fact from the test ear. Consider that both cochleas are housed within temporal bones of the same skull. When a bone vibrator, regardless of its location, sets the bones of the skull into vibration, both cochleas can be stimulated. During unmasked bone-conduction audiometry, it will be the better cochlea (or both if they are equally sensitive) that will respond. It is generally agreed that interaural attenuation for bone-conducted sound is negligible and should be considered 0 dB (e.g., Dirks, 1994; Hood, 1960; Sanders & Rintelmann, 1964; Studebaker, 1967a).

Consider the situation in which a bone vibrator is placed at the right mastoid process (see Figure 1-4). A pure-tone signal of 30 dB HL is presented. Because interaural attenuation for bone-conducted sound is considered to be zero, then 30 dB HL theoretically is reaching both cochleas. Although the vibra-

FIGURE 1–4   An example illustrating how a pure-tone signal presented through a bone vibrator placed at the mastoid process of the test ear can reach the nontest cochlea. It is generally agreed that interaural attenuation for bone-conducted sound can be as small as 0 dB. If a pure-tone signal of 30 dB HL is presented through a bone vibrator placed at the mastoid process of the test ear, theoretically 30 dB HL is reaching both cochleas.

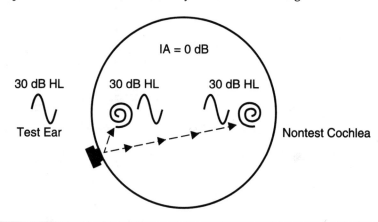

FIGURE 1–5   Expected unmasked pure-tone air-conduction thresholds in an individual with normal hearing in the right ear and no measurable hearing in the left ear. A "shadow curve" will result in the left ear; that is, unmasked thresholds in the left ear will "shadow" the bone conduction thresholds in the right ear by the amount of interaural attenuation.

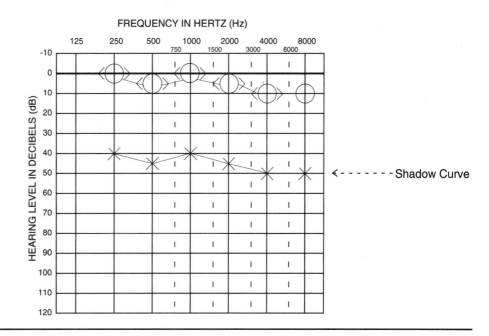

tor is placed at the right mastoid process, it cannot be assumed that the right ear is responding. In summary, a conservative estimate of interaural attenuation for bone-conducted sound, regardless of placement of the bone vibrator, is 0 dB.

As the above discussion illustrates, each ear is not always completely isolated during audiological testing. Therefore, interaural attenuation for air- and bone-conducted sound must always be considered. There will be situations when the nontest ear will contribute to the observed response. *Cross hearing* (or *cross over*) refers to the situation in which a stimulus presented to the test ear is perceived in the nontest ear; it is the consequence of limited interaural attenuation. Cross hearing occurs most frequently during audiological assessment when a substantial difference in hearing sensitivity between the two ears exists or when a stimulus is presented at high suprathreshold intensity levels (e.g., suprathreshold tests of speech recognition).

Figure 1-5 illustrates the expected *unmasked* pure-tone air-conduction thresholds in an individual with normal hearing in the right ear and no measurable hearing in the left ear (i.e., a profound sensorineural hearing loss). A *shadow curve* will result in the left ear; that is, unmasked air-conduction thresholds in the left ear "shadow" the bone-conduction thresholds in the right ear by the amount of interaural attenuation. If we assume that interaural attenuation for air-conducted sound is equal to 40 dB, then unmasked thresholds in the left ear will occur 40 dB above the bone-conduction thresholds in the right ear. The unmasked air-conduction thresholds in the left ear are not valid measures of hearing; rather, they reflect cross-hearing responses from the right ear. Assuming that interaural attenuation for bone conduction is zero, then unmasked bone-conduction thresholds obtained with the bone vibrator placed at the left mastoid process would occur at the same hearing levels for the right ear (i.e., 0 to 10 dB HL). The consequence of obtaining only unmasked thresholds in this situation should be apparent—misdiagnosis of hearing loss. Unmasked thresholds in the left ear would suggest a moderate conductive hearing loss, when in fact there is a profound sensorineural hearing impairment. Misdiagnosis of both type and degree of hearing loss would result. The solution to this situation is simple: Obtain *masked* air- and bone-conduction thresholds in the left ear. That is, masking should be applied to the better ear (i.e., right ear) to eliminate its participation while determining thresholds in the poorer ear (i.e., left ear).

Summary

A major goal of the basic audiological evaluation is the individual assessment of the auditory function of each ear. There are situations during both air-conduction and bone-conduction audiometry, however, when the nontest ear can contribute partially or totally to the observed response from the test ear.

Interaural attenuation refers to the reduction of energy between ears. Specifically, it is the decibel difference between the level of the signal at the test ear and the level at the opposite cochlea. A conservative estimate of interaural attenuation for pure-tone air-conducted sound using conventional supra-aural earphones is 40 dB. A conservative estimate of interaural attenuation for bone-conducted sound, regardless of vibrator placement, is 0 dB. *Cross hearing* occurs when a stimulus presented to the test ear is perceived in the nontest ear. Because there is limited interaural attenuation during both air- and bone-conduction testing, there will be situations in which the nontest ear can contribute to a response from the test ear. Whenever it is suspected that the nontest ear is responsive during evaluation of the test ear, a masking stimulus should be applied to the nontest ear to eliminate its participation.

Study Questions

1. Describe the two mechanisms by which an air-conducted sound presented to the test ear through a conventional supra-aural earphone can stimulate the nontest cochlea.

2. Define interaural attenuation. Is small or large interaural attenuation desirable during audiological testing? Explain why.

3. Is interaural attenuation for air-conducted sound greater for supra-aural or insert earphones? Explain your answer.

4. Interaural attenuation for air-conducted sound can be directly measured by obtaining transcranial thresholds. Briefly describe this procedure.

5. What is the range of interaural attenuation values reported for pure-tone air-conducted sound using conventional supra-aural earphones? Given this range of values, what is considered a conservative estimate of interaural attenuation for air-conducted sound?

6. What is a conservative estimate of interaural attenuation for bone-conducted sound?

7. Define cross hearing. Explain why cross hearing occurs.

8. What is a shadow curve?

9. Explain why a masking stimulus is applied to the nontest ear during an audiological evaluation.

2
Masking Theory

When we talk about masking phenomena, we are interested in how sensitivity for one sound is affected by the presence of another sound. Consider the following example. We have determined that threshold for a 1000 Hz pure-tone signal is 30 dB HL (Hearing Level). Another sound, white noise, for example, is now presented simultaneously. Pure-tone threshold is redetermined in the presence of the second stimulus. Threshold increases to 50 dB HL. Sensitivity to the pure-tone stimulus has been reduced by the presence of the white noise; it was necessary to increase the level of the pure tone to reach threshold. This increase in threshold of one sound in the presence of another is termed *masking*. The American National Standards Institute (ANSI) defines masking as follows:

1. The process by which the threshold of audibility for one sound is raised by the presence of another (masking sound)
2. The amount by which the threshold of audibility of a sound is raised by the presence of another (masking) sound

(ANSI S3.6-1989, p. 3)

In the above example, pure-tone threshold was raised from 30 dB HL (in quiet) to 50 dB HL (in the presence of the second stimulus). The threshold shift is 20 dB; the second stimulus has produced 20 dB of masking.

Masking is used clinically whenever it is suspected that the nontest ear is participating in the evaluation of the test ear. The purpose of masking is to sufficiently raise the threshold of the nontest ear so that its contribution to a response from the test ear is eliminated. Masking reduces sensitivity of the nontest ear to the test stimulus.

Masking Noise Selection

Any sound potentially can have a masking effect on another sound. Diagnostic audiometers typically provide three types of masking noise: narrow-band noise, speech spectrum noise, and white noise. Our clinical goal is to select a masker that is efficient (Hood, 1960). An efficient masker is one that produces a given effective level of masking with the least overall intensity. Stated differently, an efficient masker produces the greatest threshold shift with the least overall intensity.

A brief discussion of the classic masking experiment conducted by Fletcher in 1940 will help us to better understand this concept of masker efficiency. Recall our previous example of a 1000 Hz pure tone masked by white noise.

White noise is a broadband signal containing energy across all frequencies at approximately equal intensities. (It must be kept in mind that the acoustic spectrum of white noise will be shaped or influenced by the frequency response of the transducer.) White noise, because of its broadband spectrum, has the potential to mask pure-tone stimuli of all frequencies (Hawkins & Stevens, 1950). Which frequency components of the noise contribute to the masking of a pure-tone stimulus? Do all components contribute to the masking of the tone, or is there a certain limited or critical bandwidth of the noise that produces masking? These are the questions that Fletcher wanted to answer in his classic experiment.

Fletcher conducted what is known as a *centered masking* experiment. Initially, a very narrow band of noise was centered around a pure-tone signal. The bandwidth of the masking noise was progressively widened, and the masking effect on the pure-tone signal was measured. Fletcher observed that the masked threshold of the pure tone increased as the bandwidth of the masking noise was widened. However, once the noise band reached a certain "critical bandwidth," further widening of the band did not result in additional masking of the pure tone. Thus, Fletcher demonstrated that only a certain critical bandwidth within the white noise actually contributed to the masking of a pure tone at the center of that band.

This concept of the critical band as first described by Fletcher consists of two parts:

1. When masking a pure tone with broadband noise, the only components of the noise that have a masking effect on the tone are those frequencies included within a narrow band centered around the frequency of the tone.

2. When a pure tone is just audible in the presence of the noise, the total noise power present in the narrow band of frequencies is equal to the power of the tone.

The first part of the critical band concept has clinical implications when selecting an appropriate masker during pure-tone audiometry. White noise is an adequate masker for pure-tone stimuli. Yet it contains noise components that do not add to the effectiveness of the masker. Those additional noise components outside of the critical bandwidth only add to the overall intensity of the masking stimulus. The most efficient masker is a narrow band of noise with a bandwidth slightly greater than the critical band surrounding the tone. A narrow-band noise centered at the test frequency is the most efficient masker because it provides the greatest masking effect with the least overall intensity.

This concept is illustrated in the results of an experiment conducted by Sanders and Rintelmann (1964). Figure 2-1 presents masking audiograms obtained with three types of masking noise (sawtooth noise, white noise, and narrow-band noise) at three intensity levels (50 dB, 70 dB, and 90 dB SPL). Specifically, masked pure-tone threshold (in dB HL) is plotted as a function of pure-tone frequency; the parameter is masker type. For a given intensity level, narrow-band noise consistently produces a greater masking effect (about 10–20 dB) than does white noise. (Sawtooth noise is a complex stimulus that typically is not found on current diagnostic or portable audiometers. As the data of Sanders and Rintelmann clearly demonstrate, sawtooth noise is a very inefficient masker of pure-tone stimuli, particularly in the middle and high frequencies.) According to a recent survey of audiological practices in the United States, almost all audiologists use narrow-band noise as a masker during pure-tone audiometry (Martin, Armstrong, & Champlin, 1994).

FIGURE 2–1 Masking audiograms obtained with three types of masking noise at three intensity levels. For a given intensity level, narrow-band noise consistently produces a greater masking effect.

From "Masking in audiometry: A clinical evaluation of three methods" by J.W. Sanders and W.F. Rintelmann, 1964, *Archives of Otolaryngology, 80,* 541-556. Reprinted by permission. Copyright © 1964, American Medical Association.

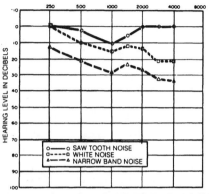

AUDIOGRAM 1 MASKED THRESHOLDS OBTAINED WITH AN OVERALL
INTENSITY LEVEL OF 50 dB SPL.

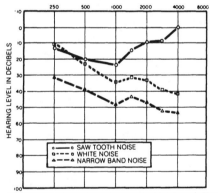

AUDIOGRAM 2 MASKED THRESHOLDS OBTAINED WITH AN OVERALL
INTENSITY LEVEL OF 70 dB SPL.

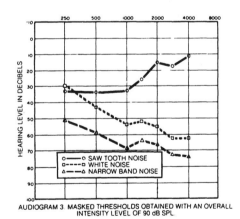

AUDIOGRAM 3. MASKED THRESHOLDS OBTAINED WITH AN OVERALL
INTENSITY LEVEL OF 90 dB SPL.

The need for masking may also arise during speech audiometry. Just as with pure-tone stimuli, speech presented monaurally through earphones can cross over from the test ear to the nontest ear once intensity is sufficiently high. Speech is a broadband signal and therefore requires a broadband masker. Although white noise is an acceptable masker, there is another type of broadband noise that is more efficient. Speech spectrum noise is white noise that has been filtered to simulate the long-term average spectrum of conversational speech. The average spectrum of speech contains the greatest energy in the low frequencies, with the spectrum level decreasing as a function of increasing frequency (Dunn & White, 1940). The American National Standards Institute (ANSI S3.6-1989) specifies that if an audiometer provides "weighted random noise for speech," the sound pressure spectrum level (i.e., energy per Hz or level per cycle) should be constant from 250 through 1000 Hz, falling off at a rate of 12 dB per octave from 1000 through 4000 Hz. Speech spectrum noise has a more limited bandwidth than white noise. It is a more efficient masker than white noise, producing a masking advantage of 8 dB (Konkle & Berry, 1983). Martin et al. (1994) reported that the majority (approximately 95 percent) of audiologists in the United States use speech spectrum noise as a masker during speech audiometry.

Calibration of Effective Masking Level

A question that needs to be addressed is how the intensity level of a masker will be specified clinically. Recall that the intensity of pure-tone and speech stimuli are specified clinically relative to average normal hearing, that is, dB HL. We could also use dB HL when specifying the intensity of a masking stimulus. However, this is not a meaningful reference. We are not interested in average normal hearing for the masking noise, rather, we are concerned with the *effect* of the masking stimulus on the test signal. When we present a masking noise to the nontest ear, we are not interested in average normal hearing for the stimulus or its sound pressure level. We are interested in how much masking a masking stimulus produces.

A direct approach involves specifying the intensity level of a masker in dB Effective Masking Level (dB EM). ANSI (1989) defines effective masking as follows:

> The level of a band of noise, whose geometric center frequency coincides with a specified pure tone, that masks the pure tone to 50% probability of detection. The hearing level reference of the masking signal is equal to that of the pure tone (ANSI S3.6-1989, p. 3).

Stated differently, effective masking refers to:

1. The dB HL to which threshold is shifted by a given level of noise, or,
2. The amount of threshold shift re 0 dB HL provided by a given level of noise.

This definition of effective masking is used relatively consistently throughout the masking literature (Hodgson, 1980; Sanders, 1972, 1978, 1991; Studebaker, 1979).

A contralateral masking paradigm is used clinically during audiological assessment. That is, the signal is presented to the test ear, and the masker is presented to the contralateral or nontest ear. An ipsilateral paradigm is created when the signal and masker are presented to the same ear. The following two examples of ipsilateral masking will help facilitate an understanding of effective masking.

Example 1: A 1000-Hz pure tone is presented through a supra-aural earphone to the right ear. Threshold is obtained at 0 dB HL. A narrow-band noise centered at 1000 Hz is then presented to the same ear; sound pressure level (SPL) of the noise is 65 dB. Pure-tone threshold is reestablished in the presence of the narrow-band noise, and threshold shifts to 50 dB HL. This given level of noise (i.e., 65 dB SPL) has produced a threshold shift of 50 dB relative to 0 dB HL; stated differently, this level of noise has shifted threshold to 50 dB HL. This level of noise can be specified, therefore, as 50 dB EM.

Example 2: A 1000-Hz pure tone is presented through a supra-aural earphone to the left ear. Threshold is obtained at 30 dB HL. A narrow-band noise centered at 1000 Hz is then presented to the same ear; sound pressure level of the noise is again 65 dB. Pure-tone threshold is reestablished in the presence of the narrow-band noise, and the threshold is shifted to 50 dB HL. As in Example 1, this given level of noise (i.e., 65 dB SPL) has produced a threshold shift of 50 dB relative to 0 dB HL. It has shifted the pure-tone threshold to 50 dB HL. This level of noise can be specified, therefore, as 50 dB EM.

The above two examples illustrate two important points.

1. A given level of effective masking will shift all unmasked thresholds to the same dB HL. For example, a masker of 75 dB EM will shift all unmasked thresholds to 75 dB HL. Unmasked pure-tone thresholds of 0 dB, 20 dB, 40 dB HL, and so on, will all be shifted to 75 dB HL in the presence of 75 dB EM. Of course, if unmasked pure-tone threshold is greater than a particular level of effective masking, then no threshold shift will occur (e.g., 75 dB EM will not have a masking effect if the unmasked pure-tone threshold is 85 dB HL).

2. Effective masking refers to the amount of threshold shift *only relative to 0 dB HL.* We know that 50 dB EM will shift the unmasked pure-tone threshold to 50 dB HL. It will produce a threshold shift of 50 dB only if the unmasked pure-tone threshold is 0 dB HL. In the above two examples, a masker of 50 dB EM shifted the threshold by 50 dB when the unmasked threshold was 0 dB HL and 20 dB when the unmasked threshold was 30 dB HL. It should be noted that when unmasked threshold was 30 dB HL, a masker of 50 dB EM did not shift threshold by 50 dB. Rather, it shifted the threshold to 50 dB HL, resulting in a 20-dB threshold shift. It is important to remember that a given level of effective masking does not always correspond to the amount of threshold shift. This will occur only when the unmasked threshold is 0 dB HL.[1]

Figure 2-2 presents hypothetical data illustrating the masking effect of two types of maskers on pure-tone threshold. The pure-tone threshold (in dB HL) is plotted as a function of the effective masking level (in dB EM) for two types of maskers—narrow-band noise and broadband noise. The sound pressure level of each masker is also noted. Pure-tone threshold in the absence of masking noise is 0 dB HL. This figure illustrates two important points about masking. First, narrow-band noise is a more efficient masker of pure-tone stimuli than broadband noise. For example, when narrow-band noise is set at 30 dB SPL, the pure-tone threshold shifts to 10 dB HL; when broadband noise is set at 45 dB SPL, the pure-tone threshold also shifts to 10 dB EM. Effective masking level for both maskers, therefore, is 10 dB EM. Narrow-band noise is the more effective (or efficient) masker because it produces the same masking effect (i.e.,

FIGURE 2–2   Hypothetical data illustrating the effect of two types of maskers on pure-tone threshold. Pure-tone threshold (in dB HL) is plotted as a function of effective masking level (in dB EM) for narrow-band and broadband noise maskers. The sound pressure level for each masker corresponding to dB effective masking is also presented.

Adapted from "Masking in speech audiometry" by D.F. Konkle and G.A. Berry, 1983. In D.F. Konkle & W. F. Rintelmann (Eds.), *Principles of Speech Audiometry* (pp. 285-319). Baltimore, MD: University Park Press. Adapted by permission.

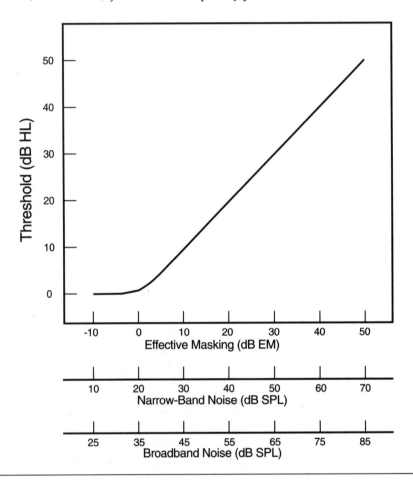

unmasked pure-tone threshold is shifted to 10 dB HL) at a lower sound pressure level. Second, masking is a linear phenomenon. That is, with every decibel increase in masker level, there is an equivalent decibel increase in the masked pure-tone threshold. For example, with every 10-dB increment in the masker level, there is a 10-dB increase in the pure-tone threshold.

Speech spectrum noise can also be calibrated in effective masking level. Just as dB HL for speech is calibrated relative to the speech recognition threshold (SRT), dB EM is also referenced to the SRT. Specifically, effective masking for speech refers to the dB HL to which the speech recognition threshold is shifted by a given level of noise. Consider the following example. An individual has an SRT of 0 dB HL. Speech spectrum noise of a given sound pressure level is presented ipsilaterally, and SRT is reestablished. The SRT shifts to 40 dB HL. The effective masking level of this given level of noise, therefore, is 40 dB EM.

The use of an effective masking level to specify contralateral masking greatly simplifies clinical masking procedures. When a masking stimulus is calibrated in effective masking, the level indicated on the masking-noise intensity dial will specify the masking effect produced in the nontest ear. The instructional manual for an audiometer will indicate the manner in which the masker intensity is calibrated. If the masking stimuli provided by an audiometer meet specifications outlined in the current American National Standards Institute specification for audiometers (ANSI S3.6-1989), then masking level will be calibrated in dB EM. Current audiometers are manufactured to meet performance specifications of this new standard.

ANSI (S3.6-1989) states that if an audiometer provides narrow-band masking, then the noise bands must be centered geometrically around the test tones. Specifically, the standard provides for each test frequency an acceptable range of upper and lower cut-off frequencies for narrow-band maskers. If the spectral density of the narrow-band noise meets the specified band limits, and the sound pressure level in each one-third octave band centered at each frequency is calibrated to a level 3 dB above the reference equivalent threshold level at the test frequency, then masking level for pure tones is calibrated in dB EM. For example, the standard reference equivalent threshold sound pressure level at 1000 Hz for a Telephonics TDH-50 supra-aural earphone is 7.5 dB. If narrow-band noise of ANSI-specified spectral density characteristics is calibrated to 10.5 dB SPL (i.e., reference level of 7.5 dB plus 3 dB), then the masker level is specified in dB EM (i.e., 0 dB EM). These recommended band limits and sound pressure levels for narrow-band maskers are based on critical band data originally reported by Fletcher (1940).

Similarly, weighted random noise used for masking speech should also meet performance specifications described by ANSI (S3.6-1989). If the speech spectrum noise has spectral density characteristics as specified by ANSI (i.e., spectrum density that is constant from 250 through 1000 Hz with spectrum level falling off at a rate of 12 dB/octave from 1000 through 4000 Hz) and if sound pressure level is calibrated to the standard reference sound pressure level for speech (i.e., 12.5 dB above the 1000 Hz standard reference sound pressure level threshold), then the masker level for speech is calibrated in dB EM (Wilber, personal communication, 1992). For example, the standard reference equivalent threshold sound pressure level at 1000 Hz for a Telephonics TDH-50 supra-aural earphone is 7.5 dB. Therefore, the standard reference sound pressure level for speech is specified as 20 dB SPL (i.e., reference level of 7.5 dB SPL at 1000 Hz plus 12.5 dB). If the speech spectrum noise of ANSI-specified spectral density characteristics is calibrated to 20 dB SPL, then the masker level is specified in dB EM.

ANSI (S3.6-1989) states that the manufacturer of current audiometers should supply data describing the spectral density characteristics of masking stimuli, the masking effect for each test signal, and the corresponding reference sound pressure levels. If the manufacturer does not provide sufficient information on the calibration of masking noise or if the masker intensity is not calibrated in effective masking, then it will be necessary for the clinician to determine the effective masking level. This can be accomplished in two ways: (1) calculation using critical band data and (2) direct measurement with normal-hearing subjects. There are advantages and disadvantages to each method. Studebaker (1979) and Sanders (1991) provide excellent reviews of these procedures. Each method will be briefly described below.

The *calculation method* involves acoustic measurement of the masking stimulus and subsequent calculation of the effective masking level (Sanders & Rintelmann, 1964). Recall that when a pure tone is just audible in the presence of a masking stimulus, the total acoustic power of the components of the masker *within the critical band* surrounding the tone is equivalent to the acoustic power of the tone. Therefore, the predicted effective masking is equal to the total energy of the masker within the critical band minus pure-tone threshold in quiet. For example, if the pure-tone threshold in quiet is 0 dB HL (i.e., a reference of average normal hearing) and the total acoustic power of the narrow-band noise within the critical band is equal to the acoustic power of the tone, then the effective masking level is equal to 0 dB EM. Similarly, if the pure-tone threshold is 0 dB HL, and the total acoustic power of the narrow-band noise within the critical band is 40 dB greater than the acoustic power of the tone, then the effective masking level is equal to 40 dB EM.

Very briefly, calculation of the effective masking level requires acoustic measurement of (1) overall sound pressure level (i.e., dB SPL) and (2) bandwidth (BW) (in Hz) of the masking stimulus. Given this information, the spectrum level or level per cycle (i.e., the energy contained within each cycle or a 1-Hz wide band) of the masker can be calculated:

$$\text{Level per cycle (in dB)} = \text{Overall dB SPL} - 10 \log_{10} \text{BW}$$

The effective masking level is subsequently determined using the critical band data of Fletcher (1940) and Hawkins and Stevens (1950). Sanders (1972, 1978, 1991) and Studebaker (1979) provide more detailed information about the calculation of effective masking levels for pure-tone and speech signals. Although the calculation method is valid and reliable (Studebaker, 1979), it does require the use of spectral analysis equipment. Fortunately, it should not be necessary today to calculate effective masking level: All currently manufactured audiometers (and those manufactured over the past few years) produce masking sounds that meet specifications outlined in the current standards (ANSI S3.6-1989).

The *real ear method* involves psychoacoustic measurement of effective masking level in ten to twelve normal-hearing young adults who are "otologically normal."[2] Specifically, a pure-tone signal and a masking noise of fixed level are presented to the *same ear*.[3] Average masked pure-tone threshold (in dB HL) is determined and represents effective masking (in dB EM) for that level of noise (Hodgson, 1981; Sanders, 1972, 1978, 1991; Studebaker, 1979). Sanders and Rintelmann (1964) have demonstrated that the actual masking obtained with normal-hearing subjects and the predicted masking determined by computation using critical band data are in very close agreement. The following procedure is recommended when using a real ear method to determine the effective masking level:

1. Deliver the pure-tone signal and the masking noise to the *same* earphone.
2. Introduce a continuous narrow-band masking noise of moderate level (approximately 50 dB on the dial).
3. Establish masked pure-tone threshold (in dB HL) for each subject using ASHA's (1978) recommended procedure for manual pure-tone audiometry.
4. Calculate the median masked threshold (in dB HL) for the ten to twelve subjects. This value represents effective masking in dB EM for the fixed level of masking noise.
5. Repeat this procedure at all audiometric frequencies for each earphone. Prepare a table of correction factors that should be applied to the masker attenuator setting. The masking stimulus is now calibrated in effective masking (dB EM).

If attenuator linearity has been verified during periodic calibration procedures, it should not be necessary to determine effective masking at more than one masker level. Hawkins and Stevens (1950) demonstrated that there is a linear relationship between masker level and masking for both pure-tone and speech stimuli (i.e., a 10-dB increase in effective masker level will result in a 10-dB increase in masked threshold). Consequently, the same correction factor can be applied throughout the entire effective masking level range.

Consider the following example. You wish to establish the effective masking level of a narrow-band noise centered at 1000 Hz. Masker level is fixed at 50 dB. Median masked pure-tone threshold at 1000 Hz for twelve normal-hearing subjects is determined to be 40 dB HL. A masker dial setting of 50 dB will shift pure-tone threshold *on the average* to 40 dB HL. Consequently, a masker level of 50 dB is equivalent to 40 dB EM. When a correction factor of –10 dB is applied to any masker dial setting at that particular frequency, the masking noise is calibrated in effective masking (i.e., dB EM).

A similar procedure can be used when determining effective masking level for speech. Recall that effective masking for speech refers to the dB HL to which the speech recognition threshold is shifted by a given level of noise. Introduce the speech signal and continuous moderate-level speech spectrum noise (approximately 50 dB on the dial) to the same earphone. Establish masked SRT (in dB HL) for each subject using ASHA's (1988) recommended procedure for speech threshold. Calculate the median masked threshold (in dB HL) for the ten to twelve subjects. This value represents effective masking in dB EM for the fixed level of masking noise.

Consider another example. When the masker level is fixed at 50 dB, median masked SRT for twelve normal-hearing subjects is determined to be 45 dB HL. A masker dial setting of 50 dB will shift the SRT *on the average* to 45 dB HL. Consequently, a masker level of 50 dB is equivalent to 45 dB EM. When a correction factor of –5 dB is applied to any masker dial setting, the speech spectrum noise will be calibrated in effective masking (i.e., dB EM).

There is considerable variability in the methods that are used by audiologists when calibrating effective masking. According to Martin's most recent survey of audiological practices in the United States (Martin et al., 1994), 35 percent of audiologists perform electroacoustic calibration using critical band data (i.e., the calculation method). Twenty-one percent of the responding audiologists use psychoacoustic calibration (i.e., the real ear method), while 33 percent use an "arbitrary reference on the hearing level dial" (p. 23).

Summary

Masking refers to the increase in threshold of one sound in the presence of another. Masking is used clinically whenever it is suspected that the nontest ear is contributing to a response from the test ear. The purpose of contralateral masking is to reduce sensitivity of the nontest ear to the test stimulus.

Masking noise selection involves finding a stimulus that is efficient. An efficient masker produces a given effective level of masking with the least overall intensity. The most efficient masker during pure-tone audiometry is a *narrow-band noise* centered at the test frequency. Specifically, the narrow-band noise should have a bandwidth slightly greater than the critical band surrounding the tone. The most efficient masker during speech audiometry is *speech spectrum noise*. This is white noise that has been filtered to simulate the long-term average spectrum of conversational speech.

Masking noise is calibrated in *effective masking level* (dB EM). Effective masking during pure-tone audiometry refers to the dB HL to which detection threshold is shifted by a given level of noise. Effective masking for speech refers to the dB HL to which the speech recognition threshold is shifted by a given level of noise. The calibration of an effective masking level can be accomplished in two ways: (1) calculation using critical band data and (2) direct measurement using normal-hearing subjects. The *calculation method* involves acoustic measurement of the masking stimulus and subsequent calculation of an effective masking level using critical band data. The *real ear method* involves psychoacoustic measurement of effective masking level in normal-hearing, young adults. Both methods yield comparable measures of effective masking level.

Study Questions

1. Define masking. What is the purpose of clinical masking?

2. Differentiate ipsilateral versus contralateral masking. Which paradigm is used during clinical masking procedures?

3. The goal clinically is to select an efficient masker. Describe how the concept of the critical band relates to the selection of an efficient masker.

4. What is the most efficient masker during pure-tone audiometry? Describe the spectrum of this masking noise.

5. What is the most efficient masker during speech audiometry? Describe the spectrum of this masking noise.

6. Define effective masking level. Briefly describe the two approaches to calibrating effective masking level.

Endnotes

1. Effective masking level is typically defined as the dB HL to which threshold is shifted by a given level of noise (e.g., ANSI, 1989; Hodgson, 1980; Sanders, 1991; Studebaker, 1979). For example, a masker of 50 dB EM will shift the air-conduction threshold of a pure-tone signal to 50 dB HL. Stated differently, a pure tone of 50 dB HL will be *just audible* in the presence of a masker of 50 dB EM. Martin (1994) has offered a slightly different definition of effective masking level. Specifically, he states that a masker of a given effective masking level will make a tone of equivalent hearing level (i.e., dB HL) *just inaudible*. For example, a masker of 50 dB EM would just mask a pure tone of 50 dB HL; the tone will not become audible again until 55 dB HL (assuming that a 5-dB step size is used to measure auditory threshold). While the standard definition of effective masking assumes that a given level of effective masking will permit a pure tone of equivalent hearing level to be "just audible," Martin's definition requires the tone to be made "just inaudible" by a given level of noise. Consequently, Martin's definition of effective masking level theoretically would require an additional 1 to 2 dB of masking to make the tone just inaudible or just masked. Although the different criteria of just audible and just masked alter the definition of effective masking level only slightly (i.e., about 1–2 dB), it is an important distinction that can sometimes

lead to some confusion when trying to understand the concept of effective masking level. The standard definition of effective masking will be used for the remainder of our discussion. First, it is the definition offered by the American National Standards Institute (ANSI S3.6-1989) and agreed upon by most authorities on clinical masking. Second, it is a definition consistent with the critical band concept (i.e., when a pure tone is *just audible* in the presence of broadband noise, the total noise power present in the narrow band of frequencies is equal to the power of the tone), which is an important component of the calibration of effective masking level.

2. ANSI (S3.6-1989) defines an otologically normal subject as an individual "in a normal state of health who is free from all signs or symptoms of ear disease and from occlusive wax in the ear canal, and has no history of ear disease or exposure to noise likely to damage hearing " (p. 3).

3. Current two-channel audiometers will allow the pure-tone and masking stimuli to be mixed in the same earphone. If it is not possible to mix the two stimuli in the same earphone (e.g., when using a portable, one-channel audiometer), then the use of a "mixing pad" will be required (see Studebaker, 1967a or Sanders, 1972, 1978, 1991 for more detailed information).

3

When to Mask: Pure-Tone Threshold Audiometry

Masking must be used whenever there is the possibility that the test signal can be perceived in the nontest ear. Most references on clinical masking present a series of equations, formulas, or statements of "When to Mask." Although these equations can be very useful clinically, it is important to understand the underlying concepts of clinical masking. Once you understand the fundamental concepts of when to mask, it becomes unnecessary to memorize a series of formulas (which, by the way, can be forgotten or remembered incorrectly). Generally, three factors must be considered when determining when to mask:

1. Intensity level of the signal at the test ear
2. Interaural attenuation
3. Hearing sensitivity in the nontest ear

Application of a common sense approach when considering the above three factors will lead to a correct decision about the need for masking.

Air Conduction: Pure-Tone Stimuli

When making a decision about the need for masking during pure-tone air-conduction testing, three factors need to be considered:

1. Unmasked air-conduction threshold in the test ear (i.e., intensity level at the test ear)
2. Interaural attenuation
3. Bone-conduction sensitivity in the nontest ear

When cross hearing occurs, the nontest ear is stimulated largely through the mechanism of bone conduction. When a decision is made about the need for masking, the unmasked *air-conduction threshold of the test ear* is compared with the *bone-conduction threshold in the nontest ear*. If the difference equals or exceeds interaural attenuation, then the air-conduction threshold in the test ear must be reestablished using masking in the nontest (i.e., contralateral) ear. If we are using supra-aural earphones, interaural attenuation is considered to be 40 dB. The rule for when to mask during pure-tone air-conduction testing can be stated as follows:

> When the air-conduction threshold obtained in the test ear exceeds the *apparent* bone-conduction threshold in the nontest ear by 40 dB or more, masking should be applied to the nontest ear.
>
> *or*
>
> The use of masking is indicated when the air-conduction threshold of the test ear is 40 dB or greater than the *apparent* bone-conduction threshold of the nontest ear.

These two statements can be written in equation form:

$$AC_T - BC_{NT} \geq 40 \text{ dB}$$

or

$$AC_T - 40 \text{ dB} \geq BC_{NT}$$

This rule is consistent with the guidelines for manual pure-tone threshold audiometry recommended by the American Speech-Language-Hearing Association (ASHA, 1978).

Note that the term "apparent" bone-conduction threshold is considered when making a decision about the need for masking. Remember that an unmasked bone-conduction threshold does not convey ear-specific information; the response can originate from either ear. When a decision is made about the need for masking, it is assumed that the bone-conduction response can be due to either ear. The unmasked bone-conduction response is therefore considered the *apparent* or *possible* threshold for each ear.

Consider the audiogram presented in Figure 3-1A. Unmasked air- and bone-conduction thresholds have been obtained. Is masking required in either ear during air-conduction testing? Remember that we will consider the unmasked bone-conduction response as a possible threshold for either ear. Use the following equation when making a decision about the need for masking:

$$AC_T - 40 \text{ dB} \geq BC_{NT}$$

Right Ear (Test Ear)		Masking Needed?
250 Hz	$60 - 40 \geq 55$?	No
500 Hz	$20 - 40 \geq 10$?	No
1000 Hz	$40 - 40 \geq 20$?	No
2000 Hz	$50 - 40 \geq 40$?	No
4000 Hz	$30 - 40 \geq 10$?	No

Contralateral masking is not required when obtaining air-conduction thresholds at any frequency in the right ear. The estimated level of the cross-hearing signal (i.e., $AC_T - 40$ dB) does not equal or exceed the apparent bone-conduction threshold in the nontest ear. Contralateral masking will be required, however, when measuring air-conduction thresholds in the left ear:

FIGURE 3–1   Audiogram A presents unmasked air- and bone-conduction thresholds. Contralateral masking is needed when obtaining air-conduction thresholds at 500, 1000, and 4000 Hz in the left ear. Audiogram B presents the same unmasked air-conduction thresholds as in Audiogram A. Although bone-conduction thresholds are not available, a comparison of the air-conduction thresholds in the two ears suggests the need for contralateral masking only when obtaining air-conduction thresholds at 500 and 4000 Hz in the left ear. See text for further discussion.

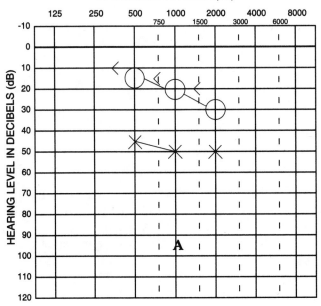

B

$$AC_T - 40\ dB \geq BC_{NT}$$

Left Ear (Test Ear)		Masking Needed?
250 Hz	70 − 40 ≥ 55?	No
500 Hz	70 − 40 ≥ 10?	Yes
1000 Hz	70 − 40 ≥ 20?	Yes
2000 Hz	70 − 40 ≥ 40?	No
4000 Hz	70 − 40 ≥ 10?	Yes

It is necessary to obtain masked air-conduction thresholds at 500, 1000, and 4000 Hz in the left ear because the estimated level of the cross-hearing signal equals or exceeds the apparent bone-conduction in the nontest (i.e., right) ear. We would have reached the same conclusions about the need for masking if the alternative equation had been used:

$$AC_T - BC_{NT} \geq 40 \text{ dB}$$

Although these equations are simple to use, it is important to understand their underlying principles. Consider the unmasked air-conduction thresholds at 1000 and 2000 Hz in the left ear.

1000 Hz: The unmasked air-conduction threshold in the left ear is 70 dB HL. A portion of that signal will be attenuated before it reaches the nontest ear. If interaural attenuation is 40 dB, then 30 dB HL is theoretically reaching the right cochlea (i.e., 70 − 40 = 30). Is bone-conduction hearing sensitive enough in the right ear to perceive the estimated cross-hearing signal of 30 dB HL? Yes, there is a possible (or apparent) bone-conduction threshold in the right ear at 20 dB HL. The unmasked air-conduction threshold of 70 dB HL in the left ear may, in fact, be a cross-hearing response from the right ear; masking should be applied to the right ear when reestablishing threshold in the left ear.

2000 Hz: The unmasked air-conduction threshold in the left ear is 70 dB HL. If interaural attenuation is 40 dB, then 30 dB HL theoretically is reaching the right cochlea (i.e., 70 − 40 = 30). Is bone-conduction hearing sensitive enough in the right ear to perceive the cross-hearing signal of 30 dB HL? No, the <u>best</u> that bone-conduction hearing sensitivity can be in the right ear is 40 dB HL. Hearing sensitivity is not good enough in the right ear to perceive the cross-hearing signal.

Note that the unmasked air-conduction threshold is 70 dB HL at both 1000 Hz and 2000 Hz. Yet masking is needed only at 1000 Hz. Why? Because bone-conduction hearing sensitivity is potentially better at 1000 than at 2000 Hz. The better that bone-conduction hearing sensitivity is in the nontest ear, the greater the potential for the nontest ear to respond to the cross-hearing signal.

A correct decision can be made about the need for masking in some situations *without* nontest ear bone-conduction thresholds. More specifically, a decision about the need for contralateral masking can be made by comparing air-conduction thresholds in the two ears:

> When the air-conduction threshold obtained in the test ear exceeds the apparent bone-conduction threshold or air-conduction threshold in the nontest ear by 40 dB or more, masking should be applied to the nontest ear.

This rule can be stated in equation form:

$$AC_T - 40 \text{ dB} \geq BC_{NT}$$
$$\textit{or}$$
$$AC_T - 40 \text{ dB} \geq AC_{NT}$$

Stated differently, contralateral masking should be applied in testing the poorer ear when the measured air-conduction threshold in that ear exceeds the air-conduction threshold in the better ear by 40 dB or more.

Consider the unmasked air-conduction thresholds at 1000 Hz and 4000 Hz in Figure 3-1*A*.

4000 Hz: The air-conduction thresholds are 30 dB HL and 70 dB HL for the right and left ears, respectively. Assume that an unmasked bone-conduction threshold has not yet been obtained. A decision about the need for masking in testing the left ear can be made using the air-conduction responses. Although we do not have a bone-conduction threshold for the right ear (i.e., the nontest ear), we can assume that the bone-conduction threshold is not poorer than the air-conduction threshold for that ear; that is , bone-conduction threshold in the right ear is 30 dB HL or better. Even if we assume that the bone-conduction threshold is the same as the air-conduction threshold in the right ear (i.e., 30 dB HL), there is at least a 40 dB or greater difference between the air-conduction threshold in the left ear (i.e., the test ear) and the bone-conduction threshold in the right ear. Masking should be applied to the right ear when testing the left ear. In this particular instance, it was not necessary to have a bone-conduction response when making a correct decision about the need for masking. A somewhat different situation occurs at 1000 Hz.

1000 Hz: Air-conduction thresholds are 40 dB HL and 70 dB HL for the right and left ears, respectively. Even without information about bone-conduction sensitivity, it can be predicted that the bone-conduction threshold in the right ear will be 40 dB HL or better in the right ear (i.e., the better ear). If we assume that the bone-conduction threshold is the same as the air-conduction threshold in the right ear (i.e., 40 dB HL), then there is less than a 40 dB difference between the two ears. There appears to be no need for contralateral masking when testing the poorer ear. However, this is only a preliminary decision. A final decision will be made when an unmasked bone-conduction threshold is obtained. In fact, when the unmasked bone conduction threshold is measured, a response is obtained at 20 dB HL (see Figure 3-1A). There is now evidence that the unmasked air-conduction threshold in the left ear can be due to cross hearing from the right ear; that is, there is a 40 dB or greater difference between air-conduction threshold in the left ear and the apparent bone-conduction threshold in the right ear.

It is conventional to obtain air-conduction thresholds prior to bone-conduction thresholds (Martin & Morris, 1989). Although a preliminary decision can be made about the need for masking, the need for masking must be reassessed *following* bone-conduction measurements. Consider the audiograms presented in Figures 3-1A and 3-1B; the audiograms are identical, with the exception that the unmasked bone-conduction thresholds are not plotted in Figure 3-1B. Assume that you have obtained only air-conduction thresholds for both ears (Figure 3-1B). Based on the air-conduction responses, contralateral masking is needed when testing the left ear at 500 and 4000 Hz (i.e., there is a 40 dB or greater difference between the air-conduction thresholds). Once unmasked bone-conduction thresholds are established (Figure 3-1A), we must reassess the need for masking. Given the unmasked bone-conduction responses, it becomes apparent that contralateral masking is also needed at 1000 Hz when testing the left ear: There is a 40 dB or greater difference between the air-conduction threshold in the left ear and the apparent bone-conduction threshold in the right ear. It will be necessary to return to earphone testing to obtain a masked air-conduction threshold in the left ear. This two-step decision-making process can be time-consuming. First, an initial decision about the need for masking is made based upon the air-conduction thresholds. Second, the need for masking is reassessed after the unmasked bone-conduction thresholds are measured. In some instances, it is necessary to then return to earphone testing to obtain masked air-conduction thresholds. An alternative (and recommend-

TABLE 3–1   Rules for when to mask during air-conduction pure-tone audiometry.

When the air-conduction threshold obtained in the test ear (AC_T) exceeds the apparent bone-conduction threshold (BC_{NT}) or air-conduction threshold (AC_{NT}) in the nontest ear by 40 dB or more, masking should be applied to the nontest ear.

$$AC_T - BC_{NT} \geq 40 \text{ dB}$$

or

$$AC_T - AC_{NT} \geq 40 \text{ dB}$$

or

The use of masking is indicated when the air-conduction threshold of the test ear (AC_T) is 40 dB or greater than the apparent bone-conduction threshold (BC_{NT}) or air-conduction threshold (AC_{NT}) of the nontest ear.

$$AC_T - 40 \text{ dB} \geq BC_{NT}$$

or

$$AC_T - 40 \text{ dB} \geq AC_{NT}$$

ed) approach involves obtaining unmasked bone-conduction thresholds *prior* to obtaining unmasked air-conduction thresholds. In this way, decisions about the need for masking during air-conduction testing can be made using the critical bone-conduction responses. The rules for when to mask during pure-tone air-conduction testing are summarized in Table 3-1.

Bone Conduction: Pure-Tone Stimuli

Remember that interaural attenuation for bone-conducted sound is considered to be zero. Theoretically, masked bone-conduction measurements are always required if ear-specific information is needed. However, consider the goal of bone-conduction testing: Determination of gross site of lesion (i.e., conductive versus sensorineural). Generally, bone-conduction measurements are useful for identifying air-bone gaps, the existence of which would suggest a conductive component. Keeping this information in mind, it will not always be necessary to obtain masked bone-conduction thresholds for each ear.

The rule for when to mask during bone-conduction testing can be stated as follows:

The nontest ear should be masked whenever the *test ear* exhibits a potential air-bone gap.

Specifically, the unmasked bone-conduction threshold (Unmasked BC) is compared to the air-conduction threshold in each ear (i.e., the test ear, AC_T). If there is evidence of an air-bone gap, contralateral masking is required. ASHA (1978) suggests that contralateral masking should be used whenever a potential air-bone gap of 10 dB or greater exists. When considering the variability inherent in bone-conduction measurements (Studebaker, 1967b), however, a criterion of 10 dB is probably too stringent. There is a certain amount of variability between air-conduction and bone-conduction thresholds, even in individuals without conductive hearing impairment. Martin (1994) suggests that a masked bone-conduction threshold should be obtained when a potential air-bone gap *greater* than 10 dB exists in the test ear. We can rewrite our rule of when to mask during bone-conduction testing as follows:

The use of masking is indicated when there exists a potential air-bone gap (AB Gap$_T$) of 15 dB or greater in the test ear.

$$AB\ Gap_T \geq 15\ dB$$

where

$$AB\ Gap_T = AC_T - Unmasked\ BC$$

What if unmasked bone-conduction thresholds suggest air-bone gaps of 10 dB or less? Although we do not know which ear is contributing to the bone-conduction responses, masking is unnecessary. Remember that the purpose of bone-conduction testing is to compare bone-conduction and air-conduction thresholds to determine whether there is a conductive component to the hearing loss. If there is no evidence of a significant air-bone gap, we have ruled out the presence of a conductive component. Our goal for bone-conduction testing has been accomplished with unmasked bone-conduction thresholds. Figure 3-2 presents three examples of the need for contralateral masking during bone-conduction testing. Unmasked air- and bone-conduction thresholds at 500, 1000, and 2000 Hz have been presented in each case.

Case A

Contralateral masking is not indicated during air-conduction testing in either ear: There are no differences of 40 dB or greater between air-conduction thresholds and unmasked bone-conduction thresholds. However, masking is required during bone-conduction testing at 500, 1000, and 2000 Hz in both ears. There are potential air-bone gaps of 15 dB or greater in both ears.

$$AB\ Gap_T \geq 15\ dB?$$
$$AC_T - Unmasked\ BC \geq 15\ dB?$$

Right Ear (Test Ear)		Masking Needed?
500 Hz	$30 - 10 \geq 15?$	Yes
1000 Hz	$35 - 0 \geq 15?$	Yes
2000 Hz	$30 - 0 \geq 15?$	Yes
Left Ear (Test Ear)		**Masking Needed?**
500 Hz	$35 - 10 \geq 15?$	Yes
1000 Hz	$30 - 0 \geq 15?$	Yes
2000 Hz	$25 - 0 \geq 15?$	Yes

Consider the unmasked bone-conduction threshold of 0 dB HL at 1000 Hz. Comparison of the unmasked bone-conduction threshold to the air-conduction thresholds suggests potential air-bone gaps of 35 dB and 30 dB in the right and left ears respectively. We know from the unmasked bone-conduction threshold that there is a significant air-bone gap *in at least one ear*. In order to obtain ear-specific information, bone-conduction thresholds must be obtained for both ears using contralateral masking.

FIGURE 3–2   Audiogram illustrating the need for contralateral masking during bone-conduction audiometry. *Case A:* Masked bone-conduction thresholds are required in both ears. *Case B:* Masked bone-conduction thresholds are not required in either ear. *Case C:* Masked bone-conduction thresholds are required only in the left ear. See text for further explanation.

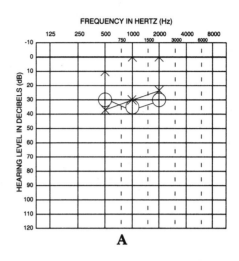

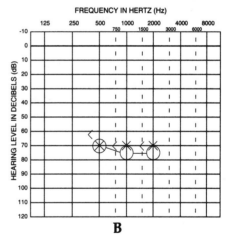

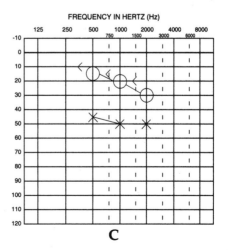

Case B

Contralateral masking is not required during air-conduction testing in either ear: There are no differences of 40 dB or greater between air-conduction thresholds and unmasked bone-conduction thresholds. Masking is also not required during bone-conduction testing in either ear. When we compare the unmasked bone-conduction threshold to the air-conduction thresholds in each ear, there are no potential air-bone gaps of 15 dB or greater.

$$\text{AB Gap}_T \geq 15 \text{ dB?}$$
$$\text{AC}_T - \text{Unmasked BC} \geq 15 \text{ dB?}$$

Right Ear (Test Ear)		Masking Needed?
500 Hz	70 − 65 ≥ 15?	No
1000 Hz	75 − 70 ≥ 15?	No
2000 Hz	75 − 70 ≥ 15?	No
Left Ear (Test Ear)		**Masking Needed?**
500 Hz	70 − 65 ≥ 15?	No
1000 Hz	70 − 70 ≥ 15?	No
2000 Hz	70 − 70 ≥ 15?	No

Consider the results at 1000 Hz. The largest air-bone gaps that can exist are 5 dB in the right ear and 0 dB in the left ear. Although we do not know which ear is contributing to the unmasked bone-conduction threshold at 70 dB HL, our measurement has given us the information we need. Bone-conduction testing suggests that there are no significant air-bone gaps in either ear; our conclusion is that the hearing loss is sensorineural in nature. The same situation occurs at 500 and 2000 Hz. We could obtain masked bone-conduction thresholds for both ears. However, it would not provide us with additional diagnostic information.

Case C

Masking is not required during air-conduction testing in either ear: There are no differences of 40 dB or greater between air-conduction thresholds and unmasked bone-conduction thresholds. Masked bone-conduction thresholds are required, however, in the left ear.

$$\text{AB Gap}_T \geq 15 \text{ dB?}$$
$$\text{AC}_T - \text{Unmasked BC} \geq 15 \text{ dB?}$$

Right Ear (Test Ear)		Masking Needed?
500 Hz	15 − 10 ≥ 15?	No
1000 Hz	20 − 15 ≥ 15?	No
2000 Hz	30 − 20 ≥ 15?	No
Left Ear (Test Ear)		**Masking Needed?**
500 Hz	45 − 10 ≥ 15?	Yes
1000 Hz	50 − 15 ≥ 15?	Yes
2000 Hz	50 − 20 ≥ 15?	Yes

When we compare the unmasked bone-conduction thresholds to the air-conduction thresholds in the right ear, there is no evidence of a significant air-bone gap at any frequency. However, there are potentially significant air-bone gaps in the left ear (i.e., 35 dB at 500 Hz and 1000 Hz, 30 dB at 2000 Hz). The unmasked bone-conduction thresholds may reflect hearing in the better ear (i.e., right ear). Bone-conduction thresholds in the left ear may, in fact, be as good as the unmasked responses; they can also be as poor as the air-conduction thresholds in that ear. We need ear-specific bone-conduction thresholds in the left ear to make a definitive statement about the gross site of lesion (i.e., conductive versus sensorineural).

Although it initially may appear that masked bone-conduction thresholds are needed in both ears, contralateral masking may be required only when testing one ear. Consider the pure-tone audiograms presented in Figure 3-3. Air- and bone-conduction thresholds have been measured at 500 Hz and 2000 Hz. It should be noted that *masked* air-conduction thresholds were required when testing the right ear. When making a decision about the need for contralateral masking during bone-conduction audiometry, it is important to remember that the *masked* air-conduction thresholds are always considered: Masked air-conduction thresholds represent true air-conduction hearing sensitivity.

500 Hz: The unmasked bone-conduction threshold of 0 dB HL suggests that there are potential air-bone gaps of 60 dB and 30 dB in the right and left ears respectively (see Figure 3-3*A*). Masked bone-conduction thresholds theoretically are required in both ears. Assuming that the unmasked bone-conduction threshold may reflect hearing sensitivity in the better ear, it is conventional to *first* obtain a masked bone-conduction threshold for the poorer ear . Narrow-band noise is applied to the left ear and a masked bone-conduction threshold of 60 dB HL is obtained in the right ear, suggesting a sensorineural hearing loss (see Figure 3-3*B*). The use of contralateral masking has established that bone-conduction threshold is 60 dB HL in the right ear; we can conclude that the *unmasked* bone-conduction threshold of 0 dB HL reflects a response from the left ear. In this case, a masked bone-conduction threshold was required only in one ear, although initially masking was indicated in both ears.

2000 Hz: The unmasked bone-conduction threshold of 0 dB HL suggests that there are potential air-bone gaps of 40 dB and 20 dB in the right and left ears respectively (see Figure 3-3*A*). Masked bone-conduction thresholds potentially are required in both ears. Narrow-band masking is applied to the left ear and a masked bone-conduction threshold of 5 dB HL is obtained in the right ear, suggesting a conductive hearing loss (see Figure 3-3*B*). In this case, the use of contralateral masking has not ruled out either ear as contributing to the unmasked bone-conduction threshold. The masked bone-conduction threshold of 5 dB HL in the right ear suggests that the unmasked threshold may be due, in fact, to the right ear; we do not have sufficient evidence that the unmasked bone-conduction response at 0 dB HL is due to the left ear. To make a statement about the gross site of lesion in the left ear, it will also be necessary to obtain a masked bone-conduction threshold. In this case, it will be necessary to obtain masked bone-conduction thresholds in both ears.

It is important to remember that the goal of bone-conduction testing is to determine the gross site of lesion. Contralateral masking is required during bone-conduction audiometry only when unmasked bone-conduction thresholds suggest the possibility of a significant air-bone gap in the test ear. The rule for when to mask during bone-conduction audiometry is summarized in Table 3-2.

FIGURE 3–3   Although unmasked bone-conduction testing initially may suggest the need for contralateral masking in both ears, it is not always necessary to obtain masked thresholds in each ear. Audiogram A presents unmasked bone-conduction thresholds at 500 Hz and 2000 Hz; Audiogram B presents the masked bone-conduction thresholds measured subsequently in the ear with poorer hearing sensitivity by air conduction (i.e., the right ear). Based on the masked bone-conduction thresholds presented in Audiogram B, a masked bone-conduction threshold is required only in the right ear at 500 Hz. Masked bone-conduction thresholds are required in both ears, however, at 2000 Hz. See text for further explanation.

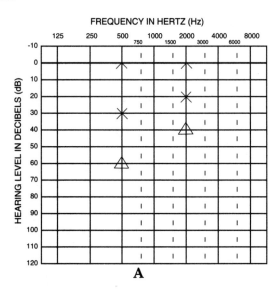

A

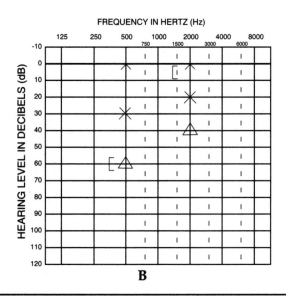

B

TABLE 3–2   The rule for when to mask during bone-conduction pure-tone audiometry.

The nontest ear should be masked whenever the test ear exhibits a potential air-bone gap of (AB Gap$_T$) 15 dB or greater.

$$AB\ Gap_T \geq 15\ dB$$

Summary

There are three factors to consider when making a decision about the need for masking during pure-tone air-conduction testing: (1) The unmasked air-conduction threshold in the test ear; (2) interaural attenuation for air-conducted sound (i.e., 40 dB); and (3) bone-conduction sensitivity in the nontest ear. Specifically, when the air-conduction threshold obtained in the test ear exceeds the apparent bone-conduction threshold (i.e., the unmasked bone-conduction response) in the nontest ear by 40 dB or more, masking should be applied to the nontest ear.

$$AC_T - BC_{NT} \geq 40\ dB$$
or
$$AC_T - 40\ dB \geq BC_{NT}$$

Many audiologists obtain air-conduction thresholds before measurement of bone-conduction responses. A correct decision about the need for contralateral masking can often be made by comparing the air-conduction thresholds of the two ears: When the air-conduction threshold in the test ear exceeds the air-conduction threshold in the nontest ear by 40 dB or more, masking should be applied to the nontest ear.

$$AC_T - AC_{NT} \geq 40\ dB$$
or
$$AC_T - 40\ dB \geq AC_{NT}$$

It is important to remember, however, that cross hearing for air-conducted sound occurs primarily through the mechanism of bone conduction. Consequently, it will be necessary to re-evaluate the need for contralateral masking during air-conduction testing following the measurement of unmasked bone-conduction responses in those cases in which the difference between the two air-conduction thresholds of the test and nontest ears does not equal or exceed interaural attenuation (i.e., 40 dB).

The major factor to consider when making a decision about the need for contralateral masking during bone-conduction audiometry is whether the unmasked bone-conduction response suggests the presence of a significant conductive component in the test ear. Specifically, the use of contralateral masking is indicated whenever the results of unmasked bone-conduction audiometry suggest the presence of an air-bone gap of 15 dB or greater in the test ear.

$$AB\ Gap_T \geq 15\ dB$$
where
$$AB\ Gap = AC_T - Unmasked\ BC$$

Study Questions

1. Generally, what are the three factors that must be considered when making a decision about the need for contralateral masking during pure-tone audiometry?

2. Specifically, what are the three factors that must be considered when making a decision about the need for contralateral masking during pure-tone air-conduction audiometry?

3. State the rule for when to mask during pure-tone air-conduction audiometry. Also express this rule in the form of an equation.

4. A decision can often be made about the need for contralateral masking by simply comparing the air-conduction thresholds of the test and nontest ears. Briefly explain.

5. Consideration of only the air-conduction thresholds of the two ears can lead to an incorrect decision about the need for contralateral masking. Briefly explain.

6. Theoretically, masked bone-conduction measurements are always required if ear-specific information is needed. Considering the goal of bone-conduction testing, why is it not always necessary to obtain masked bone-conduction thresholds for each ear?

7. State the rule for when to mask during pure-tone bone-conduction audiometry. Also express this rule in the form of an equation.

4
When to Mask: Speech Audiometry

There are four factors to consider when making a decision about the need for masking during air-conduction speech audiometry:

1. Presentation level of the speech signal (i.e., intensity level) at the test ear
2. Interaural attenuation
3. Bone-conduction sensitivity in the nontest ear
4. Type of speech measurement

The first three factors are the same as those considered during pure-tone air-conduction threshold testing. Another factor must be considered during speech audiometry—the type of speech measurement. Speech audiometry traditionally is comprised of two components:

1. Threshold measurement of speech (i.e., measures of hearing sensitivity for speech)
2. Suprathreshold measurement of speech recognition ability

The nature of the speech measurement can influence the decision about the need for contralateral masking.

Threshold Measures

Contralateral masking is indicated during speech threshold measurement whenever the presentation level of the signal at the test ear (Presentation level$_T$) equals or exceeds the pure-tone bone-conduction sensitivity in the nontest ear (BC$_{NT}$) by the amount of interaural attenuation (IA):

$$\text{Presentation level}_T - IA \geq BC_{NT}$$

The value that is used for interaural attenuation, however, will be dependent upon the nature of the threshold measurement.

There are two measures of hearing sensitivity for speech—speech recognition threshold (SRT) and speech detection threshold (SDT). ASHA (1988) defines speech recognition threshold as "the minimum hearing level for speech at which an individual can recognize 50 percent of the speech material" (p. 86). Speech detection threshold is the "minimum hearing level for speech at which an individual can just discern the presence of speech material 50 percent of the time" (ASHA, 1988, p. 86). This fundamental difference in the response required for the two speech threshold measures (i.e., recognition versus detection) may necessitate the use of a different interaural attenuation value when making a decision about the need for masking.

Interaural attenuation for speech is typically measured by obtaining speech recognition thresholds in individuals with unilateral, profound sensorineural hearing impairment and then calculating the difference in thresholds between the normal and impaired ears (without contralateral ear masking):

$$IA = Unmasked\ SRT_{impaired\ ear} - SRT_{normal\ ear}$$

Table 4-1 presents the range of interaural attenuation values reported for spondaic words presented through traditional supra-aural earphones. The smallest reported value of interaural attenuation for spondaic words is 48 dB (e.g., Martin & Blythe, 1977; Snyder, 1973). When making a decision about the need for contralateral masking during clinical practice, a single value defining the lower limit of interaural attenuation is most useful (Studebaker, 1967a). A conservative estimate of interaural attenuation for spondees, therefore, is 45 dB (Konkle & Berry, 1983). The majority (80 percent) of audiologists measure SRT using a 5-dB step size (Martin, Armstrong, & Champlin, 1994); therefore, the interaural attenuation value of 48 dB has been rounded down to 45 dB.

It has been consistently demonstrated that speech can be detected at a lower intensity than that required to reach the speech recognition threshold; specifically, the SRT requires an average of 8 to 9 dB greater intensity than the SDT (Beattie, Svihovec, & Edgerton, 1978; Chaiklin, 1959; Thurlow, Silverman, Davis, & Walsh, 1948). (It should be noted that there is considerable intersubject variability in the SRT-SDT difference. Chaiklin (1959) reported that this difference ranged from a minimum of 2 dB to a maximum of 12 to 16 dB). Given this information, a more conservative value of interaural attenuation may be needed when considering the need for contralateral masking during measurement of a speech detection threshold.

Consider the audiogram presented in Figure 4-1. Pure-tone testing reveals normal hearing at octave frequencies of 250 to 8000 Hz in the right ear; there is no measurable hearing for both air- and bone-conducted sound at equipment limits in the left ear when contralateral ear masking is applied (i.e., a profound, sensorineural hearing impairment). A speech recognition threshold of 0 dB HL

TABLE 4–1   Range of interaural attenuation values for speech (spondaic words) using conventional supra-aural earphones. The amount of interaural attenuation was calculated as follows: Interaural attenuation = Speech recognition threshold (impaired ear) – Speech recognition threshold (normal ear).

Study	Transducer (Cushion)	Number of Subjects	Range (in dB)
Martin & Blythe (1977)	TDH-49 (MX-41/AR)	N = 12	48–70
Snyder (1973)	TDH-39 (MX-41/AR)	N = 84	48–76
Sklare & Denenberg (1987)	TDH-49p (51)	N = 7	54–68

FIGURE 4–1 Audiogram showing normal hearing in the right ear and a profound, sensorineural hearing loss in the left ear. If we assume that interaural attenuation for spondaic words can be as small as 48 dB, then an unmasked speech recognition threshold of 48 dB HL theoretically will be measured in the left ear. If an unmasked speech detection threshold is measured in the left ear, it is predicted that it will occur at an intensity level about 8-9 dB lower than the unmasked SRT, that is, 39-40 dB HL.

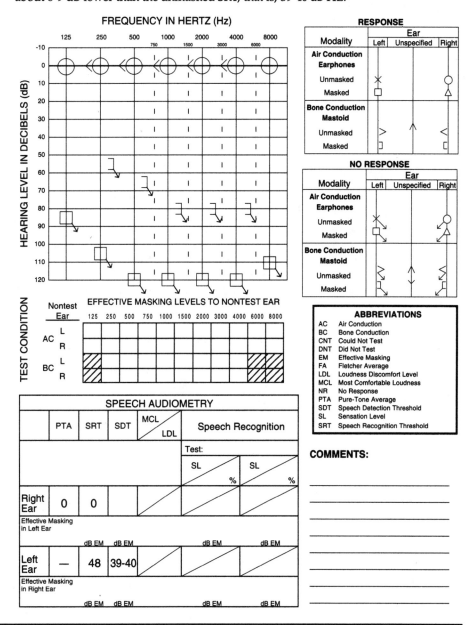

is measured in the right ear, a finding consistent with the pure-tone results. If we assume that interaural attenuation for spondaic words can be as small as 48 dB, then an unmasked SRT of 48 dB HL theoretically can be measured in the left ear. Recall that interaural attenuation for spondaic words is measured by using the SRT in the normal ear as the reference. It should also be noted that the speech *recognition* threshold and pure-tone thresholds in the normal ear should be correlated because of the manner in which standard reference threshold levels for speech and pure tones are specified (ANSI S3.6-1989).

If an *unmasked SDT* is measured in the left ear, we can predict that the threshold will occur at an intensity level about 8 to 9 dB lower than the *unmasked SRT*, that is, the unmasked speech detection threshold is expected to occur at about 39 to 40 dB HL. Comparison of the unmasked SDT in the impaired ear with the SRT (or bone-conduction thresholds predictive of the SRT) in the normal ear theoretically will result in *measured* interaural attenuation of approximately 39 to 40 dB. When an unmasked SDT is measured and the response is compared to either the SRT or the bone-conduction thresholds predictive of the SRT in the nontest (i.e., better) ear, it will be necessary to mask whenever the presentation level equals or exceeds the SRT or bone-conduction thresholds in the nontest ear by the expected interaural attenuation for spondaic words *minus approximately 8 to 9 dB*. Given that the SRT–SDT difference can be as large as 12 to 16 dB (Chaiklin, 1959) and when taking into account the clinical use of a 5-dB step size, a conservative value of interaural attenuation when measuring the SDT will be 35 dB.

It is very important to note that the actual interaural attenuation for the speech signal does not change during measurement of speech detection and speech recognition thresholds. Rather, a different response task when measuring speech threshold in each ear (i.e., detection versus recognition) can affect the *measured* interaural attenuation for the speech signal. Consider again the example presented in Figure 4-1. It was stated previously that if an SRT of 0 dB HL was measured in the normal (i.e., right) ear, an unmasked SRT would be measured at about 48 dB HL in the left ear; this would result assuming that measured interaural attenuation is 48 dB. If *unmasked SDTs* are now measured in *both* ears, the relative difference between the two speech thresholds would remain the same; theoretically, both speech thresholds would be lowered by about 8 to 9 dB because the response task has been altered in the same way for both ears. If the response task (i.e., detection versus recognition) is the same for both ears, then the measured interaural attenuation for speech should remain constant: Comparison of *SRTs between ears* or *SDTs between ears* generally should result in the same measured interaural attenuation. However, when the response task differs between ears when measuring speech thresholds, the measured interaural attenuation for speech will be altered. Consequently, when an SDT is measured in the poorer ear and compared to the SRT (or bone-conduction thresholds predictive of the SRT) in the better ear, a more conservative estimate of interaural attenuation (i.e., 35 dB) should be considered. This recommendation appears appropriate given the manner in which interaural attenuation for speech is typically determined (i.e., comparison of speech thresholds between ears which are measured using the same response task).

Just as with pure-tone air-conduction testing, the nontest ear bone-conduction thresholds must be considered when making a decision about the need for masking during the assessment of speech thresholds. Because speech is a broadband stimulus, it is necessary to consider bone-conduction hearing sensitivity at more than a single pure-tone frequency. Konkle and Berry (1983) and Sanders (1991) recommend the use of the bone-conduction pure-tone average of 500, 1000, and 2000 Hz or some other combination that is predictive of the speech recognition threshold. ASHA (1988) suggests that the bone-conduction pure-tone thresholds at either 500, 1000, 2000, or 4000 Hz should be considered. The results of a study by Martin and Blythe (1977) indicated that 250 Hz may be eliminated from any formula for determining the need for masking during establishment of the SRT. However, the nontest ear bone-conduction threshold at 250 Hz may be important when measuring a speech detection threshold. Olsen and Matkin (1991) state that the SDT may be more closely related to the best bone-conduction threshold in the 250 to 4000 Hz range when audiometric configuration sharply slopes or rises. Consequently, the most conservative approach to determining the need for masking during measurement of any speech threshold requires the consideration of the best bone-conduction threshold in the nontest ear at frequencies ranging from 250 to 4000 Hz (Coles & Priede, 1975).

In summary, contralateral masking is indicated during assessment of a speech recognition threshold when the presentation level of the speech signal at the test ear (Presentation level$_T$) exceeds the best bone-conduction threshold (from 250 to 4000 Hz) in the nontest ear (Best BC$_{NT}$) by 45 dB (i.e., interaural attenuation) or more:

$$\text{Presentation level}_T - 45\ dB \geq \text{Best BC}_{NT}$$

It is important to remember that a more conservative interaural attenuation value of 35 dB may be appropriate when establishing a speech detection threshold.

Consider the audiogram presented in Figure 4-2. We will evaluate the need for masking during assessment of speech recognition threshold. Pure-tone testing reveals a very mild, high-frequency sensorineural hearing loss in the right ear and a moderate sensorineural hearing impairment in the left ear. Unmasked speech recognition thresholds are obtained at 15 dB HL and 50 dB HL in the right and left ears, respectively. Because interaural attenuation for spondaic words is 45 dB, we generally do not become concerned about cross hearing until the presentation level of the test signal reaches approximately 45 dB HL. When a test signal of less than 45 dB HL is presented, bone-conduction hearing sensitivity in the nontest ear would have to be better than 0 dB HL for a cross-hearing response to occur. Nevertheless, let us consider the need for masking in both ears.

Right Ear: Is contralateral ear masking required when establishing the SRT in the right ear? No, there is no need for masking when assessing the SRT in the right ear. The test signal is presented at 15 dB HL; 45 dB is attenuated before it reaches the nontest cochlea (i.e., the left ear). Theoretically, a cross-hearing signal of –30 dB HL is reaching the left cochlea (i.e., 15 dB HL – 45 dB HL = –30 dB HL). Is bone-conduction hearing sensitivity in the left ear good enough to perceive the cross-hearing signal of –30 dB HL? No, the best bone-conduction threshold in the left ear is 40 dB HL.

$$\text{Presentation level}_T - 45\ dB \geq \text{Best BC}_{NT}$$
$$15\ dB\ HL - 45\ dB \geq 40\ dB\ HL\ (\text{at } 250, 500\ Hz)?$$
$$-30\ dB\ HL \geq 40\ dB\ HL?$$

Left Ear: Is contralateral ear masking required when establishing the SRT in the left ear? No, masking is not required. The unmasked SRT occurs at 50 dB HL; 45 dB is attenuated prior to reaching the nontest cochlea (i.e., the right ear). Theoretically, a cross-hearing signal of 5 dB HL is reaching the right cochlea (i.e., 50 dB HL – 45 dB HL = 5 dB HL). Is bone-conduction hearing sensitivity good enough in the right ear to contribute to a cross-hearing response when establishing SRT in the left ear? No, the cross-hearing signal of 5 dB HL is slightly less than the best bone-conduction response (i.e., 10 dB HL) in the right ear.

$$\text{Presentation level}_T - 45\ dB \geq \text{Best BC}_{NT}$$
$$50\ dB\ HL - 45\ dB \geq 10\ dB\ HL\ (\text{at } 250, 500\ Hz)?$$
$$5\ dB\ HL \geq 10\ dB\ HL?$$

FIGURE 4–2   Audiogram presenting a very mild, high-frequency sensorineural hearing loss in the right ear and a moderate sensorineural hearing impairment in the left ear. Unmasked speech recognition thresholds of 15 dB HL and 50 dB HL were obtained for the right and left ears respectively. Assuming that the spondaic words are not presented at intensity levels higher than the obtained SRTs, contralateral masking will not required when obtaining speech thresholds in either ear. However, if presentation levels are used during measurement that are higher than the obtained SRTs, contralateral masking will be required when testing the left ear. See text for further explanation.

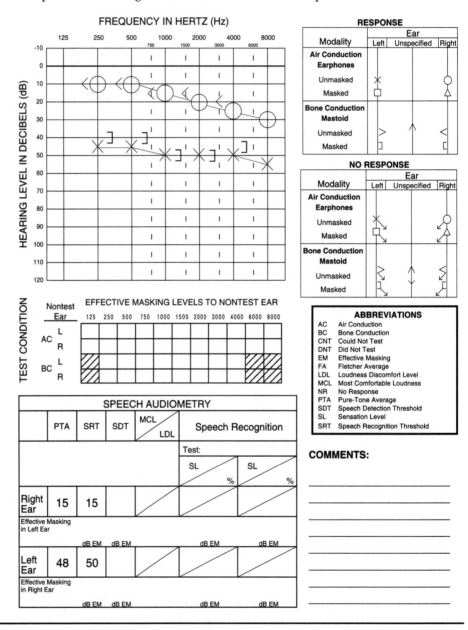

When evaluating the need for masking during assessment of the speech recognition threshold, it is very important to consider your test procedure. For example, if you are using a descending threshold determination, spondaic words will be presented at hearing levels higher than the established SRT. ASHA (1988) recommends a standardized, descending threshold technique based on the original work of Tillman and Olsen (1973). The test phase involves presenting spondaic words initially at hearing levels approximately 10 dB higher than the calculated SRT. Patient responses at these higher presentation levels contribute to the calculated SRT. This higher starting level may necessitate the need for masking.

Refer again to the audiogram in Figure 4-2. Let us assume that ASHA's recommended procedure will be used to assess SRT. This will require the use of presentation levels approximately 10 dB higher than the calculated SRTs. Is masking now required when establishing SRT? In the right ear, our starting level will be approximately 10 dB above the established SRT of 15 dB HL, that is, 25 dB HL. When taking into account the higher presentation levels used during our descending threshold technique, masking would not be required when testing the right ear.

$$\text{Presentation level}_T - 45 \text{ dB} \geq \text{Best BC}_{NT}$$
$$25 \text{ dB HL} - 45 \text{ dB} \geq 40 \text{ dB HL?}$$
$$-25 \text{ dB HL} \geq 40 \text{ dB HL?}$$

There are no bone-conduction thresholds at −25 dB HL or better in the nontest ear; the best bone-conduction threshold is 40 dB HL. Contralateral ear masking is not indicated.

A different situation occurs in the left ear. If we begin our threshold determination during the test phase at approximately 10 dB above the calculated SRT (i.e., 50 dB HL + 10 dB = 60 dB HL), cross hearing is now a possibility:

$$\text{Presentation level}_T - 45 \text{ dB} \geq \text{Best BC}_{NT}$$
$$60 \text{ dB HL} - 45 \text{ dB} \geq 10 \text{ dB HL?}$$
$$15 \text{ dB HL} \geq 10 \text{ dB HL?}$$

Theoretically, a cross-hearing signal of 15 dB HL is reaching the right ear. Because the best bone-conduction threshold occurs at 10 dB HL, contralateral masking will be needed. Again, it is important to consider the presentation levels that will be used during assessment of the SRT when determining the need for masking.

In some instances, a correct decision about the need for masking can be made without consideration of bone-conduction thresholds. Masking is required when testing the poorer ear whenever the obtained SRTs in the two ears differ by at least the amount of interaural attenuation.

$$SRT_T - SRT_{NT} \geq IA$$
or
$$SRT_T - IA \geq SRT_{NT}$$

This is comparable to the rule for when to mask during pure-tone air-conduction testing; that is, contralateral masking is needed when testing the poorer ear whenever the obtained threshold is 40 dB (i.e., interaural attenuation) or greater than the air-conduction threshold in the better ear.

Consider the following example. You have obtained speech recognition thresholds of 10 dB HL and 65 dB HL for the right and left ears, respectively. Even without information about bone-conduction hearing sensitivity, there is sufficient indication that the SRT of 65 dB HL in the left ear can reflect a cross-hearing response from the right ear; there is a difference of 55 dB between the two speech thresholds, a value that exceeds interaural attenuation (i.e., 45 dB).

$$SRT_T - SRT_{NT} \geq IA$$
$$65 \text{ dB HL} - 10 \text{ dB HL} \geq 45 \text{ dB?}$$
$$55 \text{ dB} \geq 45 \text{ dB?}$$

However, this rule of comparing the two speech thresholds when making a decision about the need for masking must be used with caution. Although the speech thresholds in the two ears may not equal or exceed interaural attenuation, there still may be the need for contralateral masking when considering the bone-conduction thresholds.

Consider the audiogram presented in Figure 4-3. Pure-tone testing reveals a mild conductive hearing loss in the right ear and a moderate sensorineural hearing impairment in the left ear. Unmasked SRTs of 35 dB HL and 50 dB HL were obtained for the right and left ears, respectively. Is contralateral masking needed when obtaining the SRT in the poorer (i.e., left) ear? If we consider the unmasked speech thresholds, there is only a 15-dB difference between the two ears; there appears to be no need for contralateral masking.

$$SRT_T - SRT_{NT} \geq IA$$
$$50 \text{ dB HL} - 35 \text{ dB HL} \geq 45 \text{ dB?}$$
$$15 \text{ dB} \geq 45 \text{ dB?}$$

Yet, when bone-conduction hearing sensitivity is considered, the need for contralateral masking when measuring SRT in the left ear becomes apparent.

Right Ear: Contralateral masking is not needed when obtaining an SRT in the right ear.

$$\text{Presentation level}_T - 45 \text{ dB} \geq \text{Best BC}_{NT}$$
$$35 \text{ dB} - 45 \text{ dB} \geq 45 \text{ dB Hz (at 250, 500 Hz)?}$$
$$-10 \text{ dB HL} \geq 45 \text{ dB HL?}$$

A cross-hearing signal of –10 dB HL theoretically is reaching the left ear. Because the best bone-conduction threshold in the nontest ear occurs at 45 dB HL, contralateral masking will not be needed. A very different situation occurs in the left ear.

Left Ear: Contralateral masking is needed when obtaining an SRT in the left ear.

$$\text{Presentation level}_T - 45 \text{ dB} \geq \text{Best BC}_{NT}$$
$$50 \text{ dB HL} - 45 \text{ dB} \geq 0 \text{ dB HL (at 500, 1000 Hz)?}$$
$$5 \text{ dB HL} \geq 0 \text{ dB HL?}$$

Contralateral masking must be applied to the right ear when measuring an SRT in the left ear. A cross-hearing signal of 5 dB HL theoretically is reaching the right cochlea (assuming that interaural attenuation is as small as 45 dB); bone-conduction hearing in the right ear is sensitive enough (i.e., 0 dB HL) to perceive this cross-hearing signal. This example demonstrates the importance of considering bone-conduction sensitivity in the nontest ear when making a decision about the need for masking during measurement of speech thresholds.

FIGURE 4–3   Audiogram presenting a mild conductive hearing loss in the right ear and a moderate sensorineural hearing impairment in the left ear. Unmasked speech recognition thresholds of 35 dB HL and 50 dB HL were obtained for the right and left ears respectively. Contralateral masking is required when measuring the SRT in the left ear.

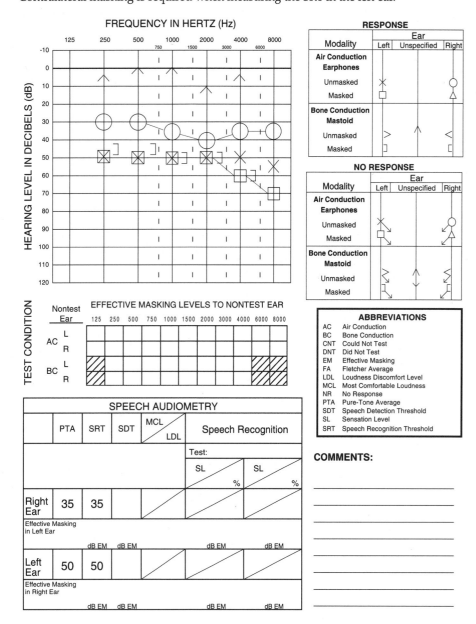

Some audiologists will not obtain an unmasked SRT in cases where pure-tone audiometry suggests that a masked SRT is indicated. Consider the audiogram in Figure 4-4. Pure-tone testing reveals normal hearing in the left ear. There is a severe, sensorineural hearing loss of relatively flat configuration in the right ear. An SRT of 10 dB HL was obtained in the left ear, a finding consistent with the pure-tone findings. Given that the pure-tone average is 77 dB HL in the right ear, it can be predicted that the SRT will be about 75 to 80 dB HL. There already is an indication that contralateral masking will be needed when

FIGURE 4–4   Audiogram presenting normal hearing in the left ear and a severe, sensorineural hearing loss of flat configuration in the right ear. Given that the pure-tone average is 77 dB HL in the right ear, it can be predicted that the SRT will be measured at approximately 75-80 dB HL. Although an unmasked SRT has not been obtained, there is sufficient indication that contralateral masking will be required when measuring the speech recognition threshold in the right ear.

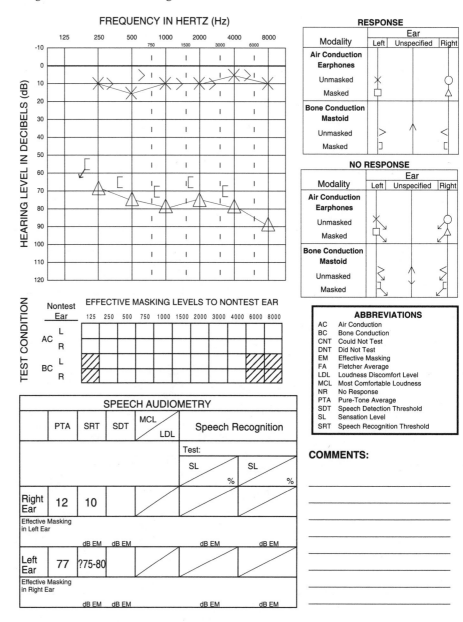

obtaining the SRT in the right ear. The estimated SRT of 75 to 80 dB HL is 45 dB greater than the best bone-conduction threshold (i.e., 5 dB) and the SRT in the left ear. Many clinicians will omit obtaining an unmasked SRT and proceed to estimating the SRT in the presence of contralateral masking.

Figure 4-5 presents an example of the need for masking when measuring a speech detection threshold. Pure-tone testing reveals a moderate-to-severe,

FIGURE 4–5 Audiogram presenting a moderate-to-severe, sensorineural hearing loss of flat configuration in the left ear. There is a profound, sensorineural hearing impairment of fragmentary configuration in the right ear. The speech recognition threshold of 60 dB HL in the right ear confirms the pure-tone findings. Contralateral masking will be required when obtaining a speech detection threshold in the right ear.

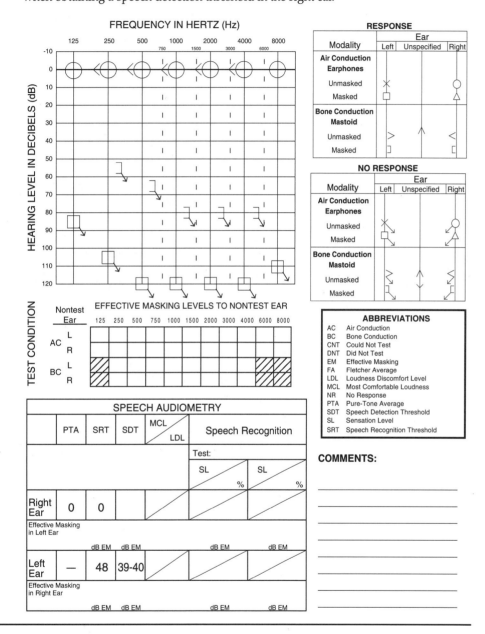

sensorineural hearing loss of flat configuration in the left ear; there is a profound, sensorineural hearing impairment of fragmentary configuration in the right ear. The SRT of 60 dB HL in the left ear confirms the pure-tone findings. Because the patient was unable to recognize spondaic words at suprathreshold levels, an SDT was obtained. An unmasked SDT of 95 dB HL is measured in the right ear. There is a 40-dB difference between presentation level of the speech signal at the test ear (i.e., 95 dB HL) and the best bone-conduction threshold in the nontest ear (i.e., 55 dB HL at 2000 Hz). If we use a conservative interaural attenuation value of 35 dB, then there is an indication for the need for contralateral masking:

$$\text{Presentation level}_T - 35 \text{ dB} \geq \text{Best BC}_{NT}$$
$$95 \text{ dB HL} - 35 \text{ dB} \geq 55 \text{ dB HL}?$$
$$60 \text{ dB HL} \geq 55 \text{ dB HL}?$$

Theoretically, a cross-hearing signal of 60 dB HL is reaching the left cochlea; bone-conduction hearing is sensitive enough (i.e., 55 dB HL) to perceive this cross-hearing signal. The SDT in the right ear should be reestablished in the presence of contralateral masking. It should be noted that we would have reached the same conclusion in this example by comparing the two speech thresholds. That is, there is a 35-dB difference between the SDT of 95 dB HL in the right ear and the SRT of 60 dB HL in the left ear. Assuming that interaural attenuation can be as small as 35 dB, contralateral masking is indicated when testing the poorer ear (i.e., the right ear).

Suprathreshold Measures

Traditionally, suprathreshold speech recognition ability is assessed by presenting a list of speech stimuli to the test ear at a fixed intensity level above threshold; the number of test items correctly recognized, reported as percent correct, is determined. The majority of audiologists present a single list of meaningful monosyllabic words, either CID W-22 or NU-6 (about 95 percent) at a fixed sensation level relative to the SRT (about 75 percent) (Martin et al., 1994). When making a decision about the need for contralateral masking during assessment of suprathreshold speech recognition, we can apply the same general rule used for speech threshold measurements. Contralateral masking is indicated during suprathreshold speech recognition measurement whenever the presentation level of the signal at the test ear equals or exceeds the best pure-tone bone-conduction threshold (from 250 to 4000 Hz) in the nontest ear by the amount of interaural attenuation:

$$\text{Presentation level}_T - \text{IA} \geq \text{Best BC}_{NT}$$

There is some evidence that it may be appropriate to apply a more conservative estimate of interaural attenuation when making a decision about the need for contralateral masking during suprathreshold speech recognition testing. Although interaural attenuation (i.e., the decibel difference between the level of the signal at the test ear and the level at the opposite cochlea) remains constant during assessment of threshold and suprathreshold measures of speech recognition, differences in performance criterion for the measurements must be taken into account when selecting a clinically appropriate value of interaural attenuation. The speech recognition threshold is specified relative to a 50 percent criterion; suprathreshold speech recognition performance, however, can range from 0 to 100 percent.

Konkle and Berry (1983) present a concise rationale for the use of a more conservative value of interaural attenuation during assessment of suprathreshold speech recognition. They state that the fundamental difference in percent correct criterion requires specification of nontest ear cochlear (i.e., bone-conduction) sensitivity in a different way than that used for threshold measurements. If suprathreshold speech recognition materials are presented at an intensity level equal to the SRT, a small percentage of the test items can be correctly recognized. The percentage of test items that can be recognized correctly at presentation levels equal to SRT depends on the type of speech stimuli, as well as on the specific talker and/or recorded version of a particular speech recognition test. For example, it has been demonstrated that the commercially available Auditec recording of NU-6 is more difficult than the Rintelmann version (Beattie, Edgerton, & Svihovec, 1977; Frank & Craig, 1984; Rintelmann and associates, 1974). Beattie et al. (1977) reported that normal-hearing listeners achieved a mean score of only 3.4 percent when the Auditec recording of NU-6 was presented at a 4-dB sensation level relative to the SRT. It is probable that mean percent correct performance would approach zero percent when test items are presented at 0 dB SL. Conversely, Rintelmann and associates (1974) reported that normal-hearing young adults achieved mean scores of approximately 17 percent (with standard deviations of almost 10 percent) when lists of NU-6 were presented to the test ear at an intensity equal to SRT (i.e., 0 dB SL). (Mean scores of approximately 4 percent were achieved when monosyllabic words were presented at –4 dB SL.) Theoretically, if NU-6 words lists were presented at an intensity sufficient to cross over to the *nontest ear* at a level equal to the nontest ear SRT (or pure-tone bone-conduction thresholds), approximately 17 percent of the test items could be recognized correctly by the nontest ear. Regardless of the type of speech stimulus (e.g., meaningful monosyllables, nonsense syllables, or sentences) and the specific version (i.e., talker/recording) of a particular speech recognition test, zero percent or chance performance (if a closed-set paradigm is used) may not be reached until about –10 dB relative to the SRT. Based on this observation, Konkle and Berry (1983) recommend that the interaural attenuation value for suprathreshold speech recognition measures should be computed as 35 dB. That is, the interaural attenuation value of 45 dB based on SRT measurement is adjusted by subtracting 10 dB. This adjustment reflects differences in percent correct criterion used for speech threshold and suprathreshold measurements.

It should be noted, however, that there is only *indirect* evidence that a more conservative estimate of interaural attenuation is needed during suprathreshold speech audiometry. The argument presented by Konkle and Berry (1983) assumes that the subject performance measured by presenting a suprathreshold speech recognition test *directly* to the nontest ear at 0 dB SL re SRT is equivalent to the performance measured *indirectly* through cross hearing (i.e., speech reaching the nontest ear through cross hearing at a sensation level of 0 dB). Theoretically, the test scores obtained in both situations would be identical if interaural attenuation across frequency was equivalent. Yet, there is considerable research indicating that interaural attenuation for air-conducted sound can vary as a function of frequency, particularly when using insert earphones (e.g., Berrett, 1973; Killion, Wilber, & Gudmundsen, 1985; Sklare & Denenberg, 1987). Consequently, a cross-hearing speech signal that has been filtered or shaped by the interaural attenuation characteristics of the particular subject and air-conduction transducer will reach the nontest ear.

For example, there is considerably greater interaural attenuation for low- than high-frequency air-conducted sound when using 3A insert earphones (see Chapter 8 for detailed information about interaural characteristics of insert receivers). Consequently, a cross-hearing speech signal will be *high-passed filtered* before it reaches the nontest ear. This undoubtedly could affect cross-hearing suprathreshold speech recognition performance, depending on the speech materials used. It may not always be possible to accurately predict cross-hearing performance on a suprathreshold speech recognition test using performance-intensity data obtained under monaural conditions in normal-hearing subjects. Unfortunately, no research studies currently available have *directly* evaluated interaural attenuation during suprathreshold speech recognition audiometry. Therefore, we must rely on indirect evidence that a more conservative estimate of interaural attenuation may be appropriate when making a decision about the use of contralateral masking during measurement of suprathreshold speech recognition.

We can restate our rule for masking during measurement of suprathreshold speech recognition as follows:

> Contralateral masking is indicated whenever the presentation level of the speech signal at the test ear exceeds the best pure-tone bone-conduction threshold in the nontest ear by 35 dB or more.

$$\text{Presentation level}_T - 35 \text{ dB} \geq \text{Best BC}_{NT}$$

It is difficult to generalize about the range of frequencies that correlates with suprathreshold speech recognition. This will vary depending on the specific speech recognition test. Because speech is a broadband stimulus, we will use a conservative approach and consider the best bone-conduction thresholds in the 250 to 4000 Hz frequency range when determining the need for masking during assessment of suprathreshold speech recognition. The rules for contralateral masking during air-conduction speech audiometry are summarized in Table 4-2.

Let us consider the need for contralateral masking during assessment of suprathreshold speech recognition ability in the audiograms presented in Figures 4-6 and 4-7. Ideally, masked air- and pure-tone bone-conduction thresholds should be obtained where indicated prior to commencement of the speech audiometry test battery.

Figure 4-6: Pure-tone testing reveals normal hearing through 1000 Hz, sloping sharply to a severe-to-profound sensorineural hearing loss in the high frequencies bilaterally. Unmasked SRTs of 10 dB HL were obtained in both ears, a finding consistent with the pure-tone findings. Masking was not required during assessment of speech recognition threshold in either ear. Suprathreshold speech recognition ability will be assessed using the California Consonant Test

TABLE 4–2	The rules for when to mask during air-conduction speech audiometry.

When the presentation level of the speech signal in the test ear (Presentation level$_T$) equals or exceeds the best pure-tone bone-conduction threshold (Best BC$_{NT}$) at either 250, 500, 1000, 2000, or 4000 Hz in the nontest ear by the amount of interaural attenuation (IA)*, masking should be applied to the nontest ear.

$$\text{Presentation level}_T - \text{IA} \geq \text{Best BC}_{NT}$$

or

$$\text{Presentation level}_T - \text{Best BC}_{NT} \geq \text{IA}$$

*IA values for speech: speech recognition threshold = 45 dB; speech detection threshold = 35 dB; suprathreshold speech recognition = 35 dB; or all speech audiometric measurements = 40 dB.

FIGURE 4–6   Audiogram presenting a moderate-to-severe, high-frequency sensorineural hearing loss bilaterally. The SRTs of 10 dB HL confirm the presence of normal hearing in the low frequencies. Contralateral masking will be required when measuring suprathreshold speech recognition in both ears.

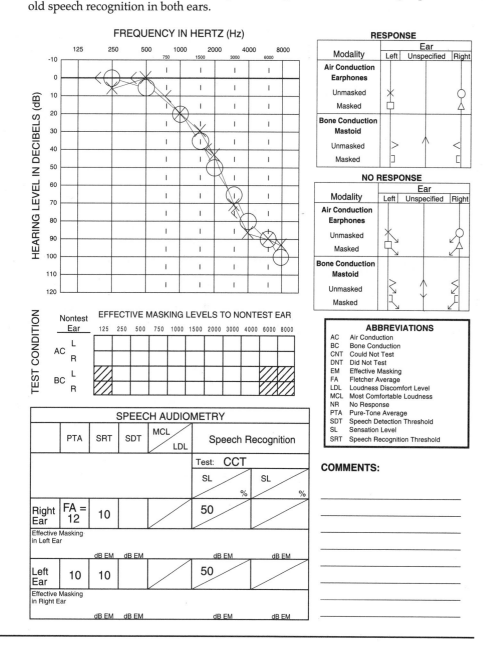

(CCT) (Owens & Schubert, 1977). This is a multiple-choice consonant recognition test that is sensitive to the speech recognition difficulties of individuals with high-frequency hearing loss. The recommended sensation level for this test is 50 dB (Schwartz & Surr, 1979). If suprathreshold speech recognition ability is assessed at 60 dB HL (i.e., 50 dB greater than the SRTs of 10 dB HL), then contralateral masking will be required in both ears.

$$\text{Presentation level}_T - 35 \text{ dB} \geq \text{Best BC}_{NT}$$
$$60 \text{ dB HL} - 35 \text{ dB} \geq 0 \text{ dB HL (at 250, 500 Hz)?}$$
$$25 \text{ dB HL} \geq 0 \text{ dB HL?}$$

Speech theoretically is reaching the nontest ear at 25 dB HL. Because there are bone-conduction thresholds at 0 dB HL, the predicted cross-hearing signal of 25 dB HL can stimulate the nontest ear. Hearing sensitivity is good enough (i.e., 0 dB HL) in the nontest ear to perceive the estimated cross-hearing signal (i.e., 25 dB HL).

Figure 4-6 illustrates an important point about contralateral masking during suprathreshold speech recognition testing. There is a common misconception that masking is not required in cases in which hearing is symmetrical. As demonstrated in the example presented here, contralateral masking is often required. The need for contralateral masking during suprathreshold speech recognition testing should be evaluated *in all cases*.

Figure 4-7: Pure-tone testing reveals normal hearing in the left ear. There is a moderate-to-severe sensorineural hearing loss of sloping configuration in the right ear. Speech recognition thresholds (i.e., 45 dB HL and 0 dB HL for the right and left ears respectively) confirm the pure-tone findings. The SRT in the right ear was obtained using contralateral masking. Consider the need for contralateral masking during assessment of suprathreshold speech recognition ability using Northwestern Auditory Test #6 (NU-6) (Tillman & Carhart, 1966). The monosyllabic words will be presented at a sensation level of 40 dB.

Is masking required during assessment of suprathreshold speech recognition in the *right ear*? If sensation level is 40 dB, then the presentation level in the right ear will be 85 dB HL (i.e., 40 dB greater than the SRT of 45 dB HL).

$$\text{Presentation level}_T - 35 \text{ dB} \geq \text{Best BC}_{NT}$$
$$85 \text{ dB HL} - 35 \text{ dB} \geq 0 \text{ dB HL?}$$
$$50 \text{ dB HL} \geq 0 \text{ dB HL?}$$

Masking will be required when assessing suprathreshold speech recognition in the right ear. Theoretically, a cross-hearing signal of 50 dB HL is reaching the nontest (i.e., left) ear. Because there are bone-conduction thresholds of 50 dB HL or better in the nontest ear, contralateral masking will be needed. It should be noted that contralateral masking was needed during assessment of the speech recognition threshold in the right ear. Therefore, we can assume that masking also will be required during any suprathreshold speech measurement.

Contralateral masking will not be required, however, during assessment of suprathreshold speech recognition in the left ear. If a sensation level of 40 dB is used, then presentation level in the left ear will be 40 dB HL (i.e., 40 dB greater than the SRT of 0 dB HL).

$$\text{Presentation level}_T - 35 \text{ dB} \geq \text{Best BC}_{NT}$$
$$40 \text{ dB HL} - 35 \text{ dB} \geq 35 \text{ dB HL (at 250 Hz)?}$$
$$5 \text{ dB HL} \geq 35 \text{ dB HL?}$$

A cross-hearing signal of 5 dB HL is reaching the nontest ear. Because the best bone-conduction threshold in the nontest ear is 35 dB HL, we are not concerned about the occurrence of cross hearing. Hearing sensitivity is not good enough (i.e., 35 dB HL) to perceive the estimated cross-hearing signal (i.e., 5 dB HL).

FIGURE 4–7 Audiogram presenting normal hearing in the left ear. There is a moderate-to-severe, sensorineural hearing loss of sloping configuration in the right ear. Speech recognition thresholds (45 dB HL and 0 dB HL for the right and left ears respectively) confirm the pure-tone findings. Contralateral masking will be required when measuring suprathreshold speech recognition in the right ear.

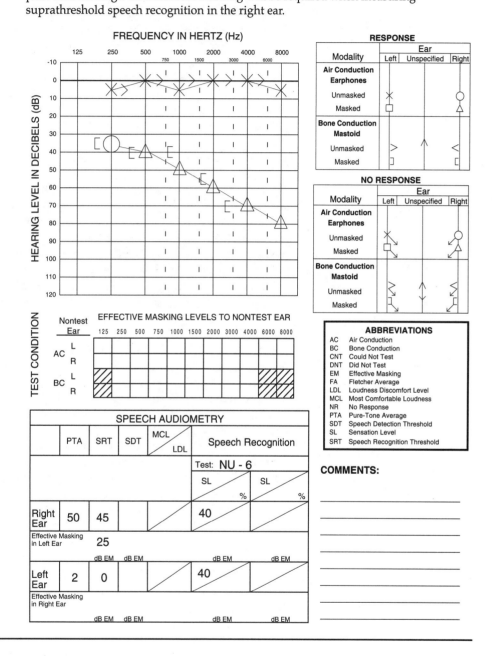

It is important to remember that the use of an interaural attenuation value of 35 dB for measurement of suprathreshold speech recognition is very conservative. In fact, the majority of audiologists will use an interaural attenuation value of 40 dB for *all* air-conduction measurements, both pure tones and speech, when making a decision about the need for contralateral masking (Martin et al., 1994; Martin & Morris, 1989). The use of a single interaural attenuation value of 40 dB for all speech audiometric measurements (threshold and suprathreshold) is suggested by Martin (1994). It is an approach that can be justified based on empirical and theoretical data. Recall that the smallest reported value of interaural attenuation for spondaic words (i.e., SRT) is *48 dB*. Because the speech detection threshold (i.e., SDT) requires an average of 8 to 9 dB less intensity than the SRT, it may be appropriate to use a more conservative interaural attenuation value of *39-40 dB* for the SDT (i.e., 48 dB – 8 or 9 dB). Finally, given the fundamental difference in percent correct criterion when measuring the speech recognition threshold versus suprathreshold speech recognition, it has been suggested that the interaural attenuation value used for SRT be adjusted during suprathreshold speech recognition testing by subtracting 10 dB (Konkle & Berry, 1983; Studebaker, 1979). A more conservative interaural attenuation value of *38 dB* (i.e., 48 dB – 10 dB) would result. Based on this data, the use of interaural attenuation values of 45 dB for the SRT, 35 dB for the SDT, and 35 dB for measurement of suprathreshold speech recognition is recommended.

The use of a single interaural attenuation value of 40 dB for *all* threshold and suprathreshold speech measures, however, can also be supported. Although use of an interaural attenuation value of 40 dB is somewhat too conservative during assessment of speech recognition threshold, it probably would prove adequate in most cases during assessment of the speech detection threshold and suprathreshold speech recognition. If the Auditec recorded versions of either NU-6 or W-22 are used to assess suprathreshold speech recognition, for example, a less conservative estimate of interaural attenuation than 35 dB would be needed. Beattie et al. (1977) reported that normal-hearing listeners achieved an average percent correct performance of about 3 percent when either W-22 or NU-6 was presented at 4 dB SL. We can estimate that close to 0 percent correct performance would be achieved at 0 dB SL. Thus, we could easily justify using a less conservative correction factor of either 0 dB or 5 dB rather than the general correction factor of 10 dB. In this instance, an adjusted interaural attenuation value of either 45 dB (i.e., IA of 45 dB 0 dB) or the more conservative 40 dB (i.e., IA of 45 dB – 5 dB) would be appropriate. Given that the majority (80 percent) of audiologists use a monitored live-voice presentation during assessment of suprathreshold speech recognition using either W-22 or NU-6 (Martin et al., 1994), however, it is not possible to know the performance-intensity characteristics of a particular live-voice speech recognition test. The conservative interaural attenuation estimate of 35 dB for suprathreshold speech recognition can be easily supported, particularly during monitored live-voice presentation. Although the use of different interaural attenuation values for each test of the speech audiometric test battery is recommended, it is not the only "correct" approach. Any decision on the need for masking that is based on both empirical/theoretical data and clinical experience is appropriate and "correct."

Summary

There are four factors to consider when making a decision about the need for contralateral masking during air-conduction speech audiometry:

1. Presentation level of the speech signal (i.e., intensity level) at the test ear

2. Interaural attenuation

3. Bone-conduction sensitivity in the nontest ear

4. Type of speech measurement (i.e., speech threshold versus suprathreshold speech recognition)

Generally, contralateral masking is indicated during speech threshold measurement whenever the presentation level of the speech signal at the test ear (Presentation level$_T$) equals or exceeds the pure-tone bone-conduction sensitivity in the nontest ear (BC$_{NT}$) by the amount of interaural attenuation (IA):

$$\text{Presentation level}_T - \text{IA} \geq \text{BC}_{NT}$$

Because speech is a broadband stimulus, it is necessary to consider bone-conduction hearing sensitivity at more than a single pure-tone frequency. The most conservative approach involves considering the best bone-conduction threshold in the 250 to 4000 Hz frequency range when determining the need for masking during measurement of any speech threshold.

The smallest reported value of interaural attenuation for spondaic words is 48 dB. Consequently, a conservative estimate of interaural attenuation when measuring the speech recognition threshold using spondaic words is 45 dB. Given the intensity relationship between speech detection and speech recognition thresholds, a more conservative interaural attenuation value of 35 dB may be appropriate when measuring the speech detection threshold.

There is some evidence that a more conservative value of interaural attenuation should also be used during assessment of suprathreshold speech recognition. The fundamental difference in percent correct criterion during suprathreshold testing requires specification of nontest ear bone-conduction sensitivity in a different way than that used for speech recognition threshold measurement. A conservative estimate of interaural attenuation during measurement of suprathreshold speech recognition is 35 dB (i.e., the interaural attenuation value of 45 dB based on speech recognition threshold measurement is adjusted by subtracting 10 dB).

In summary, contralateral masking should be applied to the nontest ear whenever the presentation level of the speech stimulus in the test ear equals or exceeds the best pure-tone bone-conduction threshold from 250 to 4000 Hz in the nontest ear by the amount of interaural attenuation.

$$\text{Presentation level}_T - \text{IA} \geq \text{Best BC}_{NT}$$

or

$$\text{Presentation level}_T - \text{Best BC}_{NT} \geq \text{IA}$$

A conservative approach involves using different interaural values for each test of the speech audiometric test battery:

Speech recognition threshold	45 dB
Speech detection threshold	35 dB
Suprathreshold speech recognition	35 dB

An alternative approach involves using a single interaural attenuation value of 40 dB for all speech audiometric measures. Consideration of the suprathreshold speech recognition materials used, as well as the mode of presentation (i.e., recorded versus monitored-live voice), will influence the selection of an appropriate value of interaural attenuation.

Study Questions

1. List the four factors that must be considered when making a decision about the need for masking during air-conduction speech audiometry.

2. Briefly describe how interaural attenuation for speech is typically measured.

3. What is a conservative estimate of interaural attenuation when measuring the speech recognition threshold using spondaic words?

4. A more conservative value of interaural attenuation than 45 dB may be appropriate when measuring the speech detection threshold. Briefly explain.

5. Bone-conduction thresholds in the nontest ear must be considered when making a decision about the need for contralateral masking during the assessment of speech threshold. Which test frequencies should be considered? Provide your rationale.

6. State the rule for when to mask during air-conduction speech audiometry. Also express this rule in the form of an equation.

7. A decision can often be made about the need for contralateral masking by simply comparing the speech thresholds of the test and nontest ears. Briefly explain.

8. Consideration of only the speech thresholds of the two ears can lead to an incorrect decision about the need for contralateral masking. Briefly explain.

9. There is some evidence that it may be appropriate to apply a more conservative estimate of interaural attenuation when making a decision about the need for contralateral masking during suprathreshold speech recognition testing. Briefly discuss.

10. When making a decision about the need for contralateral masking during speech audiometry, interaural attenuation must be considered. A conservative approach involves using different interaural attenuation values for each test of the speech audiometric test battery. An alternative approach involves using a single interaural attenuation value for all speech audiometric measures. Which of the two approaches is the most appropriate? Briefly discuss.

5

Clinical Masking Procedures: Pure-Tone Threshold Audiometry

Whenever it is suspected that the nontest ear is responsive during evaluation of the test ear, a masking stimulus must be applied to the nontest ear to eliminate its participation. Although there are many different approaches to clinical masking, all procedures address two basic questions. First, what is the minimum level of noise that is needed to just mask the cross-hearing signal in the nontest ear? Stated differently, this is the minimum masking level (or minimum effective masking level) that is needed to avoid *undermasking* (i.e., the test signal continues to be perceived in the nontest ear). Second, what is the maximum level of noise that can be presented to the nontest ear that will not shift or change the true threshold in the test ear? Stated differently, this is the maximum masking level (or maximum effective masking level) that can be used without *overmasking*. Not only can cross hearing occur for the test signal, it can also occur for the masking stimulus as well. Once the masking stimulus in the nontest ear reaches sufficient intensity, it can cross to the test ear and produce a masking effect in the test ear (i.e., overmasking). The purpose of masking is to make the test tone inaudible in the nontest ear without changing the true threshold in the test ear. The primary goal of any clinical masking procedure is to avoid both undermasking and overmasking.

Studebaker (1979) has identified two major approaches to clinical masking—psychoacoustic and acoustic. The psychoacoustic procedures are "those based upon observed shifts in the measured threshold as a function of suprathreshold masker effective levels in the nontest ear" (p. 82). These methods are also referred to as shadowing or threshold shift procedures. The acoustic procedures are "those based upon calculating the approximate acoustic levels of the test and masker signals in the two ears under any given set of conditions and on this basis deriving the required masking level" (p. 82). The acoustic procedures are also known as formula or calculation methods. Generally, the psychoacoustic methods are considered appropriate for threshold measurement while the acoustic methods prove most efficient for suprathreshold procedures.

A number of authorities (e.g., Liden, Nilsson, & Anderson, 1959; Martin, 1967, 1974; Studebaker, 1962, 1964) have presented formulas or equations for the calculation of minimum and maximum masking levels during pure-tone audiometry. A discussion of these formulas will facilitate an understanding of how appropriate levels of masking are selected during clinical masking procedures.

Minimum Masking Level

Four factors influence minimum masking level during pure-tone threshold audiometry:

1. Presentation level of the test signal
2. Interaural attenuation of the test signal
3. The presence of an air-bone gap in the nontest (i.e., masked) ear
4. The occlusion effect (only during bone-conduction audiometry)

Air Conduction

Liden, Nilsson, and Anderson (1959) offered the following formula for calculating minimum masking level (M_{min}) during pure-tone air-conduction audiometry:

$$M_{min} = A_t - 40 + (A_m - B_m)$$

where A_t is equal to the air-conduction threshold in the test ear, 40 (dB) is a conservative estimate of interaural attenuation, A_m is equal to air-conduction threshold of the masked ear, and B_m is equal to bone-conduction threshold of the masked ear. The factor $(A_m - B_m)$ is a measure of an air-bone gap in the masked ear (AB Gap_m). Therefore, we can simplify this equation as follows:

$$M_{min} = A_t - 40 + AB\ Gap_m$$

A similar formula for calculation of minimum masking level was described by Studebaker (1964). He states that minimum masking level (Min_{HL}) equals the level of the test signal reaching the masked ear (i.e., level of the signal at the test ear, T_T, minus interaural attenuation, IA), plus the air-conduction threshold in the masked (i.e., nontest) ear (AC_m), minus the bone-conduction threshold in the masked ear (AC_m), plus the minimum masking levels for subjects with normal hearing (Min_N):

$$
\begin{aligned}
Min_{HL} &= (T_T - IA) + AC_m - BC_m + Min_N \\
&= (T_T - IA) + (AC_m - BC_m) + Min_N \\
&= T_T - IA + AB\ Gap_m + Min_N
\end{aligned}
$$

If the masking noise level is calibrated in dB EM and if we assume that the minimum masking level for normals (Min_N) is equal to 0 dB EM (Martin, 1967), then Studebaker's formula can be simplified as follows:

$$
\begin{aligned}
Min_{HL} &= T_T - IA + AB\ Gap_m + Min_N \\
&= T_T - IA + AB\ Gap_m
\end{aligned}
$$

It should be apparent that the minimum masking level formulas described by Liden and associates (1959) and Studebaker (1964) are essentially identical. We can summarize the formula for minimum masking level as follows:

$$M_{min} = AC_T - IA + AB\ Gap_{NT}$$

where AC_T is the unmasked air-conduction threshold of the test ear, IA is inter-aural attenuation, and $AB\ Gap_{NT}$ is the air-bone gap in the nontest (i.e., masked) ear.

Consider the hypothetical example presented in Figure 5-1. Unmasked pure-tone testing at 1000 Hz reveals air-conduction thresholds of 25 dB HL and 65 dB HL in the right and left ears respectively. Unmasked bone-conduction threshold is 0 dB HL. Because there is a 40-dB difference between the air-conduction thresholds in the right and left ears (or a 40 dB or greater difference between the air-conduction threshold in the left ear and the unmasked bone-conduction threshold), contralateral masking is indicated when measuring air-conduction threshold in the left ear. Let us calculate the minimum masking level using the above formula:

$$
\begin{aligned}
M_{min} &= AC_T - IA + AB\ Gap_{NT} \\
&= 65 - 40\ (\text{conservative estimate of IA}) + 25 \\
&= 25 + 25 \\
&= 50\ \text{dB EM}
\end{aligned}
$$

FIGURE 5–1 An example illustrating calculation of minimum masking level during air-conduction audiometry. Unmasked pure-tone testing at 1000 Hz reveals that contralateral ear masking will be required when measuring air-conduction threshold in the left ear. (1) Calculation of initial minimum masking level in the right ear using the "formula" approach. $M_{min} = AC_T - IA + AB\ Gap_{NT} = 65 - 40 + 25 = 50$ dB EM. If we assume that 65 dB is a more accurate estimate of interaural attenuation in this particular case, then minimum masking level is calculated as follows: $M_{min} = AC_T - IA + AB\ Gap_{NT} = 65 - 65 + 25 = 25$ dB EM. (2) Calculation of initial minimum masking level in the right ear using Martin's (1967, 1974) approach. $M_{min} = AC_{NT} = 25$ dB EM.

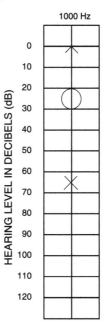

The *initial* minimum masking level needed in the nontest (i.e., right) ear is 50 dB EM. If the test signal is presented at 65 dB HL and if we assume that interaural attenuation can be as small as 40 dB, then theoretically a cross-hearing signal of 25 dB HL is reaching the nontest ear. A masker level of 25 dB EM will be needed to just mask the cross-hearing signal of 25 dB HL in the nontest ear. However, there is a potential air-bone gap of 25 dB in the nontest ear. This will reduce the intensity (and effectiveness) of the masker by the size of the air-bone gap (i.e., 25 dB). Therefore, the minimum masking level must be increased by the size of the air-bone gap. We must compensate for the presence of an air-bone gap in the masked ear by increasing the minimum masking level.

Although the "formula" approach for calculating the minimum masking level is accurate (and necessary during administration of suprathreshold auditory tests), it proves to be disadvantageous during threshold audiometry. First, it can be somewhat time-consuming. Second, the clinician may not have the required information to calculate minimum masking level at that time. For example, the formula approach requires information about an air-bone gap in the nontest ear. Yet a decision about the need for masking during air-conduction audiometry often can be made by comparing the air-conduction thresholds of the two ears (i.e., a 40 dB or greater difference between the air-conduction thresholds). Martin (1967, 1974) has suggested that such formulas are unnecessary during threshold audiometry and has simplified the calculation of the minimum masking level. Martin states that the initial minimum masking level is simply equal to the air-conduction threshold of the nontest ear:

$$M_{min} = AC_{nontest\ ear}$$
$$= AC_{NT}$$

Consider again the hypothetical example presented in Figure 5-1. Recall that it is necessary to introduce contralateral masking to the right ear while retesting the air-conduction threshold in the left ear. According to Martin, the initial minimum masking level is equal to the air-conduction threshold of the nontest ear—25 dB EM. There is no need to consider the presence of an air-bone gap in the nontest ear. Martin explains the derivation of this equation in two ways.

First, a signal detected *at threshold* (without contralateral masking) is assumed to have a sensation level (SL) of 0 dB, regardless of whether it is perceived in the test or nontest ear. Given this assumption, the initial minimum masking required is a level of noise that will just mask a signal of 0 dB SL. Martin (1967) argues that if cross hearing is suspected and the air-conduction threshold in the nontest ear is 0 dB HL, then the minimum masking level is equal to 0 dB EM. If the air-conduction threshold in the nontest ear is 30 dB HL, then 30 dB EM is required to just mask the cross-hearing signal of 0 dB SL in the nontest ear, and so on.

Second, Martin (1974) states that the use of formulas for calculating minimum masking should result in the same level of masking noise. Consider again the formula approach for calculation of minimum masking level:

$$M_{min} = AC_T - IA + AB\ Gap_{NT}$$

Given certain assumptions, M_{min} calculated using the formula approach will result in a level of masking equal to air-conduction threshold of the nontest ear. Refer again to Figure 5-1. Using the formula approach, we calculated M_{min} to be equal to 50 dB EM. Martin argues that this patient's interaural attenuation could not be equal to 40 dB as shown in the formula: 60 – 40 (IA) + 25 = 50 dB EM. If we assume that (1) the unmasked bone-conduction threshold of 0 dB HL could reflect a response from the right (i.e., nontest) ear and (2) interaural attenuation is equal to 40 dB, then an unmasked air-conduction threshold theoretically would be obtained in the left ear at a level 40 dB greater than the bone-conduction response (0 dB HL). That is, unmasked air-conduction threshold in the left ear would be equal to 40 dB HL. Yet an unmasked air-conduction threshold occurred at 65 dB HL, a level 65 dB greater than the assumed bone-conduction threshold in the right ear. In this particular case, the patient's interaural attenuation is at least 65 dB. Let us recalculate minimum masking level substituting 65 dB for 40 dB as our estimate of interaural attenuation:

$$M_{min} = AC_T - IA + AB\ Gap_{NT}$$
$$= 65 - 65\ (\text{estimate of IA}) + 25$$
$$= 0 + 25$$
$$= 25\ dB\ EM$$

The minimum masking level of 25 dB EM calculated from our formula is equal to the air-conduction threshold of the nontest ear. Martin's simplified equation for minimum masking level supports the theoretical foundations of the formula approach. We often cannot estimate interaural attenuation for a particular patient. It is assumed, therefore, that interaural attenuation can be as small as 40 dB. However, Martin's simplified approach for the calculation of the minimum masking level does not require information about either interaural attenuation or an air-bone gap in the nontest ear.

Martin (1974) recommends that approximately 10 dB should be added to the initial minimum masking level to account for intersubject variability with respect to effectiveness of masking levels. Recall that dB effective masking refers to the dB HL to which threshold is shifted by a given level of noise. Calibration of effective masking level is based on the *averaged* responses of a group of normal-hearing subjects. A given effective masking level will not prove equally effective for all subjects. Studebaker (1979) explains that if we assume that masked thresholds are normally distributed around the average effective level and that the standard deviation of the distribution is approximately 5 dB, then a safety factor of 10 dB added to the initial minimum masking level should prove sufficient in 98 percent of all cases. Although the cautious audiologist may decide to add 15 or 20 dB to the initial staring level, Studebaker recommends that a safety factor of not less than 10 dB should be added to the calculated minimum masking level. We can rewrite Martin's simplified equation for the initial minimum masking level as follows:

$$M_{min} = AC_{NT} + 10\ dB\ (\text{safety factor})$$

It is important to differentiate the terms *minimum masking level* and *initial minimum masking level* (or *initial masking level* as described by Martin in 1994). These terms are not always used consistently in the literature. Generally, the minimum masking level is the minimum level of noise needed to just mask the test signal reaching the nontest (i.e., masked) ear. During pure-tone threshold audiometry using contralateral masking, however, it is often necessary to increase the intensity of the signal in order to reach threshold in the test ear. Consequently, it is also necessary to increase the intensity of the masker in the nontest ear. The minimum masking level required to establish threshold in the test ear is often greater than the initial level calculated based on unmasked pure-tone thresholds. The important point to remember is that the minimum masking level initially presented to the nontest ear may need to be increased during the course of clinical masking to measure the true threshold in the test ear.

Bone Conduction

Studebaker (1964) offered the same minimum masking level formula for both air- and bone-conduction audiometry. Recall his simplified formula from above:

$$\text{Min}_{HL} = T_T - IA + AB\ \text{Gap}_m$$

In the case of bone-conduction audiometry, T_T is equal to bone-conduction threshold of the test ear. If we assume that interaural attenuation for bone conduction can be as small as 0 dB, then we can further simplify Studebaker's formula as follows:

$$\text{Min}_{HL} = T_T - IA + AB\ \text{Gap}_m$$
$$= T_T - 0 + AB\ \text{Gap}_m$$
$$= T_T + AB\ \text{Gap}_m$$

Liden and associates (1959) offered a similar formula for calculating the minimum effective masking level during bone-conduction measurements:

$$M_{min} = B_t + (A_m + B_m)$$

where B_t is equal to bone-conduction threshold of the test ear, A_m is air-conduction threshold of the masked (i.e., nontest) ear, and B_m is equal to bone-conduction threshold of the masked ear. Because the factor $(A_m + B_m)$ corresponds to an air-bone gap in the masked ear, we can simplify this formula as follows:

$$M_{min} = B_t + AB\ \text{Gap}_m$$

This formula is similar to that offered by Liden and associates (1959) for air-conduction, with the exception that interaural attenuation does not factor into the equation. The assumption is that interaural attenuation for bone conduction is zero. It should be clear that the formulas offered by Studebaker (1964) and Liden and associates (1959) are essentially the same. We can summarize the formula for the minimum masking level for bone conduction as follows:

$$M_{min} = BC_T + AB\ \text{Gap}_{NT}$$

where BC_T is the unmasked bone-conduction threshold when testing at the "test" ear and $AB\ \text{Gap}_{NT}$ is the air-bone gap in the nontest (i.e., masked) ear.

Consider the hypothetical example presented in Figure 5-2. Unmasked air-conduction thresholds at 2000 Hz were obtained at 30 dB HL and 55 dB HL in the right and left ears respectively. With the bone vibrator placed at the left mastoid, an unmasked bone-conduction threshold was measured at 20 dB HL. There is no need for contralateral masking during air-conduction audiometry because there is not a difference of 40 dB or more between the unmasked bone-conduction threshold and either unmasked air-conduction threshold. Howev-

FIGURE 5–2   An example illustrating calculation of minimum masking level during bone-conduction audiometry. Unmasked bone-conduction testing at 2000 Hz reveals that contralateral masking will be required when measuring bone-conduction threshold in the left ear (i.e., potential air-bone gap ≥ 15 dB). (1) Calculation of initial minimum masking level using the "formula" approach. $M_{min} = BC_T + AB\ Gap_{NT} = 20 + 10 = 30$ dB EM. (2) Calculation of initial minimum masking level using Martin's (1967, 1974) approach. $M_{min} = AC_{NT} = 30$ dB EM.

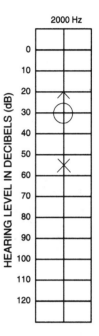

er, contralateral masking will be needed when testing bone conduction in the left ear because of a potential air-bone gap of 35 dB. We will use the above formula to determine the initial minimum masking level:

$$M_{min} = BC_T + AB\ Gap_{NT}$$
$$= 20 + 10$$
$$= 30\ dB\ EM$$

A test signal of 20 dB HL is presented. Because it is assumed that interaural attenuation can be as small as 0 dB, a cross-hearing signal of 20 dB HL theoretically can be reaching the left (i.e., nontest) cochlea. A masker level of 20 dB EM will be needed to just mask the cross-hearing signal of 20 dB HL in the nontest ear. However, the potential air-bone gap of 10 dB in the nontest ear will reduce the effectiveness of the masker. Therefore, the minimum masking level must be increased by the size of the air-bone gap. The minimum masking level is calculated to be 30 dB EM, a level equal to the air-conduction threshold in the nontest ear.

The formula approach for determination of minimum masking levels during bone-conduction threshold audiometry is not clinically practical. It has been presented to illustrate that formulas for minimum masking levels for both air- and bone-conduction audiometry are derived from the same theoretical constructs.

As with air-conduction audiometry, Martin's simplified approach to calculating the minimum masking level will prove more useful clinically. Specifically, the initial minimum masking level is equal to the air-conduction threshold of the nontest ear. This has already been demonstrated in Figure 5-2. Again, we see that the use of formulas for calculating initial minimum masking level for threshold bone-conduction audiometry is not necessary. When testing by bone conduction, however, the *occlusion effect* must be added to the minimum masking level to compensate for covering (i.e., occluding) the nontest ear with an earphone (Martin, 1967, 1974; Studebaker, 1964).

The *occlusion effect* is the apparent improvement in low-frequency bone-conduction thresholds that occurs when the external auditory meatus is covered or occluded. The contribution of the external auditory meatus to bone-conduction thresholds is discussed by Tonndorf (1968, 1972). When sound is applied to the skull through a bone vibrator, the osseous and cartilaginous walls of the ear canal will vibrate. Sound waves subsequently are generated within the ear canal and reach the cochlea through the normal air-conduction route (i.e., the osseotympanic component of bone-conduction hearing). When the ear canal is uncovered or unoccluded, it functions as a high-pass filter. High-frequency sound waves pass through the ear canal to the tympanic membrane while low-frequency sounds are dissipated through the outer opening. During unmasked bone-conduction threshold testing, some sound energy radiated through the walls of the ear canal will escape, particularly in the lower frequencies. If the ear canal is covered by a supra-aural earphone during bone-conduction testing, however, the high-pass filter effect is eliminated. The outcome is the increased transmission of low frequency bone-conducted sound. Studebaker (1979) points out that the occlusion effect does not actually affect hearing sensitivity of the occluded ear, but rather increases the intensity of the signal reaching the cochlea. It should be noted that the occlusion effect is present only in ears with normal hearing and sensorineural hearing loss; the effect is decreased or absent in ears with conductive hearing impairment.

Bone-conduction thresholds are always obtained with the test ear *unoccluded*. However, when an earphone is placed over the nontest ear during masked bone-conduction audiometry, an occlusion effect may be created in the nontest ear. Consequently, there is increased probability that the nontest ear will respond when obtaining a masked bone-conduction threshold in the test ear. The nontest ear, in effect, becomes more sensitive to the cross-hearing bone-conducted sound. Therefore, the initial masking level must be increased by the amount of the occlusion effect. Unfortunately, if the occlusion effect is not appropriately corrected for, this increased level of noise may increase the probability of overmasking.

It is agreed that the occlusion effect must be considered when determining the initial minimum masking level during bone-conduction threshold audiometry. Failure to do so can result in undermasking. We can restate Martin's (1967, 1974, 1994) equation for initial minimum masking level during bone-conduction audiometry as follows:

$$M_{min} = AC_{NT} + \text{Occlusion effect} + 10 \text{ dB (safety factor)}$$

This equation is essentially the same as that recommended for air-conduction threshold audiometry, the difference being the addition of the occlusion effect.

There are two basic approaches to adding the occlusion effect to the initial minimum masking level. The clinician can use either *average* or *individual* occlusion effect values. The first approach involves using a constant number for the occlusion effect that is based on *average* or typical data reported in the literature. Table 5-1 presents mean occlusion effects (in dB) reported by various investiga-

TABLE 5-1 Mean occlusion effects in decibels (dB) for normal-hearing subjects. The occlusion effect was calculated by subtracting the occluded bone-conduction threshold (ear covered by a supra-aural earphone and cushion) from the unoccluded bone-conduction threshold. Bone-conduction thresholds were measured with the bone vibrator placed either at the frontal bone[1] (i.e., forehead) or mastoid process.[2]

Study	Earphone (Cushion)	Frequency (in Hz)				
		250	500	1000	2000	4000
Berger & Kerivan (1983)[1]	TDH-50 (MX-41/AR)	20.3	21.6	7.5	-1.3	—
Berrett (1973)[1]	TDH-39 (MX-41/AR)	19.0	17.7	9.0	0.9	—
Dirks & Swindeman (1967)[1]	TDH-39 (MX-41/AR)	23.7	19.3	7.5	-0.6	—
Elpern & Naunton (1963)[1]	TDH-39 ("firm rubber cushion")	28.0	20.0	9.0	0	0
Goldstein & Hayes (1965)[2]	TDH-39 (MX-41/AR)	19.4	12.6	5.7	1.1	-4.1
Goldstein & Hayes (1965)[1]	TDH-39 (MX-41/AR)	12.2	13.1	4.9	0	0
Hodgson & Tillman (1966)[1]	TDH-49 (MX-41/AR)	22.0	19.0	7.0	0	0

tors. The size of the occlusion effect is determined by subtracting the occluded bone-conduction threshold from the unoccluded bone-conduction threshold.

It should be noted that the occlusion effect occurs only in the lower frequencies (1000 Hz and below). Based on the average occlusion effects reported in the literature, the following values are recommended for clinical use: 30 dB at 250 Hz, 20 dB at 500 Hz, 10 dB at 1000 Hz, and 0 dB at frequencies above 1000 Hz. These values are summarized in Table 5-2. Studebaker (1967a) cautions, however, about the use of average occlusion effect values. He recommends that the value used be the largest occlusion effect reported across individuals.

Remember that the occlusion effect should be added to the initial minimum masking level only if the nontest ear exhibits normal hearing or a sensorineural hearing loss. There is no need to compensate for the occlusion effect if there is a conductive hearing loss in the nontest ear. The increase in sound pressure level created by the occlusion is attenuated by the conductive hearing loss. Studebaker (1979) states that an air-bone gap as small as 20 dB can eliminate the occlusion effect. This statement is supported by the research of Martin, Butler, and Burns (1974). They measured occlusion effects at 250 and 500 Hz in subjects with normal hearing, conductive hearing loss, and sensorineural hearing impairment. All subjects with conductive hearing impairment exhibited air-bone gaps of at least 20 dB. At both 250 and 500 Hz, the modal occlusion effect was 0 dB in the conductive group. The largest occlusion effect measured did not exceed 5 dB. We can conclude that if the *nontest ear* (i.e., the masked ear) exhibits a potential air-bone gap of 20 dB or more, the occlusion effect should not be added to the initial minimum masking level.

In a variation of this first approach, Martin and colleagues (1974) described a procedure in which standard occlusion effects are added to initial masking levels. However, no assumptions are made about the effect of a potential air-bone gap on the occlusion effect. Rather, the occlusion effect for the individual subject is measured in the nontest ear at 250 Hz. If the difference in threshold between the occluded and unoccluded states exceeds 10 dB or more, it is assumed that a conductive component does not exist. A standard occlusion effect is subsequently added to the initial masking level.

Figure 5-3 illustrates the calculation of initial minimum masking levels during bone-conduction threshold audiometry. Unmasked air- and bone-conduction thresholds have been obtained at 500, 1000, and 2000 Hz. Masked bone-conduction thresholds are needed only in the left ear. When we compare the unmasked bone-conduction thresholds to the air-conduction thresholds in the right ear, there is no evidence of a significant air-bone gap at any frequency. However, there are potentially significant air-bone gaps in the left ear (i.e., 35 dB at 500 and 1000 Hz, 25 dB at 2000 Hz). We will calculate the initial minimum masking levels needed in the right ear when measuring bone-conduction thresholds in the left ear. The average occlusion effect values recommended in Table 5-2 will be used in our calculations:

$$M_{min} = AC_{NT} + \text{Occlusion effect} + 10 \text{ dB (safety factor)}$$
$$500 \text{ Hz} \qquad M_{min} = 10 + 20 + 10 = 40 \text{ dB EM}$$
$$1000 \text{ Hz} \qquad M_{min} = 20 + 10 + 10 = 40 \text{ dB EM}$$
$$2000 \text{ Hz} \qquad M_{min} = 40 + 0 + 10 = 50 \text{ dB EM}$$

Because there was no evidence of a conductive hearing loss in the masked ear, the occlusion effect was added to the initial minimum masking levels.

The use of a fixed value for the occlusion effect based on average data has

TABLE 5–2   Occlusion effect values in decibels recommended for clinical use during masked bone-conduction audiometry. These values are considered appropriate when contralateral masking is delivered through a traditional supra-aural earphone.

Frequency (in Hz)				
250	500	1000	2000	4000
30	20	10	0	0

disadvantages. First, considerable intersubject variability for the occlusion effect has been reported (e.g., Dirks & Swindemann, 1967; Elpern & Naunton, 1963; Goldstein & Hayes, 1965; Hodgson & Tillman, 1966). The use of a single correction value for all subjects could result in the use of either too little or too much masking when compensating for the occlusion effect in a particular case. Second, determination of the presence of a potential air-bone gap in the nontest ear is often based on unmasked bone-conduction thresholds. Failure to compensate for the occlusion effect because of an incorrect assumption about a con-

FIGURE 5–3   An example illustrating calculation of initial minimum masking level during bone-conduction audiometry. Unmasked bone-conduction testing at 500, 1000, and 2000 Hz reveals that contralateral masking will be required when measuring bone-conduction thresholds in the left ear (i.e., potential air-bone gaps ≥ 15 dB). Because there is no evidence of a conductive component in the masked ear, the occlusion effect should be added to initial masking levels.

$$M_{min} = AC_{NT} + \text{Occlusion effect} + 10 \text{ dB (safety factor)}$$

500 Hz $M_{min} = 10 + 20 + 10 = 40$ dB EM

1000 Hz $M_{min} = 20 + 10 + 10 = 40$ dB EM

2000 Hz $M_{min} = 40 + 0 + 10 = 50$ dB EM

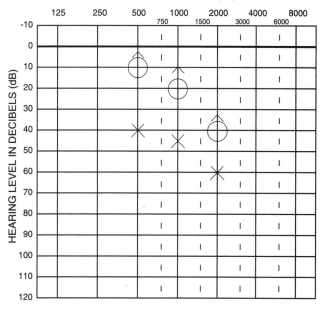

ductive component in the nontest ear could result in undermasking. Third, it is difficult to predict the effect of minimal conductive hearing loss on the magnitude of the occlusion effect. Consequently, the occlusion effect may not be corrected for appropriately when determining initial minimum masking level.

The second major approach to correcting for the occlusion effect avoids the disadvantages associated with using average values. Martin and colleagues (1974) first described a method by which the occlusion effect of the patient's masked ear is determined and subsequently added to the initial minimum masking level. The patient's unoccluded bone-conduction thresholds are measured initially at 250, 500, and 1000 Hz. Occluded thresholds are redetermined by placing the supra-aural earphone over the nontest ear *without* masking noise present. The patient's occlusion effect in the nontest ear is determined by subtracting at each frequency the occluded threshold from the unoccluded threshold. This value is then added to the initial minimum masking level. The use of individually measured occlusion effects when determining required masking levels is recommended by other investigators (Silman & Silverman, 1991; Studebaker, 1979).

There is a limitation, however, to the method by which individual occlusion effects are determined. Diagnostic audiometers typically permit selection of a lower intensity limit of –10 dB HL. Thus, it may not be possible to measure a valid occlusion effect in individuals whose unoccluded bone-conduction thresholds approach the lower limit of intensity (i.e., –10 dB HL).

Consider the following example. Your patient has normal hearing in the better ear. An unmasked (and unoccluded) bone-conduction threshold of 0 dB HL is measured at 250 Hz. It may not be possible to estimate an accurate occlusion effect in this individual. If an occluded bone-conduction threshold is measured at –10 dB HL (i.e., the lower output limit), then it can only be stated that the occlusion effect is ≥ 10 dB. Remember that demonstration of the occlusion effect requires the ability to measure an improvement in bone-conduction sensitivity. The presence of unmasked bone-conduction thresholds within the normal range may restrict valid measurement of the occlusion effect. The accurate determination of individual occlusion effects often requires unoccluded bone-conduction thresholds that fall outside the normal range of hearing (i.e., > 20 dB HL). This is particularly true in the very low frequencies where the occlusion effect is the greatest. Consequently, it may be necessary to use *average* rather than *individual* occlusion effect values during bone-conduction audiometry when masking an ear with very good hearing sensitivity.

The occlusion effect and air conduction   Our discussion of the occlusion effect has been limited to the selection of appropriate masking levels during bone-conduction audiometry. However, the occlusion effect has clinical implications during both bone-conduction and air-conduction audiometry.

Interaural attenuation for air-conducted sound typically is determined with both ears covered or occluded. There is considerable evidence that occlusion of the nontest ear (i.e., normal ear) will affect the measured interaural attenuation for air-conducted sound (Berrett, 1973; Chaiklin, 1967; Feldman, 1963; Killion, Wilber, & Gudmundsen, 1985; Littler, Knight, & Strange, 1952; Van Campen, Sammeth, & Peek, 1990; Zwislocki, 1953). Consider that cross hearing for air-conducted sound is primarily a bone-conduction phenomenon (e.g., Zwislocki, 1953). When the nontest ear is covered or occluded by an air-conduction transducer, an occlusion effect is introduced in that ear. Consequently, the occlusion effect is exhibited by decreased low-frequency interaural attenuation in the occluded condition (i.e., both ears occluded) versus the unoccluded condition (i.e., nontest ear unoccluded) (e.g., Berrett, 1973; Killion et al., 1985; Van Campen et al., 1990).

Berrett (1973) studied the relationship between interaural attenuation for air-conducted sound and the occlusion effect. He reported that there were no statistically significant differences between the magnitude of the difference between interaural attenuation values measured in the occluded and unoccluded conditions and the magnitude of the occlusion effect. Berrett concluded that if the opposite ear is unoccluded and exhibits a normal occlusion effect, then interaural attenuation will be increased in magnitude by the size of the occlusion effect. This latter finding does not have clinical implications during air-conduction audiometry because both ears traditionally are covered or occluded. The audiologist simply uses reported interaural attenuation values measured in the occluded condition.

Because the test ear is unoccluded during masked bone-conduction audiometry, however, interaural attenuation for the air-conducted masker signal will be increased when compared to the values measured in the occluded air-conduction condition for normal ears. Consequently, maximum masking level will be increased. Unfortunately, the net effect of this increased interaural attenuation is negligible when using a traditional supra-aural earphone for introducing contralateral masking. If both ears exhibit a normal occlusion effect in the low frequencies (i.e., ears with normal hearing or a sensorineural hearing loss), then the increased interaural attenuation that results by not occluding the test ear is offset by the increased masking required when occluding the nontest (i.e., masked) ear with a supra-aural earphone. Both minimum and maximum masking levels are increased by an equivalent amount in the low frequencies. The important point to remember is that the use of higher levels of masking to compensate for the occlusion effect during bone-conduction audiometry will not necessarily increase the probability of overmasking.

Summary

The minimum masking level is the minimum amount of noise required to just mask the cross-hearing signal in the nontest ear. A number of authorities have presented formulas for calculation of minimum masking level. Martin (1967, 1974) has simplified the calculation of initial minimum masking level during air- and bone-conduction threshold audiometry. Generally, initial minimum masking level is equal to air-conduction threshold of the nontest ear. Martin's equations are recommended for clinical use during masked pure-tone threshold audiometry and are summarized in Table 5-3.

TABLE 5–3 Formulas for determining initial minimum masking level and maximum masking level during pure-tone threshold audiometry.

Initial Minimum Masking Level

$$AC_{NT} + 10 \text{ dB safety factor (Air Conduction)}$$
$$AC_{NT} + OE + 10 \text{ dB safety factor (Bone Conduction)}$$

Maximum Masking Level

$$BC_T + IA - 5 \text{ dB (Air Conduction)}$$
$$BC_T + IA - 5 \text{ dB (Bone Conduction)}$$

Maximum Masking Level

Maximum masking level refers to the maximum level of noise that can be used in the nontest ear that will not shift or change the true threshold in the test ear. Calculation of maximum masking level helps the clinician evaluate the possibility of overmasking. Two factors influence maximum masking level during pure-tone threshold audiometry: (1) The bone-conduction threshold of the test ear and (2) the interaural attenuation of the air-conducted masking stimulus.

Liden and associates (1959) offered the following formula for calculating maximum masking level (M_{max}) during pure-tone air- and bone-conduction audiometry:

$$M_{max} = B_t + 40$$

where B_t is equal to bone-conduction threshold of the test ear and the number 40 (dB) is equal to interaural attenuation for air-conducted sound. The equation for maximum masking level is the same for both air- and bone-conduction audiometry: Masking noise is delivered through an air-conduction transducer regardless of the transducer used for measuring pure-tone threshold. Because we are concerned about an undesired masking effect in the test ear, bone-conduction sensitivity in the test ear must be considered. As a result, overmasking is more of a potential problem when bone-conduction sensitivity is very good in the test ear. The poorer hearing sensitivity is by bone conduction in the test ear, the progressively greater levels of masking that can be used without overmasking. It is always assumed that the maximum masking level does not exceed the patient's loudness discomfort level.

The original equation described by Liden, Nilsson, and Anderson requires two modifications. First, a value of 5 dB must be subtracted from the level calculated to result in overmasking. If $B_t + 40$ is just sufficient to produce overmasking, then clinically we want to use a masking level that is slightly less than the calculated value. Because dB HL and dB EM are calibrated in 5-dB increments, maximum masking level is now calculated as $B_t + 40 - 5$ dB. Second, Liden and associates assumed that interaural attenuation for air-conducted sound could be as small as 40 dB. However, a less conservative estimate of interaural attenuation can often be substituted into the equation. A more general equation for calculation of maximum masking level (M_{max}) can be stated as follows:

$$M_{max} = B_T + IA - 5 \text{ dB}$$

Consider the example presented in Figure 5-4. Pure-tone testing at 1000 Hz revealed unmasked air-conduction thresholds of 60 dB HL and 10 dB HL in the right and left ears respectively. Unmasked bone-conduction threshold is 5 dB HL. Contralateral masking will be required when establishing both air- and bone-conduction thresholds in the right ear. (Masked thresholds for the right ear are also indicated. We will consider this information later.) Let us calculate the maximum masking level during pure-tone threshold audiometry. Remember that maximum masking level is the same during both air- and bone-conduction audiometry.

$$M_{max} = B_T + IA - 5 \text{ dB}$$
$$= 5 + 55 - 5$$
$$= 55 \text{ dB EM}$$

FIGURE 5–4   An example illustrating calculation of maximum masking level during pure-tone threshold audiometry. Contralateral masking will be required when measuring air- and bone-conduction thresholds in the right ear. The maximum masking level that can be used in the left ear is estimated using the following formula: $M_{max} = B_T + IA - 5$ dB. A very conservative estimate of maximum masking level typically will result when an unmasked bone-conduction threshold is used in the masking equation: $M_{max} = 5 + 55 - 5$ dB $= 55$ dB EM. The actual bone-conduction threshold in the right ear is 80 dB HL (determined subsequently using contralateral masking). When the masked bone-conduction threshold is substituted for the unmasked threshold of 5 dB HL, a more accurate and higher maximum masking level results: $M_{max} = 80 + 55 - 5 = 130$ dB EM.

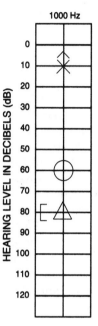

Because only an unmasked bone-conduction threshold is available at the time that masking requirements are determined, we assume that bone-conduction threshold in the test ear can be as good as 5 dB HL. Rather than using the very conservative estimate of 40 dB for interaural attenuation, we will use the more accurate estimate of 55 dB. If bone-conduction threshold in the left (i.e., nontest) ear is assumed to be 5 dB HL (i.e., the *unmasked* bone-conduction threshold) and unmasked air-conduction threshold in the right (i.e., test) ear is 60 dB HL, then interaural attenuation is estimated to be at least 55 dB. Given these assumptions, the maximum masking level is calculated as 55 dB EM. If bone-conduction hearing sensitivity in the test (i.e., right) ear is 5 dB HL and interaural attenuation is equal to 55 dB, then overmasking will occur when masker level in the nontest (i.e., left) ear exceeds 55 dB EM.

It is important to remember that the estimated maximum masking level during pure-tone threshold audiometry is typically very conservative. The actual maximum masking level that can be employed without overmasking is generally higher than the estimated value because an unmasked bone-conduction threshold is used when calculating the formula. This is true particularly when there is a sensorineural hearing loss in the test ear. Refer again to Figure 5-4. The true air- and bone-conduction thresholds obtained with contralateral masking are plotted for the right ear. Note that the actual bone-conduction threshold in the right ear is 80 dB HL. When this value is substituted for the unmasked bone-conduction threshold of 5 dB HL, a more accurate and considerably higher maximum masking level results:

$$M_{max} = B_T + IA - 5 \text{ dB}$$
$$= 80 + 55 - 5$$
$$= 130 \text{ dB EM}$$

Although it was originally estimated that the maximum masking level could be as low as 55 dB EM, the actual level based on the true bone-conduction threshold of the test ear was 130 dB EM. If there had been a conductive hearing loss in the test ear (i.e., the unmasked bone-conduction threshold of 5 dB HL actually reflected hearing in the test ear), then the estimated maximum masking level of 55 dB EM would have been correct.

Many beginning clinicians incorrectly conclude that the estimated maximum masking level cannot be exceeded during clinical masking procedures. This frequently is not the case. Because an unmasked bone-conduction threshold is used during determination of maximum masking level, the resultant value is often much smaller than the masking level that will actually result in overmasking. This was illustrated in the above example. The calculation of maximum masking level during masked pure-tone threshold audiometry is often of limited use. However, consideration of maximum masking level will caution the audiologist about the possibility of overmasking, particularly in cases of conductive hearing impairment. The equation for calculation of maximum masking level during pure-tone air- and bone-conduction threshold audiometry is summarized in Table 5-3.

Recommended Clinical Procedures

When it is suspected that a pure-tone signal presented to the test ear is actually being detected by the nontest ear, contralateral masking must be presented to the nontest ear. The most popular method (Martin, Armstrong, & Champlin, 1994) for obtaining masked pure-tone thresholds was first described by Hood in 1957 (Hood, 1960; Hood's original paper was reprinted in the United States in 1960). The Hood method, also referred to as the *plateau, shadowing,* or *threshold shift* procedure, is a psychoacoustic technique that relies on observations about the relationship between masker level in the nontest ear and measured threshold in the test ear.

Consider the example presented in Figure 5-5. Unmasked pure-tone testing reveals air-conduction thresholds of 10 dB HL and 70 dB HL in the right and left ears respectively (Figure 5-5A). Contralateral masking will be required when testing the left ear because there is a 40 dB or greater difference between the two air-conduction thresholds. The initial minimum masking level that will be applied to the nontest (i.e., right) ear is 20 dB EM:

$$M_{min} = AC_{NT} + 10 \text{ dB}$$
$$= 10 + 10$$
$$= 20 \text{ dB EM}$$

FIGURE 5–5 Audiogram illustrating the need for contralateral masking when measuring pure-tone threshold in the left ear (A). Contralateral masking is required when testing the left ear because there is a 40 dB or greater difference between the two air-conduction thresholds. The initial masking level presented to the right (i.e., nontest) ear is 20 dB EM. That is, $M_{min} = AC_{NT} + 10$ dB = 10 dB HL + 10 = 20 dB EM. There are two possible outcomes that can occur when pure-tone threshold is re-established in the left ear: (1) No measured threshold shift (B) suggests that the pure-tone signal was originally perceived in the test ear; (2) A measured threshold shift (C) suggests that the pure-tone signal was originally perceived in the nontest ear.

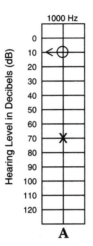

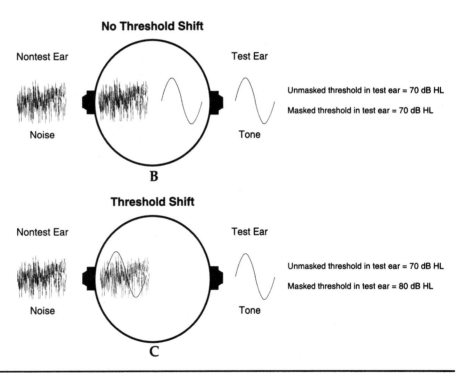

Recall that the purpose of masking is to raise the threshold of the nontest ear sufficiently to eliminate its contribution to a response from the test ear. If we assume that overmasking is not occurring, then the masking noise should have an effect only on the responsiveness of the nontest ear.

There are two possible outcomes that can occur when pure-tone threshold is re-established in the presence of contralateral masking: (1) no measured threshold shift or (2) a measured threshold shift. If the pure-tone stimulus was originally perceived in the test ear, then the introduction of contralateral masking should have no effect on the measured threshold. Conversely, if the pure tone was originally perceived in the nontest ear, then the presence of a masking stimulus in the nontest ear will produce a masking effect and a threshold shift will be measured.

The first outcome is illustrated in Figure 5-5B. A pure-tone signal is presented at 70 dB HL to the left ear. A masking stimulus of 20 dB EM (initial masking level) is presented to the nontest ear and pure-tone threshold is re-established. Because pure-tone threshold remains unaffected with the presence of contralateral masking, it is concluded that the measured response of 70 dB HL reflects hearing in the left ear. A masking effect (i.e., a threshold shift) will occur when the masking stimulus is presented to the ear that is responsive to the tone.

Figure 5-5C illustrates the outcome where the presence of contralateral masking does produce a masking effect. When the initial making level of 20 dB EM is presented to the nontest ear, the subject no longer can perceive the pure tone presented at 70 dB HL (unmasked threshold). It is necessary to increase the signal to 80 dB HL for the subject to respond again. The presence of masking in the nontest ear produced a masking effect, that is, a shift from the originally measured threshold. It is concluded, therefore, that the unmasked threshold of 70 dB HL was a result of cross hearing in the nontest ear. When the unmasked pure-tone signal is perceived in the nontest ear, the subsequent application of a masking stimulus will raise the threshold of the nontest ear, resulting in a measured threshold shift.

The underlying concept of the Hood procedure is that the introduction of masking to the nontest ear will produce a threshold shift for the signal only if the nontest ear is contributing to the observed response. Decisions about which ear (i.e., test or nontest) is contributing to a measured threshold are based on whether a threshold shift occurs when masking is introduced to the nontest ear. Although Hood described a masking procedure for threshold measurement during bone-conduction audiometry, the technique is equally effective during air-conduction testing. The major components of Hood's shadowing technique can be described as follows:

1. An unmasked pure-tone threshold is obtained.
2. Masking noise is introduced to the nontest ear at an effective level 10 dB above air-conduction threshold (i.e., initial masking level).
3. Pure-tone threshold is re-established in the presence of masking in the nontest ear.
4. If there is no change in pure-tone threshold (5 dB or less) with the presence of masking in the nontest ear (i.e., no measured threshold shift), the unmasked threshold is accepted as the true threshold of the test ear.
5. If there is an increase in pure-tone threshold with the presence of masking, masker level is increased in successive 10-dB steps. Pure-tone threshold is re-established with each increase in masker level. True threshold of the test ear is reached when measured threshold remains unchanged with further increases in masker level.

Hood (1960) outlined two essential steps of the test procedure:

1. The demonstration of the shadowing effect
2. The identification of the changeover point (also known as the *plateau*.)

The hypothetical example presented in Figure 5-6 illustrates the concepts of shadowing and changeover point. Unmasked pure-tone testing at 1000 Hz reveals air-conduction thresholds of 0 dB HL and 50 dB HL in the right and left ears, respectively. Unmasked bone-conduction threshold is 0 dB HL (Figure 5-6*A*). Because there is a 40 dB or greater difference between the two air-conduction thresholds, contralateral masking will be required when measuring air-conduction threshold in the left ear. We will use the Hood or shadowing procedure to establish a masked air-conduction threshold in the left ear. Figure 5-6*B* presents pure-tone air-conduction threshold in the left (i.e., test) ear as a function of effective masking level (dB EM) in the right (i.e., nontest) ear.

1. Unmasked pure-tone threshold in the right ear is equal to 50 dB HL.

2. Masking noise is introduced to the nontest ear at an effective level 10 dB above air-conduction threshold (i.e., initial masking level). This is equal to 10 dB EM (i.e., AC_{NT} + 10 dB safety factor, 0 dB HL + 10 dB = 10 dB EM).

3. Pure-tone threshold is re-established and shifts to 60 dB HL. As the effective level of noise is raised sequentially to 20 dB EM and 30 dB EM, the pure-tone threshold continues to shift by 10 dB. There is a shadowing effect or a "step by step correlation" between the intensities of the pure-tone threshold and the masking noise. Stated differently, the masked pure-tone threshold "shadows" the threshold of the nontest (i.e., masked) ear by the effective level of the noise. Because threshold shifts occur when masking is introduced, it is concluded that the masking noise and the test tone are restricted to the nontest ear. Masker levels of less than 30 dB EM are considered *undermasking*—there is insufficient masking present to establish the true threshold in the test ear.

4. A different phenomenon occurs as the intensity of the masking noise is further increased. When the masking noise is changed in 10-dB increments from 30 dB EM to 80 dB EM, pure-tone threshold remains unchanged at 80 dB HL. A "plateau" (i.e., a condition of stability) has been reached in the masking function. Studebaker (1964, p. 29) defines plateau as "a threshold value in the tested ear which is relatively unaffected by changes in noise intensity in the opposite ear." Hood refers to the initial point on the masking function at which pure-tone threshold remains unchanged with further increments in masker level as the "changeover point." In this particular example, the changeover point occurs at 80 dB HL, which corresponds to the true threshold of the test ear. Because there is no additional masking effect as the masker intensity is increased, it is concluded that the nontest ear is no longer contributing to the observed threshold response. The threshold of the test ear has been reached. The intensity range of masker levels from 30 dB through 80 dB EM represents *adequate masking*. The true air-conduction threshold (i.e., 80 dB HL) obtained in the left ear with contralateral masking is plotted on the audiogram presented in Figure 5-6*A*.

5. When the masker level exceeds 80 dB EM, we again observe a pure-tone threshold shift. In fact, the threshold shift corresponds directly to increments in masking level. That is, the pure-tone threshold shifts 10 dB with each 10-dB increment in the masking level. *Overmasking* is now occurring. Because of cross hearing, the masking noise is now reaching the *test ear* with sufficient intensity to produce a masking effect (i.e., a threshold shift) in that ear. Both the *plateau* and *overmasking* portions of the masking function represent responses from the test ear.

The masking plateau represents a range of masking levels. The lower and upper boundaries of the plateau represent minimum masking and maximum

FIGURE 5–6 Hypothetical example illustrating the concepts of "shadowing" and "changeover point." (A) Unmasked pure-tone testing at 1000 Hz reveals air-conduction thresholds of 0 dB HL and 50 dB HL in the right and left ears respectively. Unmasked bone-conduction threshold is 0 dB HL. Contralateral masking is required when measuring air-conduction threshold in the left ear. (B) Masking noise is introduced to the nontest ear at an effective level 10 dB above air-conduction threshold (i.e., 10 dB EM, initial masking level). As the effective level of noise is raised sequentially to 20 dB EM and 30 dB EM, a shadowing effect occurs. Because the masked pure-tone threshold "shadows" the threshold of the nontest ear by the effective level of noise, it is concluded that a nontest ear response is occurring. When the masking noise is raised sequentially in 10-dB increments from 30 dB to 80 dB EM, pure-tone threshold remains unaffected. A "plateau" has occurred in the masking function, suggesting that pure-tone threshold of the test ear has been reached. The point on the masking function where pure-tone threshold remains stable with further increments in masker level is the "changeover point." When masker level exceeds 80 dB EM, pure-tone threshold once again begins to shift, a phenomenon suggesting that overmasking is occurring.

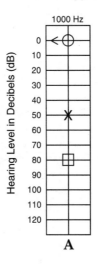

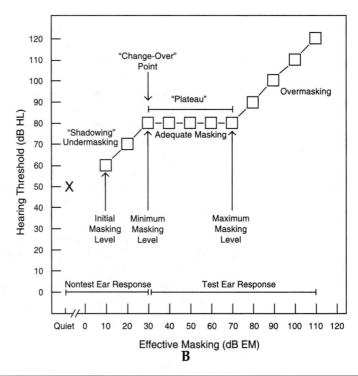

masking levels. In this context, we can define minimum masking level as the minimum amount of noise required to establish true threshold in the test ear. Recall from the above example that although the initial masking level was 10 dB EM, it was not sufficient to eliminate the participation of the nontest ear. The maximum masking level is the maximum amount of noise that can be used without producing a threshold shift in the test ear (i.e., overmasking).

Martin (1994) states that the width of the masking plateau is influenced by three factors: (1) interaural attenuation, (2) air-conduction threshold of the nontest ear, and (3) bone-conduction threshold of the test ear. *Interaural attenuation* affects minimum and maximum masking levels equally. The use of a transducer with increased interaural attenuation (i.e., insert receivers) will reduce the minimum masking level yet increase the maximum masking level. A wide masking plateau is advantageous because it reduces the probability of overmasking. Although the air-conduction threshold of the nontest ear and the bone-conduction threshold of the test ear both affect the width of the masking plateau, each variable influences the minimum and maximum masking levels in different ways. The *air-conduction threshold of the nontest ear* affects minimum masking level. The poorer the air-conduction threshold of the nontest ear, the higher the minimum masking level that is required. Conversely, the *bone-conduction threshold of the test ear* affects the maximum masking level. The better the bone-conduction threshold in the test ear, the lower the maximum masking level that is permissible. Each of these three factors can reduce the width of the masking plateau—the outcome is increased probability of overmasking.

Clinically, it is neither necessary nor time efficient to measure the entire masking plateau. The goal of the plateau procedure is to establish that the pure-tone threshold remains unchanged as the masker level is increased. In his original paper, Hood (1960) did not specify the number of masking increments needed to measure a masking plateau. It is generally agreed that a masking plateau has been established when the masker level can be increased over a range of at least 15 to 20 dB without shifting pure-tone threshold (Kaplan, Gladstone, & Lloyd, 1993; Martin, 1980; Sanders, 1991; Silman & Silverman, 1991).

Although Hood (1960) originally recommended that the masker level be changed in increments of 10 dB, others have suggested that the noise level be increased using a 5-dB step size. Silman and Silverman (1991) recommend an increment size of 5 dB because the clinical procedure for pure-tone threshold measurement also uses 5-dB increments. Martin (1980) states that although many clinicians use 10-dB masker increments to increase speed, accuracy is increased slightly by using a 5-dB step size. This can be important when the width of the masking plateau is narrow (e.g., a bilateral conductive hearing loss). The use of a 10-dB step size may be too large to precisely measure a masking plateau of only 10 to 15 dB. Although masker increment size (i.e., 5 or 10 dB) is somewhat arbitrary, the clinician should consider such issues when making a decision about the step size used during the plateau procedure.

The recommended clinical procedure for use of the plateau method during pure-tone threshold audiometry is summarized in Table 5-4. It is important to note that either the level of the tone or noise is increased by 5 dB depending on the patient's response. If there is a response to the tone in the presence of the noise, the level of the noise is increased by 5 dB. The patient's response to the tone is measured again. If a response to the tone occurs at the same level, the level of the noise is increased again by 5 dB, and so on. If the patient does not continue to respond to the tone in the presence of the noise, the level of the tone is raised in 5-dB steps until a response is obtained. The goal of the plateau procedure is to establish the hearing level (i.e., dB HL) at which pure-tone threshold remains

TABLE 5–4   Summary of the masking plateau procedure used during pure-tone threshold audiometry.

1. Introduce masking noise to the nontest ear at initial minimum masking level:

   AC_{NT} + 10 dB safety factor (Air Conduction)

   AC_{NT} + Occlusion effect + 10 dB (Bone Conduction)

2. Level of the tone or noise is increased by 5 dB. If there is a response to the tone in the presence of the noise, the level of the noise is increased by 5 dB. If there is no response to the tone in the presence of the noise, the level of the tone is raised in 5-dB steps until a response is obtained.

3. A plateau has been reached when the level of the noise can be raised 15 to 20 dB without an upward shift in the threshold of the tone. This corresponds to a response to the tone at the same level (i.e., dB HL) at three to four consecutive masking levels.

4. Masked threshold for the tone has been reached and corresponds to the level of the tone at which a masking plateau is established.

unchanged with increments in masker level. Figure 5-7 provides three examples that illustrate the use of the plateau method for obtaining masked pure-tone air-conduction thresholds. The unmasked air- and bone-conduction thresholds are the same in each example; the outcomes of the plateau procedure, however, are different. Unmasked air-conduction thresholds were obtained at 70 dB HL and 20 dB HL for the right and left ears respectively. An unmasked bone-conduction threshold was obtained at 10 dB HL. Because of the 40 dB or greater difference between the two air-conduction thresholds, it will be necessary to re-establish the air-conduction threshold in the right ear with contralateral masking. Masking will be introduced to the nontest (i.e., left) ear at the initial minimum masking level. This is equivalent to 30 dB EM:

$$M_{min} = AC_{NT} + 10 \text{ dB}$$
$$= 20 + 10$$
$$= 30 \text{ dB EM}$$

The plateau procedure will be used to establish masked air-conduction threshold in the right ear.

Case A

The initial minimum masking is introduced to the nontest ear at 30 dB EM. The pure tone is presented at a level equal to unmasked threshold. Because the patient continues to respond to the tone at 70 dB HL, the masker is then increased to 35 dB EM. The tone still remains audible when presented at 70 dB HL. The masker level is again increased by 5 dB to 40 dB EM; the patient still responds to the tone at 70 dB HL. Because the masker can be increased in 5-dB steps over a 20-dB range (from 30 dB through 50 dB EM) and pure-tone threshold remains stable, a plateau has been reached. Masked pure-tone threshold in the right ear is recorded as 70 dB HL. In this case, contralateral masking confirmed that the unmasked pure-tone threshold of 70 dB HL was not a result of cross hearing.

It has been suggested that it is not necessary to establish a masking plateau in cases in which the introduction of the initial minimum masking level does

FIGURE 5–7   Three examples illustrating the use of the plateau method for obtaining masked pure-tone air-conduction thresholds. Contralateral masking is required when measuring air-conduction threshold in the right ear. The unmasked air- and bone-conduction thresholds are the same in each example; however, the outcomes of the plateau procedure differ.

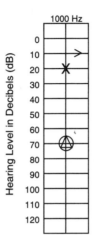

dB EM	dB HL
--	70
30	70
35	70
40	70
45	70
50	70

Threshold = 70 dB HL

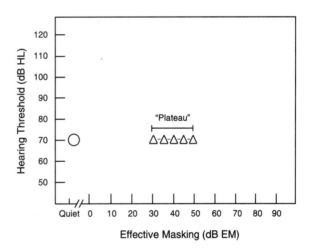

Case A: Unmasked pure-tone threshold (i.e., 70 dB HL) remains unaffected with increasing masker level. Contralateral masking has demonstrated that the unmasked pure-tone threshold is the true threshold of the test ear. Because unmasked pure-tone threshold is equal to the true (i.e., masked) threshold, "shadowing" and a "changeover" point are not observed on the masking function.

not shift the unmasked pure-tone threshold (Silman & Silverman, 1991). In Figure 5-7A, the introduction of minimum masking did not produce a threshold shift when compared to the unmasked threshold condition. It is concluded that the unmasked threshold of 70 dB HL reflects hearing in the test ear. This screening procedure reduces the need for additional levels of masking. Studebaker (1967a) and Coles and Priede (1970), however, wisely caution about the use of only one masking level when establishing pure-tone threshold. When

FIGURE 5–7   Continued

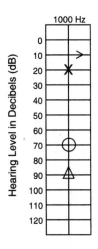

dB EM	dB HL
--	70
30	80
35	85
40	90
45	90
50	90
55	90
60	90

Threshold = 90 dB HL

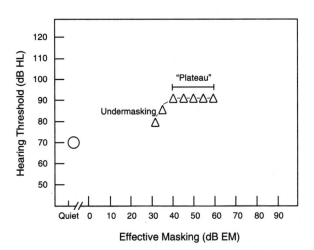

Case B: Unmasked pure-tone threshold is shifted initially with increasing masker level. A masking plateau is reached when masker level is increased from 40 dB through 60 dB EM (i.e., a 20 dB-wide masking plateau). Because pure-tone threshold remains unaffected at 90 dB HL with increasing masker level, pure-tone threshold in the right ear is recorded as 90 dB HL.

low effective masking levels are used, intersubject variability of effective masking level and the occlusion effect (in the case of bone-conduction audiometry) can result in undermasking in individual cases. Studebaker recommends the use of at least two levels of masking to ensure that the initial minimum masking level is sufficient.

Refer again to *Case A* presented in Figure 5-7. Because the introduction of initial minimum masking level does not produce a threshold shift from the unmasked condition, we can abbreviate the plateau procedure. To ensure that undermasking does not occur, we can present one additional level of masking to the nontest ear rather than the three to four consecutive levels needed to establish a plateau. For example, a second masking level of 40 dB EM confirms

FIGURE 5–7 Continued

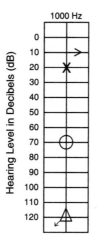

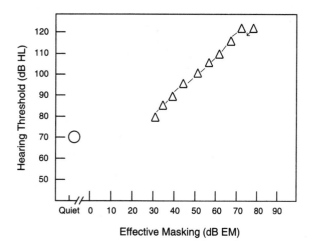

dB EM	dB HL
--	70
30	80
35	85
40	90
45	95
50	100
55	105
60	110
65	115
70	120
75	--

No response at 120 dB HL

Case C: Unmasked pure-tone threshold continues to shift to the output limits of the audiometer with increasing masker level. A masking plateau cannot be obtained. Consequently, it is concluded that there is no measurable hearing in the right ear at equipment limits (i.e., 120 dB HL).

that the pure-tone threshold remains unchanged when masking is introduced. The validity of the unmasked pure-tone threshold as a response from the test ear is more firmly established when at least two masking levels are used.

Case B

Again we will introduce the initial minimum masking level to the nontest ear at 30 dB EM. A different situation occurs than does in Case A. The patient no longer responds to the tone at 70 dB HL; it is necessary to increase the level of the tone to 80 dB HL in order to reach audibility. Because a threshold shift has occurred, it is concluded that the nontest ear contributed to the unmasked pure-tone threshold. We will now determine whether a masking plateau exists with the pure tone presented at 80 dB HL. The masker is increased by 5 dB to a level of 35 dB EM. However, the patient no longer responds to the tone at 80 dB HL; the tone must be increased to 85 dB HL to elicit a response. The shadowing effect is observed through masker levels of 40 dB EM. The change-over point does not occur until the tone reaches a level of 90 dB HL. When the masker is increased in 5-dB steps from 40 dB through 60 dB EM, pure-tone threshold remains unchanged at 90 dB HL. The masking plateau has been reached. The masked pure-tone threshold in the right ear is recorded as 90 dB HL.

Case C: Case C is similar to *Case B* in that a threshold shift occurs with introduction of the initial minimum masking level. However, a masking plateau is never achieved. Note that as masker level is increased by 5 dB, the pure-tone threshold is raised by an equivalent amount. The demonstration of the shadowing effect suggests that the tone and noise are confined to the nontest ear. When a masker level of 75 dB EM is presented, there is no response to the tone at equipment limits (i.e., 120 dB HL). This is recorded on the audiogram using the "no response" symbol. Assuming that overmasking is not occurring, it is concluded that there is no measurable hearing at equipment limits in the test ear. The hearing loss exceeds the pure-tone output limits.

Occasionally, a plateau cannot not be measured because of the output limits of the masking noise. The pure-tone threshold continues to shift with increments in masker level. However, the maximum masking level generated by the audiometer has been reached and a response to the tone can still be obtained. In this situation, the masker level cannot be further increased to measure a masking plateau. In effect, the clinician has "run out" of masking. In this case, it can only be stated that the true threshold equals or exceeds the last measured level (Studebaker, 1964).

Recall that the plateau procedure does not require that the pure-tone threshold be formally re-established each time that the masker level is increased. Rather, the tone is presented at the same level as the previous response. If no response occurs, the tone is raised in 5-dB steps until audibility is achieved. Keep in mind that a decision is made about raising the level of the tone based on only one response from the patient. Yet, the pure-tone threshold is defined clinically using a 50 percent response criterion and a minimum of three responses at a single level (ASHA, 1978). Variability in response to the tone can occur when testing at threshold. On occasion, the level of the tone may be increased inappropriately because of a decision-making process based on a single response. This can lead to imprecision when estimating the masked threshold. It is not time-efficient, however, to formally re-establish the pure-tone threshold each time that the masker level is raised. A compromise involves formally re-establishing the pure-tone threshold using a standardized procedure (e.g., ASHA, 1978) in the presence of the final level of masking noise that is used to establish the plateau. This often leads to a 5-dB improvement in the masked pure-tone threshold. Re-establishment of masked pure-tone threshold at the end of the plateau procedure is optional; it is a decision typically based on time considerations.

Central Masking

The introduction of contralateral masking can produce a small threshold shift in the test ear even when masker intensity is insufficient to produce overmasking (i.e., peripheral masking). Wegel and Lane (1924) referred to this phenomenon as "central masking." Liden and associates (1959) suggested that threshold shifts in the presence of low levels of masking are mediated through a central nervous system mechanism. Central masking has been reported to affect thresholds during both pure-tone and speech audiometry (e.g., Dirks & Malmquist, 1964; Liden et al., 1959; Martin, 1966; Martin, Bailey, & Pappas, 1965; Martin & DiGiovanni, 1979; Studebaker, 1962). Although the threshold shift produced by central masking is generally considered to be about 5 dB during pure-tone and speech threshold audiometry (Konkle & Berry, 1983; Martin, 1966, 1994), variable results have been reported across subjects and studies. There is also some evidence that the magnitude of the central masking effect increases with increasing masker intensity (e.g., Dirks & Malmquist, 1964; Martin et al., 1965; Studebaker, 1962).

Currently there is no generally accepted procedure that accounts for the effect of central masking during threshold audiometry. In a recent survey of audiologic practices in the United States conducted by Martin and colleagues (1994), 77 percent of responding audiologists indicated that they did not account for central masking (e.g., subtract 5 dB from the obtained masked threshold) during threshold pure-tone and speech audiometry. .

Generally, it is not recommended that the effect of central masking be subtracted from masked thresholds. Because of reported intersubject variability in the magnitude of the effect, it is difficult to determine an appropriate threshold correction. In addition, the effect generally is about 5 dB, the magnitude of which is considered to be within good test-retest reliability during threshold measurement. It is important, however, that the clinician always indicate where and how much contralateral masking is used. This information is useful in audiogram interpretation because it alerts the clinician to the possibility of central masking effects.

Martin (1966, 1994) suggests that it may appropriate to compensate for central masking during assessment of suprathreshold speech recognition. If contralateral masking is required during assessment of suprathreshold speech recognition, but not for the speech recognition threshold, the sensation level of the speech may be decreased effectively by 5 dB because of a central masking effect. In such cases, Martin recommends that the presentation level of the speech signal should be increased by 5 dB above the level customarily used in order to compensate for the central masking effect. It should be noted, however, that the effect of central masking on suprathreshold speech recognition performance is equivocal (e.g., Martin, 1966; Spencer & Priede, 1974).

The Masking Dilemma

Situations can occur in which the introduction of the initial minimum masking level can result in overmasking. Consider the example presented in Figure 5-8. Unmasked air- and bone-conduction pure-tone thresholds are presented in Figure 5-8*A*. Because there is a 40 dB or greater difference between the air-conduction thresholds and the unmasked bone-conduction thresholds in both ears, it will be necessary to re-establish air-conduction thresholds bilaterally using contralateral masking. In addition, masked bone-conduction thresholds will be required in both ears because of potential air-bone gaps of 15 dB or greater. The true pure-tone thresholds obtained with contralateral masking are presented in Figure 5-8*B*: There is a moderate, conductive hearing loss bilaterally. Unfortunately, in this particular case it may be impossible to obtain valid masked air- and bone-conduction thresholds because of overmasking.

Consider the unmasked air-conduction thresholds at 1000 Hz. We first will re-establish pure-tone air-conduction threshold in the right ear; contralateral

FIGURE 5–8   The classic example of a masking dilemma is demonstrated with a bilateral conductive hearing loss that exceeds approximately 40 dB. (A) Because there is a 40 dB or greater difference between the unmasked air-conduction threshold and the unmasked bone-conduction thresholds in both ears, contralateral masking will be required bilaterally during air-conduction threshold measurement. Masked bone-conduction thresholds will be required in both ears because of potential air-bone gaps of 15 dB or greater. (B) It may not be possible to obtain the true masked air- and bone-conduction thresholds in this particular case because of overmasking.

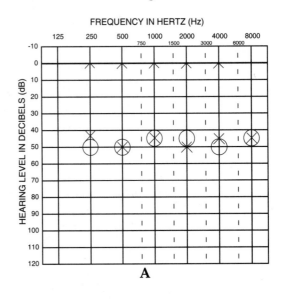

A

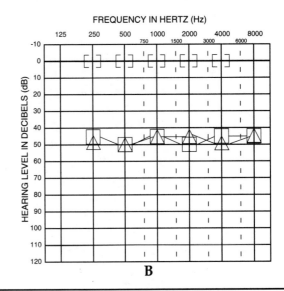

B

masking will be presented to the left ear. Initial minimum masking level is equal to 55 dB EM:

$$M_{min} = AC_{NT} + 10 \text{ dB}$$
$$= 45 + 10$$
$$= 55 \text{ dB EM}$$

Because the unmasked bone-conduction threshold is equal to 0 dB HL and the unmasked air-conduction threshold is equal to 45 dB HL, we know that interaural attenuation is not less than 45 dB. We will use this value of interaural attenuation (rather than the more conservative value of 40 dB) when estimating maximum masking level:

$$M_{max} = BC_T + IA - 5 \text{ dB}$$
$$= 0 + 45 - 5$$
$$= 40 \text{ dB EM}$$

If we assume that interaural attenuation is equal to 45 dB, then a situation has occurred where M_{min} (i.e., 60 dB EM) *exceeds* M_{max} (i.e., 45 dB EM). Our masking dilemma is clear: The initial minimum masking level needed to just mask a cross-hearing signal in the nontest ear may be sufficient to produce overmasking. The same situation would occur when obtaining a masked air-conduction threshold in the left ear. Theoretically, the introduction of initial masking will produce a threshold shift of the test signal. As masker intensity is subsequently increased in the nontest ear, an equivalent shift in the measured pure-tone threshold will occur in the test ear. It will not be possible to obtain a masking plateau. A masking dilemma exists because it may not be possible to determine whether overmasking is occurring or whether the maximum output for the pure-tone signal has been reached before a masking plateau has been established. The latter situation would occur when obtaining a masked pure-tone threshold in an individual with a profound hearing loss that exceeds output limits of the audiometer.

Studebaker (1979) explains that a masking dilemma occurs when the width of the masking plateau diminishes to or near 0 dB. Recall that the width of the masking plateau is partly related to both minimum and maximum masking levels. Generally, a masking dilemma will occur whenever there is a significant hearing loss in the nontest ear and a conductive hearing loss in the test ear. The existence of a significant hearing loss in the nontest ear requires higher initial masking levels; the presence of a conductive hearing loss in the test ear (i.e., normal bone-conduction hearing sensitivity) decreases the maximum masking level (i.e., maximum permissible masking). The consequence is a reduced or nonexistent masking plateau.

The classic example of a masking dilemma is demonstrated with a bilateral conductive hearing loss that exceeds approximately 40 dB (e.g., the case presented in Figure 5-8). The possibility exists for overmasking to occur when obtaining masked air- and bone-conduction thresholds in both ears. Naunton (1960) states that in some subjects with bilateral conductive hearing loss it is impossible to mask the nontest ear without masking the hearing of the test ear at the same time. In fact, Naunton demonstrated in two clinical cases of otosclerosis that a masking stimulus presented to the nontest ear produced a greater masking effect *in the test ear* than in the ear that received the masking stimulus directly. Konkle and Berry (1983, p. 301) state that "whenever the combined magnitude of the conductive components for each ear equals or exceeds two times the interaural attenuation value for either the test signal or masker, it will not be possible to use contralateral masking to mask the nontest ear and obtain valid test ear responses because a plateau will not occur." If we assume that interaural attenuation can be as small as 40 dB, then the use of contralateral masking in cases of bilateral conductive hearing loss that equals or exceeds 40 dB will produce a masking dilemma.

The consequence of overmasking is that the clinician will obtain thresholds in the test ear that are poorer than the actual thresholds. Consider the audiogram presented in Figure 5-9. This example illustrates how overmasking affects masked bone-conduction thresholds in an individual with bilateral conductive hearing impairment. The unmasked bone-conduction threshold (i.e., 0 dB HL) suggests a potential air-bone gap of 35 dB bilaterally; it will be necessary to obtain masked bone-conduction thresholds in both ears. Because air-conduction thresholds are the same bilaterally, the initial masking level will be equivalent in both ears. When calculating inital masking level, it is not necessary to add a correction factor for the occlusion effect because of evidence suggesting a significant conductive component bilaterally.

$$M_{min} = AC_{NT} + 10 \text{ dB}$$
$$= 35 + 10$$
$$= 45 \text{ dB EM}$$

If we assume that the unmasked bone-conduction threshold of 0 dB HL can reflect hearing in either ear, then the estimated maximum masking level will also be the same in both ears. We will assume that interaural attenuation can be as small as 40 dB.

$$M_{max} = BC_T + IA - 5 \text{ dB}$$
$$= 0 + 40 - 5$$
$$= 35 \text{ dB EM}$$

If interaural attenuation is in fact 40 dB, then overmasking will occur with the introduction of the initial masking level: M_{min} (i.e., 45 dB EM) exceeds M_{max} (i.e.,

---

FIGURE 5–9   Audiogram illustrating how overmasking affects masked bone-conduction thresholds in an individual with bilateral conductive hearing loss. Overmasking can occur with the introduction of initial masking level. Assuming that interaural attenuation can be as small as 40 dB, then initial masking level theoretically can exceed maximum masking level. The consequence is that masked bone-conduction threshold can be shifted to a hearing level equal to or greater than the air-conduction threshold without the establishment of a masking plateau.

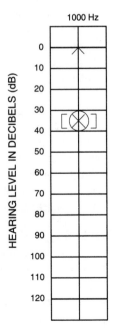

35 dB EM). When contralateral masking is applied to either ear, masked bone-conduction threshold theoretically will shift with each increment in masker intensity. Masked pure-tone threshold eventually is shifted to a hearing level equal to or greater than the air-conduction threshold without establishing a masking plateau. This would occur when measuring masked bone-conduction thresholds in both ears. It should be clear that overmasking is occurring in this situation. Given that unmasked bone-conduction threshold is equal to 0 dB HL, we know that there is a conductive hearing loss in at least one ear. Consequently, we should have been able to obtain a masked bone-conduction threshold of 0 dB HL in at least one ear. In such a situation, it will be necessary to indicate on the audiogram that valid masked bone-conduction thresholds could not be obtained because of overmasking.

A major advantage of the plateau procedure is that observations about the relationship between the masker level in the nontest ear and the measured threshold in the test ear can rule out the occurrence of overmasking in some instances. Consider the examples presented in Figure 5-10. Unmasked air-conduction thresholds at 2000 Hz were obtained at 45 dB HL and 35 dB HL in the right and left ears respectively; the unmasked bone-conduction threshold is

---

FIGURE 5–10   Example illustrating how establishment of a masking plateau can rule out the occurrence of overmasking. (A) Unmasked pure-tone air-conduction thresholds at 2000 Hz were obtained at 45 dB HL and 35 dB HL in the right and left ears respectively. It will be necessary to re-establish air-conduction threshold in the right ear using contralateral masking. Initial masking level is equal to 45 dB EM (i.e., AC_{NT} + 10 dB = 35 + 10 = 45 dB EM). Assuming that interaural attenuation is at least 45 dB, then maximum masking is estimated to be 40 dB EM (i.e., BC_T + IA − 5 dB = 0 + 45 − 5 = 40 dB EM). A situation has resulted where initial masking level exceeds the estimated maximum level. (B) In the first outcome, masking can be increased over a range of 20 dB without shifting the initial pure-tone threshold of 45 dB HL. Masked threshold is equal to the unmasked response (i.e., 45 dB HL). Although overmasking was a possibility in this case, the establishment of a masking plateau ruled out the occurrence of overmasking. (C) In the second outcome, pure-tone threshold shifts with each increment in masker intensity. The occurrence of overmasking cannot be ruled out because a masking plateau could not be established.

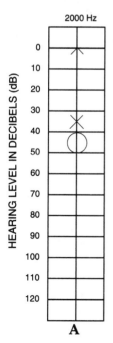 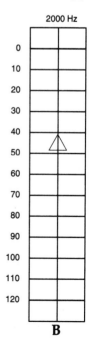 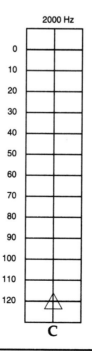

equal to 0 dB HL (Figure 5-10*A*). It will be necessary to re-establish air-conduction threshold in the right ear using contralateral masking.

We will consider the measurement of masked air-conduction threshold in the right ear. Initial minimum masking level is equal to 45 dB EM:

$$M_{min} = AC_{NT} + 10 \text{ dB}$$
$$= 35 + 10$$
$$= 45 \text{ dB EM}$$

Because the unmasked bone-conduction threshold is 0 dB HL and the unmasked air-conduction threshold is equal to 45 dB HL, it can be concluded that interaural attenuation for the air-conducted sound is not less than 45 dB. If we assume that interaural attenuation is at least 45 dB, then the maximum masking level is estimated to be 40 dB EM:

$$M_{max} = BC_T + IA - 5 \text{ dB}$$
$$= 0 + 45 - 5$$
$$= 40 \text{ dB EM}$$

A situation has resulted where M_{min} (i.e., 45 dB HL) exceeds the estimated M_{max} (i.e., 40 dB EM). There is the possibility of overmasking when measuring masked air-conduction threshold in the right ear. It is important to keep in mind that estimates of M_{max} are often very conservative. If interaural attenuation is in fact greater than 45 dB, then the maximum permissible masking will be increased. If such is the case, then it may be possible to establish a masking plateau.

There are two possible outcomes that can occur when measuring masked air-conduction threshold in the right ear. In the first case (Figure 5-10*B*), the introduction of initial masking does not result in a threshold shift in the right ear. In fact, when masking is increased by another 20 dB, this pure-tone threshold remains unchanged at 45 dB HL. Because there is no measured threshold shift when masking is introduced, we can conclude that the true threshold of the right ear is equal to 45 dB HL. There is no evidence that overmasking is occurring. It can be concluded that the actual interaural attenuation for this patient was greater than the estimated value of 45 dB that was used when the maximum masking level was calculated. Although overmasking may be predicted in a particular case, in many instances a masking plateau can be established. Whenever pure-tone threshold remains unchanged with increases in masker intensity, it can be concluded that overmasking is not occurring.

A different situation results in the second case (Figure 5-10*C*). The introduction of initial masking does produce a threshold shift from the unmasked condition at the test ear. In fact, the pure-tone threshold continues to shift each time that masker intensity is increased. The pure-tone threshold eventually is shifted to the output limits of the audiometer (e.g., 120 dB HL) without the establishment of a masking plateau. In this particular example, the occurrence of overmasking cannot be ruled out.

Fortunately, other audiologically relevant information available at the time of pure-tone threshold audiometry can alert the audiologist to the possibility of bilateral conductive hearing loss (e.g., case history, otologic report, prior audiologic report). The results of acoustic immittance measurements (e.g., tympanometry, static acoustic immittance, and ipsilateral/contralateral acoustic reflex studies) are particularly important and can help establish the presence of conductive pathology prior to pure-tone threshold audiometry. Such information can alert the audiologist to the possibility of a masking dilemma and the need for alternate testing strategies during threshold audiometry.

One solution to the masking dilemma is the use of insert receivers or earphones (e.g., Coles & Priede, 1970; Studebaker, 1962, 1964). Partly because of their smaller contact area with the skull, insert earphones result in significantly increased interaural attenuation values for air-conducted sound when compared to the traditional supra-aural earphone, particularly in the low frequencies (e.g., Killion et al., 1985; Sklare & Denenberg, 1987). The use of insert earphones greatly reduces the probability of overmasking because of increased interaural attenuation. The use of a transducer with increased interaural attenuation effectively increases the range between the minimum and maximum masking levels, thereby increasing the width of the masking plateau and the range of permissible masking (Studebaker, 1962). The use of insert earphones during clinical masking procedures is discussed in greater detail in Chapter 8.

Audiogram Interpretation

It is typical to graphically record both unmasked and masked pure-tone thresholds on the same audiogram. Consequently, audiogram interpretation will involve consideration of both unmasked and masked responses. Consider the following two examples.

Figure 5-11 presents an example in which contralateral masking was required when obtaining both air- and bone-conduction pure-tone thresholds in the left ear. Pure-tone testing reveals normal hearing in the right ear. Masked air- and bone-conduction responses in the left ear indicate a severe, sensorineural hearing loss of flat configuration. It should be noted that the unmasked air-conduction thresholds in the left ear are disregarded when interpreting hearing status in the left ear. Because a significant threshold shift occurred with the introduction of contralateral masking, it can be concluded that the unmasked air-conduction thresholds in the left ear reflected cross-hearing responses from the better (i.e., right) ear. Consequently, the *unmasked* air-conduction symbols should not be connected by lines. To avoid "clutter" on the audiogram, some audiologists do not report the unmasked air-conduction responses. In cases in which contralateral masking is required, it is acceptable to record only the masked thresholds (ASHA, 1990).

It is traditional to report the effective masking levels used when obtaining masked air- and bone-conduction thresholds. If the clinician uses the recommended psychoacoustic procedure for measuring masked pure-tone thresholds, then a range of masker levels will be used when establishing the masking plateau. The *final* masking level used to obtain masked threshold at each frequency should be reported for the *nontest* ear (ASHA, 1990). Refer again to Figure 5-11. Contralateral masking was used when obtaining both air- and bone-conduction thresholds in the left ear; masking levels are reported for the right (i.e., nontest) ear in a table provided on the audiogram form. For example, a masked air-conduction threshold at 500 Hz was obtained at 75 dB HL in the left ear; this masked air-conduction response was measured with a final masking level of 50 dB EM in the right ear. A masked bone-conduction threshold at 500 Hz was obtained at 65 dB HL in the left ear; the final masking level used in the right ear was 90 dB EM.

Figure 5-12 presents an example in which contralateral masking was

FIGURE 5–11	An example where contralateral masking was required when obtaining both air- and bone-conduction pure-tone thresholds in the left ear. Masked air- and bone-conduction thresholds indicate a severe, sensorineural hearing impairment of flat configuration in the left ear. The effective masking levels used in the nontest ear when obtaining masked pure-tone thresholds are provided on the audiogram form.

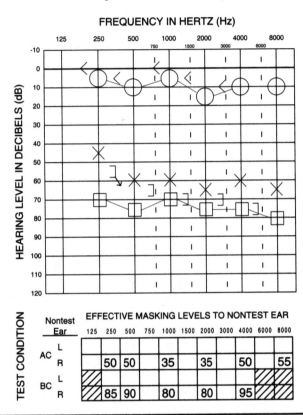

EFFECTIVE MASKING LEVELS TO NONTEST EAR

Test Condition	Nontest Ear	125	250	500	750	1000	1500	2000	3000	4000	6000	8000
AC	L											
	R		50	50		35		35		50		55
BC	L											
	R		85	90		80		80		95		

required when obtaining both air- and bone-conduction thresholds in the right ear. Masked air-conduction thresholds were obtained across frequency at the same hearing levels as the unmasked air-conduction responses in the right ear. Contralateral masking simply has confirmed that the unmasked responses reflect hearing in the test ear. Masked bone-conduction thresholds do not suggest the presence of significant air-bone gaps in the right ear. Our conclusion is that there is a moderate, sensorineural hearing loss of flat configuration in the right ear.

Although the results of unmasked bone-conduction audiometry suggested that masked bone-conduction thresholds were indicated in both ears because of potential air-bone gaps, masking was only required when assessing the right ear. Masked bone-conduction thresholds were measured first in the poorer (i.e., right) ear. Because masked bone-conduction responses were obtained in the right ear at levels ranging from 40 to 45 dB HL, we can assume that the unmasked responses of 0 to 5 dB HL reflect hearing in the left ear. Our conclusion is that there is a mild, conductive hearing loss of flat configuration in the left ear.

The previous examples illustrated two important points about interpretation of masked and unmasked audiometric responses. First, in cases in which contralateral masking is required, only *masked* air-conduction thresholds are

FIGURE 5–12   An example where contralateral masking was required when obtaining both air- and bone-conduction pure-tone thresholds in the right ear: Masked thresholds indicate a moderate, sensorineural hearing loss of flat configuration. Pure-tone testing suggests the presence of a mild, conductive hearing impairment of flat configuration in the left ear. Because masked bone-conduction responses were obtained in the right ear at hearing levels ranging from 40-45 dB HL, it can be assumed that the unmasked bone-conduction thresholds of 0-5 dB HL reflect responses in the left ear.

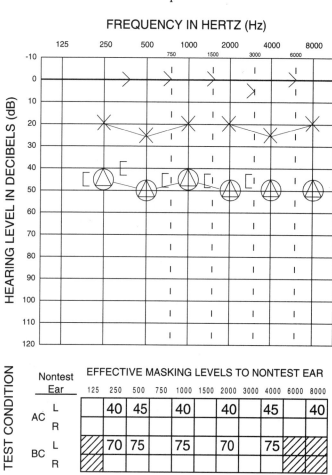

used in audiogram interpretation. Second, ear-specific information can be inferred from unmasked bone-conduction responses in some situations. Additional examples of audiogram interpretation are presented in Chapter 9.

Summary

Although there are many different approaches to clinical masking, each addresses two basic questions. First, what is the minimum level of noise that is needed to just mask the cross-hearing signal in the nontest ear (i.e., the minimum masking level)? Second, what is the maximum level of noise that can be presented to the nontest ear that will not affect the true threshold in the test ear (i.e., maximum masking level)? Studebaker (1979) describes two basic approaches to clinical masking. The *psychoacoustic procedure* relies on observations of the relationship between the measured threshold in the test ear and the masker level in the nontest ear. It is an approach that is considered appropriate for *threshold* measurement. The *acoustic procedure* involves deriving the required masking level by calculating the estimated acoustic levels of the test and masker signals in the test and nontest ears. This latter approach proves most efficient during suprathreshold procedures.

A number of authorities have discussed formulas or equations for calculating the minimum and maximum masking levels during pure-tone audiometry. Four factors influence minimum masking levels during pure-tone threshold audiometry:

(1) Presentation level of the test signal
(2) Interaural attenuation of the test signal
(3) The presence of an air-bone gap in the nontest (i.e., masked) ear
(4) The occlusion effect (only during bone-conduction audiometry)

Martin (1967, 1974) has suggested that formulas are unnecessary during threshold audiometry and has simplified the calculation of minimum masking level. The initial minimum masking level (M_{min}) during pure-tone air-conduction audiometry is equal to the air-conduction threshold of the nontest ear (AC_{NT}) plus a safety factor of at least 10 dB:

$$M_{min} = AC_{NT} + 10 \text{ dB (safety factor)}$$

The initial masking level during pure-tone bone-conduction audiometry is also equal the to air-conduction threshold of the test ear plus a safety factor of 10 dB. However, it is also necessary to consider the occlusion effect (OE) when determining the initial masking level during bone-conduction threshold audiometry:

$$M_{min} = AC_{NT} + OE + 10 \text{ dB (safety factor)}$$

Whenever an earphone is placed over the nontest ear during masked bone-conduction audiometry, an occlusion effect may be created in the nontest ear. Thus the nontest ear can become more sensitive to the cross-hearing bone-conducted sound. The initial masking level must be increased by the amount of the occlusion effect. The clinician can use either *average* or *individual* occlusion effect values when adding the occlusion effect to the initial minimum masking level.

The maximum masking level alerts the clinician to the possibility of over-masking. Two factors affect maximum masking level during pure-tone audiometry: (1) The bone-conduction threshold of the test ear (B_T) and (2) interaural attenuation (IA) of the air-conducted masking stimulus. A general equation for calculation of the maximum masking level (M_{max}) that can be used during both air- and bone-conduction pure-tone audiometry can be stated as follows:

$$M_{max} = B_T + IA - 5 \text{ dB}$$

The most popular method for obtaining masked pure-tone threshold was first described by Hood. The Hood method is also referred to as the *plateau, shadowing,* or *threshold shift* procedure. It is a psychoacoustic technique that relies on observations about the relationship between the masker level in the nontest ear and the measured threshold in the test ear. The masking plateau represents a range of masking levels (e.g., 15 to 20 dB) over which the measured pure-tone threshold remains unchanged. The goal of the plateau procedure is to establish the hearing level (i.e., dB HL) at which pure-tone threshold remains unchanged with increments in masker level. The recommended clinical procedure for use of the plateau method is summarized in Table 5-4.

Central masking is a phenomenon whereby introduction of contralateral masking can produce a small threshold shift in the test ear even when masker intensity is insufficient to produce overmasking. The threshold shift produced by central masking is generally about 5 dB during pure-tone and speech threshold audiometry. There currently is no accepted procedure that compensates for the effect of central masking during threshold audiometry. Although some audiologists will correct for the central masking effect by subtracting 5 dB from the measured masked threshold, the majority of clinicians do not (Martin et al., 1994).

A *masking dilemma* can occur whenever the introduction of the initial minimum masking level equals or exceeds the maximum masking level (i.e., overmasking). The classic example of a masking dilemma is demonstrated with a bilateral conductive hearing loss that exceeds about 40 dB. The consequence of overmasking is that measured thresholds in the test ear are poorer than the true thresholds. One solution to the masking dilemma is the use of insert earphones, which greatly increase interaural attenuation for air-conducted sound.

Study Questions

1. Differentiate minimum versus maximum masking level.

2. Briefly describe the two major approaches to clinical masking.

3. What are the four factors that influence the minimum masking level during pure-tone threshold audiometry?

4. Summarize the formula for calculating minimum masking level during pure-tone air-conduction audiometry. What are the disadvantages of the formula approach for calculating the minimum masking level?

5. Martin has simplified the calculation of the initial masking level during pure-tone air-conduction audiometry. Describe this approach.

6. It is generally recommended that at least 10 dB should be added to the initial masking level. Explain why.

7. Differentiate the terms minimum masking level and initial minimum masking level.

8. Describe Martin's approach to determining initial masking level during pure-tone bone-conduction audiometry.

9. Define occlusion effect. Why is the occlusion effect added to the initial masking level during pure-tone bone-conduction audiometry?

10. The occlusion effect should not be added to the initial masking level in all cases. Explain why.

11. Describe the two approaches to adding the occlusion effect to the initial minimum masking level during pure-tone bone-conduction audiometry. What are the advantages and disadvantages of each approach?

12. Briefly describe the relationship between interaural attenuation for air-conducted sound and the occlusion effect.

13. What are the two factors that influence the maximum masking level during pure-tone threshold audiometry?

14. Summarize the equation for calculation of the maximum masking level. Why can the same equation be used during both air- and bone-conduction audiometry?

15. Explain why the estimated maximum masking level during pure-tone threshold audiometry is often very conservative.

16. Two possible outcomes can occur when the pure-tone threshold is re-established in the presence of contralateral masking: *no threshold shift* and a *measured threshold shift*. What does each outcome suggest about the responsiveness of the test and nontest (i.e., masked) ears? Explain.

17. Hood's masking procedure is comprised of two major steps: (1) Demonstration of the shadowing effect and (2) Identification of the change-over point. Describe each of these steps. How does each step relate to the responsiveness of the test and nontest (i.e., masked) ears?

18. Define the masking plateau. What three factors affect the width of the masking plateau?

19. What is generally considered to be the minimum width of a clinically acceptable masking plateau?

20. The masker level can be changed in increments of either 5 dB or 10 dB during the plateau procedure. What is the advantage of using a masker increment of 5 dB? 10 dB?

21. Summarize the recommended clinical procedure for use of the plateau procedure during pure-tone threshold audiometry.

22. Define central masking. What is the clinical significance of central masking?

23. What is the masking dilemma? Why does use of the plateau procedure prove advantageous in cases in which overmasking is suspected?

24. How are unmasked and masked air-conduction thresholds used in audiogram interpretation?

25. Can ear-specific information be inferred from unmasked bone-conduction thresholds? Explain.

6

Clinical Masking
Procedures:
Speech Audiometry

While the psychoacoustic masking approach (i.e., threshold shift procedure) proved more efficient for pure-tone threshold measurement, acoustic masking procedures will be required during speech audiometry, particularly during suprathreshold speech recognition testing. Recall that the acoustic procedures are based upon calculating the estimated acoustic levels of the test and masker stimuli present in the two ears during a particular test condition and on this basis selecting an appropriate masking level (Studebaker, 1979). A major weakness of the acoustic or formula methods is that their application requires prior information about air-bone gaps in both the test and nontest ears (Konkle & Berry, 1983; Studebaker, 1979). Use of the formula-based acoustic methods requires knowledge about an air-bone gap in the nontest ear in order to calculate minimum masking level. In addition, information about bone-conduction sensitivity in the test ear is needed to calculate the maximum masking level. Although unmasked bone-conduction thresholds can be used to estimate the required masking levels during pure-tone threshold audiometry, incorrect assumptions about the origin of a bone-conducted response can lead to the use of inappropriate levels of masking. Assuming that pure-tone threshold data are available prior to performing speech audiometry, the use of acoustic masking procedures for calculating required masking levels can be employed effectively during both threshold and suprathreshold speech audiometric measures. Studebaker (1979, p. 89) states: "Armed with a knowledge of the conductive loss in each ear gained from the initial threshold test, it is possible to proceed with assurance to contralateral masking during any subsequent hearing tests using purely calculated levels."

Acoustic Masking Procedures

Studebaker (1979) states that one of the goals of the acoustic or formula method is to use rules that will place the masking level at approximately the middle of the range of correct values (i.e., the middle of the masking plateau). This concept was originally discussed by Luscher and König in 1955 (as cited by Studebaker, 1979). Recall that the lower and upper boundaries (i.e., range) of the masking plateau represent minimum and maximum masking levels. Studebaker (1962) described a formula to determine a mid-masking level during bone-conduction testing. This level was originally defined as the arithmetic mean *between* the maximum and minimum masking levels:

$$M_0 = (M_{max} - M_{min}) / 2$$

where M_0 is equal to the mid-masking level, M_{max} is equal to the maximum masking level, and M_{min} is equal to the minimum masking level. For example, if M_{min} is equal to 20 dB EM and M_{max} is equal to 80 dB EM, then the masker level that occurs at the middle of the range (i.e., midplateau) is 50 dB EM:

$$M_0 = (M_{max} - M_{min}) / 2$$
$$= (80 - 20) / 2$$
$$= 60 / 2$$
$$= 30 \text{ dB}$$

The mid-masking level will occur 30 dB above the minimum masking level, yet 30 dB below the maximum, that is, 50 dB EM. A more direct approach to calculating the mid-masking level (M_{mid}) involves determining the arithmetic mean of the minimum and maximum masking levels. We can restate Studebaker's original equation as follows:

$$M_{mid} = (M_{max} + M_{min}) / 2$$

Using the previous example, the mid-masking level can now be calculated directly:

$$M_{mid} = (M_{max} + M_{min}) / 2$$
$$= (80 + 20) / 2$$
$$= 100 / 2$$
$$= 50 \text{ dB EM}$$

Studebaker (1962) states that at the mid-masking level, the risk of insufficient masking (i.e., masking levels less than the required minimum) or overmasking (i.e., masking levels greater than the permissible maximum) is minimized. Although Studebaker originally described the midplateau procedure for use in bone-conduction audiometry, the basic goal of the method will prove equally effective during both threshold and suprathreshold speech audiometry.

Minimum Masking Level

Three factors influence minimum masking levels during air-conduction speech audiometry: (1) Presentation level of the test signal, (2) interaural attenuation of the test signal, and (3) the presence of an air-bone gap in the nontest (i.e., masked) ear. Recall that these same factors also influenced the minimum masking levels during pure-tone air-conduction audiometry.

Liden and co-workers (1959) offered the following formula for calculating minimum masking level (M_{min}) during speech audiometry:

$$M_{min} = S_t - 40 + (AA_m + AB_m)$$

where S_t is equal to presentation level of the speech signal at the test ear, 40 (dB) is equal to interaural attenuation, and $(AA_m - AB_m)$ is equal to the average air-bone gap in the nontest ear (i.e., the difference between average hearing loss for air-conducted sound, AA_m, and average loss for bone-conducted sound, AB_m). This is virtually identical to the formula for minimum masking level offered by Liden and co-workers for pure-tone air-conduction audiometry with one exception: *Average* air-bone gap in the nontest ear must be considered. Because speech is a broadband signal, it is no longer appropriate to consider bone-conduction sensitivity at only a single frequency in the nontest ear as is the case during pure-tone audiometry. Liden and co-workers recommended that "average hearing loss" should be calculated using pure-tone frequencies of 500, 1000, and 2000 Hz.

A similar formula for calculation of minimum masking level is described by Coles and Priede (1975). Their approach is more conservative, however. Rather than using an *average* air-bone gap, they recommend that the *maximum* air-bone gap in the nontest ear at any frequency in the range from 250 to 4000 Hz be considered. The presence of an air-bone gap in the nontest ear will reduce the effectiveness of the masking stimulus. There is the assumption that the largest air-bone gap will have the greatest effect on masker intensity. Consequently, it is the largest air-bone gap that must be compensated for when calculating the minimum masking level.

Ideally, our equation for the minimum masking level should be applicable to all speech audiometric measurements, both threshold and suprathreshold. We can rewrite the formula for the minimum masking level as originally described by Liden and co-workers as follows:

$$M_{min} = PL_T - IA + Max\ AB\ Gap_{NT}$$

where PL_T is the presentation level of the speech signal in dB HL at the test ear, IA is the interaural attenuation value for the particular speech measurement, and Max AB Gap$_{NT}$ is the maximum air-bone gap in the nontest ear in the frequency range from 250 to 4000 Hz. Two modifications of the original formula described by Liden and co-workers (1959) should be noted. First, the specific value of interaural attenuation is not specified. Liden and co-workers (1959) and Coles and Priede (1975) recommended the use of an interaural attenuation value of 40 dB. However, it was discussed earlier that the use of a single value of interaural attenuation for all speech audiometric measurements may not be appropriate in all clinical situations (e.g., Konkle & Berry, 1983). The use of *different* interaural attenuation values for each speech audiometric test can be supported. Specifically, the use of interaural attenuation values of 45 dB for the speech recognition threshold, 35 dB for the speech detection threshold, and 35 dB for the measurement of suprathreshold speech recognition was recommended (see Chapter 4). Second, following the recommendation of Coles and Priede (1975), the maximum air-bone gap in the frequency range from 250 to 4000 Hz is considered when determining the minimum masking level. This is consistent with an earlier recommendation that the best bone-conduction threshold in the 250 to 4000 Hz frequency range should be considered when determining the need for masking during all speech audiometric measurements.

Maximum Masking Level

Two factors influence maximum masking level during speech audiometry: (1) The bone-conduction hearing sensitivity of the test ear and (2) the interaural attenuation (IA) of the air-conducted masking stimulus. Again, these same factors influenced maximum masking levels during pure-tone audiometry.

Liden and co-workers (1959) offered the following formula for calculating maximum masking level (M_{max}) during speech audiometry:

$$M_{max} = AB_t + 40$$

where AB_t is the test ear's average bone-conduction threshold (i.e., average of 500, 1000, and 2000 Hz) and 40 (dB) is equal to interaural attenuation. Martin (1994) states that overmasking has occurred when the effective masking level in the nontest ear (EM_{NTE}) minus the patient's interaural attenuation (IA) is equal or greater than the *best* bone-conduction threshold of the test ear (Best BC_{TE}):

$$EM_{NTE} - IA \geq Best\ BC_{TE}$$

There is the assumption that the best bone-conduction threshold in the test ear is most susceptible to the effects of overmasking and must be considered when determining maximum masking levels.

Our equation for maximum masking level should be applicable to all speech audiometric measurements. We can rewrite the formula for maximum masking level as originally described by Liden and co-workers as follows:

$$M_{max} = Best\ BC_T + IA - 5\ dB$$

where Best BC_T is equal to the best bone-conduction threshold in the test ear in the frequency range from 250 to 4000 Hz and IA is equal to the interaural attenuation value for the particular speech measurement. The same interaural attenuation values used to determine the minimum masking level should also be used when calculating the maximum masking level (i.e., 45 dB for speech recognition threshold, 35 dB for speech detection threshold and suprathreshold speech recognition, or 40 dB for all speech audiometric tests). If Best BC_T + IA is just sufficient to produce overmasking, then clinically a slightly lower masking level than the calculated value must be used. A value of 5 dB is subsequently subtracted from the calculated value.

Selection of Appropriate Masking Levels

The optimal masking level during speech audiometry is one that falls above the minimum effective masking and below the maximum permissible masking levels (Konkle & Berry, 1983; Liden et al., 1959; Studebaker, 1979). Given that the minimum and maximum masking levels, respectively, represent the lower and upper limits of the masking plateau, then our goal is to select a masker level that occurs at the middle of the range (i.e., midplateau). Table 6-1 summarizes formulas for calculating the minimum, maximum, and mid-masking levels during speech audiometry. Consider the following three examples that demonstrate the application of the midplateau masking method for measuring the speech recognition threshold, the speech detection threshold, and suprathreshold speech recognition.

Speech Recognition Threshold

Figure 6-1A presents an example of the midplateau masking method when assessing speech recognition threshold. Pure-tone testing revealed a very mild

TABLE 6–1 Formulas for determining the minimum, maximum, and mid-masking levels during speech audiometry.

Minimum Masking Level

$$M_{min} = PL_T - IA + \text{Max AB gap}_{NT}^*$$

Maximum Masking Level

$$M_{max} = \text{Best BC}_T^* + IA - 5 \text{ dB}$$

Mid-Masking Level

$$M_{mid} = (M_{max} + M_{min}) / 2$$

*Bone-conduction thresholds in the frequency range from 250 to 4000 Hz.

conductive hearing loss of flat configuration in the right ear. There is a severe, sensorineural hearing loss of flat configuration in the left ear; air- and bone-conduction responses were measured with contralateral masking in the right ear. Speech recognition threshold (SRT) was measured at 20 dB HL in the right ear, a finding that is consistent with the pure-tone results. Based upon pure-tone findings in the left ear, we can predict that the true SRT will be measured at about 65 dB HL. If we assume that interaural attenuation for the speech recognition threshold can be as small as 45 dB, then it will be necessary to introduce contralateral masking to the right ear when measuring the SRT in the left ear. Recall the equation for determining the need for contralateral masking when assessing the SRT:

$$\text{Presentation level}_T - IA \geq \text{Best BC}_{NT}$$
$$PL_T - IA \geq \text{Best BC}_{NT}$$
$$65 \text{ dB HL} - 45 \text{ dB} \geq 0 \text{ dB HL (at 250, 500, 2000 Hz)?}$$
$$20 \text{ dB HL} \geq 0 \text{ dB HL?}$$

Theoretically, 20 dB HL is reaching the nontest (i.e., right) cochlea. Because of bone-conduction responses of 0 dB HL in the right ear, cross hearing is a possibility when measuring the SRT in the left ear.

The first step in selecting an appropriate masking level in this case involves determining the minimum and maximum masking levels. The minimum masking level (M_{min}) is calculated as follows:

$$M_{min} = PL_T - IA + \text{Max AB gap}_{NT}$$
$$= 65 \text{ dB HL} - 45 \text{ dB} + 20 \text{ dB}$$
$$= 40 \text{ dB EM}$$

If spondees will be presented at intensity levels no greater than 65 dB HL when measuring the SRT, and if interaural attenuation is equal to 45 dB, then theoretically 20 dB HL is reaching the nontest cochlea. However, there is a maximum air-bone gap of 20 dB in the right ear for which we must compensate by adding 20 dB to the effective masking level. The minimum masking level is calculated to be 40 dB EM. This is the minimum masking level needed to obtain the true SRT of 65 dB HL in the left ear.

FIGURE 6–1   Example illustrating the midplateau method when measuring the speech recognition threshold (SRT). (A) Pure-tone testing reveals a mild conductive hearing loss in the right ear; there is a severe, sensorineural hearing loss in the left ear. The SRT of 20 dB in the right ear confirms the pure-tone findings. Based on pure-tone results in the left ear, we can predict that an SRT will be measured at about 65 dB HL. Given this assumption, contralateral masking will be required when measuring SRT in the left ear. The first step in selecting an appropriate masking level involves estimating minimum and maximum masking levels. $M_{min} = PL_T - IA + Max\ AB\ gap_{NT} = 65 - 45 + 20 = 40\ dB\ EM$. $M_{max} = Best\ BC_T + IA - 5\ dB = 60 + 45 - 5\ dB = 100\ dB\ EM$. Mid-masking level is calculated as follows: $M_{mid} = (M_{max} + M_{min})/2 = (100 + 40)/2 = 70\ dB\ EM$. (B) The theoretical contralateral masking function that would result in the present example. Speech threshold (in dB HL) is plotted as a function of effective masking level (dB EM) in the nontest ear.

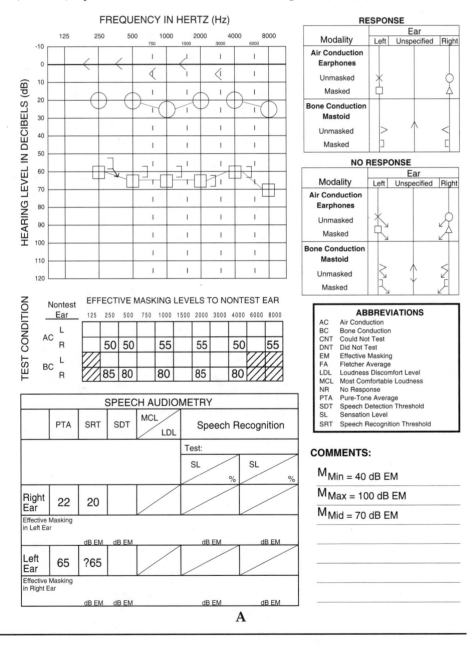

A

FIGURE 6–1   Continued

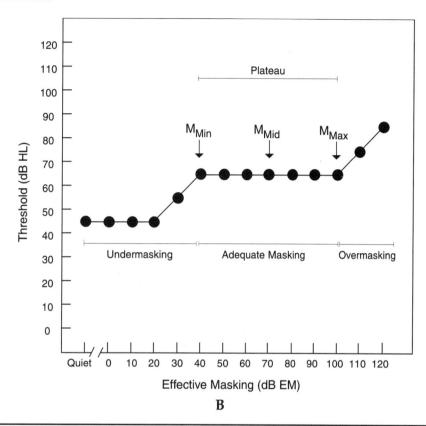

B

The maximum masking level (M_{max}) is calculated as follows:

$$M_{max} = \text{Best BC}_T + \text{IA} - 5 \text{ dB}$$
$$= 60 \text{ dB HL} + 45 \text{ dB} - 5 \text{ dB}$$
$$= 100 \text{ dB EM}$$

If interaural attenuation is equal to 45 dB, then the maximum permissible masking level that we can use when measuring the SRT is 100 dB EM.

Recall that the minimum and maximum masking levels delineate the boundaries of the masking plateau. If the minimum masking level is equal to 40 dB EM and the maximum masking level is equal to 100 dB EM, then the mid-masking level (i.e., midplateau) is equal to 70 dB EM:

$$M_{mid} = (M_{max} + M_{min}) / 2$$
$$= (100 \text{ dB EM} + 40 \text{ dB EM}) / 2$$
$$= 140 \text{ dB EM} / 2$$
$$= 70 \text{ dB EM}$$

Figure 6-1*B* presents the theoretical contralateral masking function that would result in the present example. Speech threshold (in dB HL) is plotted as a function of the effective masking level (dB EM) in the nontest ear. Effective masking levels less than 40 dB EM would result in undermasking, while levels greater than 100 dB EM would produce overmasking. An effective masking level of 70 dB EM is considered appropriate because the midpoint of the masking plateau has been reached.

When selecting an appropriate masking level, it is very important to consider the presentation levels of the spondees during threshold measurement. When calculating the minimum masking level, the audiologist should consider the highest presentation levels used during threshold assessment. For example, if the clinician uses the standardized, descending threshold technique recommended by ASHA (1988), then spondaic words will be presented initially at hearing levels approximately 10 dB higher than the calculated SRT. This higher starting level will necessitate the need for higher levels of masking. The audiologist may choose to use the higher presentation levels in the formula for calculation of minimum masking level. For example, rather than using the predicted SRT of 65 dB HL as the presentation level in the minimum masking formula, a value of 75 dB HL could be substituted. This would result in a slightly higher (i.e., 10 dB) minimum masking level of 50 dB EM (rather than the originally calculated 40 dB EM). The effect on the mid-masking level, however, will be minimal: The midplateau would be shifted to a higher level by only 5 dB.

In the above example, the midplateau masking method has proven to be efficient in two ways. First, recall that effective masking levels are based on average data obtained from a number of individuals. As in the case with pure-tone audiometry, a safety factor of at least 10 dB should be added to the minimum masking level to account for intersubject variability (Martin, 1974; Studebaker, 1979). Stated differently, the selected masking level should be at least 10 dB greater than the calculated minimum masking level. Second, spondees may be presented at levels approximately 10 dB above the measured SRT during the assessment procedure. Consequently, somewhat higher minimum masking levels (approximately 10 dB) will be required. In the example presented in Figure 6-1, the midplateau procedure resulted in the selection of a masking level that accounted for both factors. Specifically, a masking level that is 30 dB greater than the calculated minimum is sufficient to account for both intersubject variability and the higher presentation levels often required during the threshold measurement.

Speech Detection Threshold

Figure 6-2 presents an example illustrating the application of the midplateau masking procedure when measuring a speech detection threshold (SDT). Pure-tone testing revealed a mild, sensorineural hearing loss of flat configuration in the left ear. There is a profound, sensorineural hearing impairment of relatively flat configuration in the right ear; both air- and bone-conduction thresholds were measured with contralateral masking. An SRT was obtained at 35 dB HL in the left ear, a finding consistent with the pure-tone results. Because the patient could not recognize spondees at suprathreshold levels in the right ear, a speech detection threshold was obtained. Based upon pure-tone findings in the right ear, we can predict that the true SDT will be measured at about 90 to 100 dB HL. Given this assumption, contralateral masking will be required when measuring a SDT in the right ear:

$$\text{Presentation level}_T - \text{IA} \geq \text{Best BC}_{NT}$$
$$100 \text{ dB HL} - 35 \text{ dB} \geq 30 \text{ dB HL (at 250 Hz)?}$$
$$65 \text{ dB HL} \geq 30 \text{ dB HL?}$$

FIGURE 6–2 Example illustrating the use of the midplateau masking procedure when measuring the speech detection threshold (SDT). Pure-tone testing reveals a mild, sensorineural hearing loss in the left ear; there is a profound, sensorineural hearing loss in the right ear. An SRT of 35 dB HL was measured in the left ear, a finding consistent with the pure-tone results. Because the patient could not correctly recognize any spondees at suprathreshold levels in the right ear, an SDT will be measured. Based on pure-tone findings, it is predicted that an SDT will be measured at levels ranging from about 90-100 dB HL. Given this assumption, contralateral masking will be required when measuring SDT in the right ear. Selecting an appropriate masking level using the midplateau procedure will involve a three-step procedure. (1) $M_{min} = PL_T - IA + $ Max AB Gap$_{NT} = 100 - 35 + 0 = 65$ dB EM. (2) $M_{max} = $ Best BC$_T$ + IA $- 5$ dB $= 95 + 35 - 5 = 125$ dB EM. (3) $M_{mid} = (M_{max} + M_{min}) / 2 = (125 + 65) / 2 = 95$ dB EM. Using the midplateau masking procedure, an appropriate level of contralateral masking is 95 dB EM.

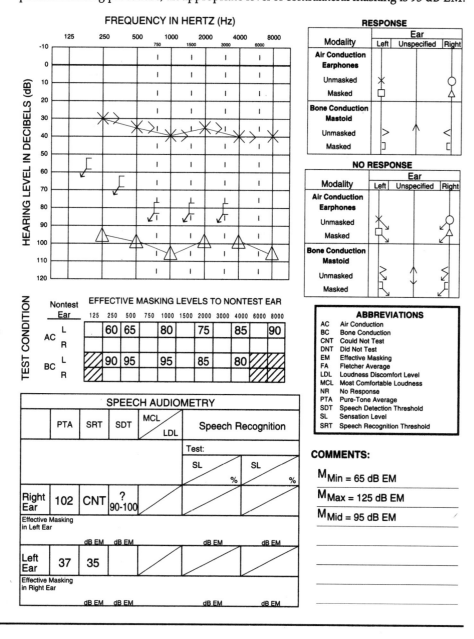

If we assume that speech can be presented to the test ear at levels as high as 100 dB HL and if interaural attenuation for the SDT can be as small as 35 dB, then theoretically a cross-hearing signal can reach the nontest ear at a level of 65 dB HL. Because of a bone-conduction threshold of 30 dB HL in the left (i.e., nontest) ear, cross hearing is a possibility when measuring the SDT in the right ear.

A comment is needed about the value used for Best BC_T when calculating M_{max}. Because no responses to bone-conducted stimuli were obtained in the right ear at output limits of the audiometer, the assumption is that there is a sensorineural hearing impairment. Stated differently, masked bone-conduction testing did not demonstrate the presence of air-bone gaps in the right ear; thus, our conclusion is that the hearing impairment is sensorineural in nature. Given that there were no responses to bone-conducted stimuli at output limits of the audiometer, what is the best bone-conduction threshold in the right ear?

There are two approaches to estimating the best bone-conduction threshold in the right ear. First, because our conclusion is that the hearing impairment is sensorineural, we can assume that the best bone-conduction threshold in the right ear is equal to the best air-conduction threshold in the 250 to 4000 Hz range (i.e., 95 dB HL at 250 Hz). Second, we can take a more conservative approach and assume that the best bone-conduction threshold may be as little as 5 dB greater than the lowest hearing level at which a "no response" to bone-conducted sound occurred. Because the lowest output limit for bone-conducted sound (for this particular audiometer) was 55 dB HL at 250 Hz, we can assume that the Best BC_T can be no better than 60 dB HL. Consequently, a very conservative estimate of Best BC_T would be 60 dB HL.

Which of the two approaches for estimating Best BC_T is correct? Because clinical masking is not an exact science, it is often necessary to make assumptions about relevant variables (e.g., interaural attenuation, bone-conduction sensitivity). Ideally, a case history and acoustic immittance measurements should be conducted before audiometric testing. Such information can alert the audiologist to the possibility of conductive pathology and is useful when developing testing strategies during clinical masking procedures. For example, if there is no history of middle ear disorders and the results of tympanometry are normal, then it may be reasonable to assume that the site of lesion in the profoundly impaired right ear is probably *sensorineural* in nature. Consequently, we can use the best air-conduction threshold of 95 dB HL at 250 Hz as our estimate of Best BC_T.

$$M_{max} = \text{Best } BC_T + IA - 5 \text{ dB}$$
$$= 95 \text{ dB HL} + 35 \text{ dB} - 5 \text{ dB}$$
$$= 125 \text{ dB EM}$$

Conversely, if the patient reports a history of middle ear disorders and the results of tympanometry are abnormal, then the more conservative approach to estimating Best BC_T is recommended. This patient may exhibit a conductive component that cannot be demonstrated through bone-conduction audiometry. Consequently, the more conservative estimate of Best BC_T (i.e., 60 dB HL) would be used when calculating M_{max}.

$$M_{max} = \text{Best } BC_T + IA - 5 \text{ dB}$$
$$= 60 \text{ dB HL} + 35 \text{ dB} - 5 \text{ dB}$$
$$= 90 \text{ dB EM}$$

In this particular example, let us assume that the results of tympanometry are normal (i.e., a finding that suggests normal middle ear function). Thus, we will use the less conservative estimate of M_{max} (i.e., using 95 dB HL as the estimate of Best BC_T) when calculating the mid-masking level (i.e., M_{mid}). The result will be a higher mid-masking level. Assuming that the SDT may occur at a hearing level as high as 100 dB HL, we will select an appropriate masking level using the midplateau procedure. Again, our selection will involve a three-step procedure:

1. M_{min} = PL_T – IA + Max AB gap_{NT}

          = 100 dB HL – 35 dB + 0 dB

          = 65 dB EM

2. M_{max} = Best BC_T + IA – 5 dB

          = 95 dB HL + 35 dB – 5 dB

          = 125 dB EM

3. M_{mid} = $(M_{max} + M_{min})$ / 2

          = (125 + 65) / 2

          = (190) / 2

          = 95 dB EM

If the SDT is measured at approximately 100 dB HL (or less) in the right ear, then an appropriate masking level in the left ear is 95 dB EM.

It is important to remember that when using the midplateau procedure, you want to select a masking level that falls *within the vicinity* of midplateau. The midplateau should be considered a small range of values surrounding the mid-masking level (i.e., ±10 dB). Depending on the particular case and the selected audiological procedures, the audiologist can justify using either a slightly higher or lower masking level. Ideally, the selected masking level should fall at least 10 dB above M_{min} to account for intersubject variability in the calibration of the effective masking level (i.e., a 10-dB safety factor). In addition, the selected masking level should not exceed M_{max} to avoid overmasking. In the above example (Figure 6-2), the mid-masking level was calculated as 95 dB EM. This intensity level is high and may be uncomfortable for the patient. A slightly lower masker level of 85 dB EM can be easily justified because it falls within the vicinity of the midplateau (i.e., 95 dB HL) and is at least 10 dB above M_{min} (i.e., 65 dB HL), thus meeting the goals of the procedure.

Suprathreshold Speech Recognition

The example presented in Figure 6-3 illustrates use of the acoustic masking procedure during assessment of suprathreshold speech recognition. Pure-tone testing revealed a mild, sensorineural hearing loss of relatively flat configuration in the right ear. There is a mild-to-moderate, sensorineural hearing loss of flat configuration in the left ear; contralateral masking was required when measuring bone-conduction thresholds. Speech recognition thresholds were obtained at 25 dB HL and 40 dB HL in the right and left ears respectively, a finding consistent with the pure-tone results; contralateral masking was not required when measuring SRT in either ear. Suprathreshold speech recognition will be assessed at a 40-dB sensation level using NU-6 monosyllabic word lists. Contralateral masking will be required when evaluating suprathreshold speech recognition in the left ear only:

FIGURE 6-3   Example illustrating the use of the midplateau procedure during assessment of suprathreshold speech recognition. Pure-tone testing reveals a mild, sensorineural hearing loss in the right ear; there is a mild-to-moderate, sensorineural hearing impairment in the left ear. SRTs of 25 dB HL and 40 dB HL in the right and left ears respectively confirm the pure-tone results. Although contralateral masking was not required during assessment of speech recognition thresholds, masking will be needed when measuring suprathreshold speech recognition in the left ear. If presentation level of the speech signal is equal to 80 dB HL and if a conservative estimate of interaural attenuation is 35 dB, then cross hearing becomes a possibility. Selecting an appropriate masking level using the midplateau procedure will involve a three-step procedure. (1) $M_{min} = PL_T - IA + Max\ AB\ Gap_{NT} = 80 - 35 + 5 = 50$ dB EM. (2) $M_{max} = Best\ BC_T + IA - 5$ dB $= 40 + 35 - 5 = 70$ dB EM. (3) $M_{mid} = (M_{max} + M_{min})/2 = (70 + 50)/2 = 60$ dB EM. Using the midplateau masking procedure, an appropriate level of contralateral masking is 60 dB EM.

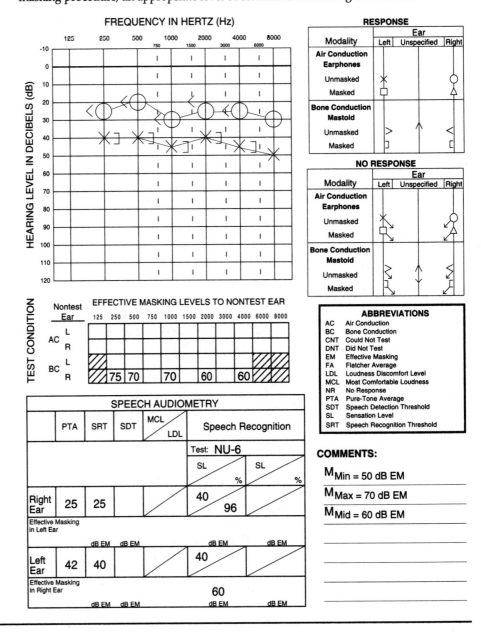

$$\text{Presentation level}_T - IA \geq \text{Best BC}_{NT}$$
$$(40 \text{ dB HL} + 40 \text{ dB SL}) - 35 \text{ dB} \geq 20 \text{ dB HL (at 500, 2000 Hz)}?$$
$$80 \text{ dB HL} - 35 \text{ dB} \geq 20 \text{ dB HL}?$$
$$45 \text{ dB HL} \geq 20 \text{ dB HL}?$$

If the presentation level of the speech signal is equal to 80 dB HL (i.e., SRT of 40 dB HL + 40 dB SL) and if a conservative estimate of interaural attenuation is 35 dB, then theoretically a cross-hearing signal of 45 dB HL can reach the right (i.e., nontest) ear. Because of bone-conduction responses of 20 dB HL, cross hearing is a possibility when measuring suprathreshold speech recognition in the left ear.

Again, we will use the midplateau masking method for selecting an appropriate masking level in the right ear. If M_{min} is equal to 50 dB EM and M_{max} is equal to 70 dB EM, then the mid-masking level (M_{mid}) is calculated to be 60 dB EM.

$$
\begin{aligned}
1.\ M_{min} \ &= PL_T - IA + \text{Max AB gap}_{NT} \\
&= 80 \text{ dB HL} - 35 \text{ dB} + 5 \text{ dB (at 2000 Hz)} \\
&= 50 \text{ dB EM} \\
2.\ M_{max} \ &= \text{Best BC}_T + IA - 5 \text{ dB} \\
&= 40 \text{ dB HL} + 35 \text{ dB} - 5 \text{ dB} \\
&= 70 \text{ dB EM} \\
3.\ M_{Mid} \ &= (M_{max} + M_{min}) / 2 \\
&= (70 + 50) / 2 \\
&= (120) / 2 \\
&= 60 \text{ dB EM}
\end{aligned}
$$

It should be noted that the width of the masking plateau is very narrow (i.e., 20 dB). This is not uncommon during suprathreshold speech recognition testing. Because higher presentation levels are used during suprathreshold tests, the minimum masking level is increased. The maximum masking level, however, remains unaltered. Consequently, the width of the masking plateau is reduced. In this particular example, the mid-masking level is 10 dB greater than the minimum (i.e., M_{min}), which is considered an adequate safety factor.

There are two important advantages of the midplateau masking procedure. First, the midplateau method eliminates interaural attenuation as a source of error when selecting an appropriate masking level. The value of interaural attenuation used when determining the minimum and maximum masking levels does not affect the calculated mid-masking level. Interaural attenuation has equal yet opposite effects on minimum and maximum masking levels. Recall that it is traditional to use a conservative estimate of interaural attenuation when determining contralateral masking requirements. Although the use of a conservative value of interaural attenuation will underestimate the width of the masking plateau, the calculated mid-masking level (i.e., the midpoint of the masking plateau) remains unaffected. The midplateau procedure will always result in the selection of an appropriate masking level, regardless of the value of interaural attenuation used.

Second, the mid-masking level can be predicted for both threshold and suprathreshold measures by using the same formula (Konkle & Berry, 1983). Specifically, the midplateau method avoids a potential problem inherent in suprathreshold speech recognition testing that is related to calibration of effective masking level and percent correct response criterion. Recall that calibration of the effective masking level for speech typically is based upon the level that produces 50 percent correct performance for spondaic words. For example, 60 dB effective masking (dB EM) is the level of noise that will shift the speech recognition threshold to 60 dB HL. Studebaker (1979) points out that during suprathreshold speech recognition testing, some test words presented below the SRT can be correctly recognized. If the goal of contralateral masking during suprathreshold speech recognition testing is to completely eliminate the participation of the nontest ear, then it will be necessary to increase the masker level by approximately 10 dB above that level producing masking of the nontest ear SRT. Stated differently, the minimum masking level must be increased by 10 dB.

Studebaker (1979) has also noted that overmasking during suprathreshold speech recognition testing can occur whenever performance of the test ear is reduced by the masker by any amount. Specifically, overmasking may occur at noise levels 10 dB below the level that would affect the SRT. Stated differently, the same masker level theoretically can produce 10 dB greater masking during suprathreshold speech recognition than during measurement of the SRT. Consequently, maximum masking level must be decreased by 10 dB during suprathreshold speech recognition testing. The overall effect is that the width of the masking plateau is reduced by 20 dB during assessment of suprathreshold speech recognition. This is accounted for clinically by using a 10-dB smaller value of interaural attenuation for suprathreshold speech recognition (i.e., 35 dB) than for the speech recognition threshold (i.e., 45 dB). Because the extremes of the masking plateau (i.e., minimum and maximum masking levels) are modified equally, the location of the masking plateau midpoint remains unchanged. Konkle and Berry (1983) state that one of the primary advantages of the mid-plateau procedure is that the plateau midpoint is not affected by different listener response criteria (e.g., speech recognition threshold versus suprathreshold speech recognition).

Studebaker (1979) has described an alternate acoustic masking procedure for use during all speech audiometric testing that is consistent with the goal of selecting a masker level that occurs at the midpoint of the masking plateau. He states that the recommended effective masking level (dB EM) is equal to the level of the speech signal in the test ear, adjusted for the difference in the air-bone gaps exhibited in the two ears. If there is a larger air-bone gap in the non-test ear, minimum masking level will be increased by the size of the air-bone gap; thus, the midpoint of the masking plateau will be shifted upward by one-half of the air-bone gap. If there is a larger air-bone gap in the test ear, the maximum masking level will be decreased by the size of the air-bone gap; consequently, the midpoint of the masking plateau will be shifted downward by one-half of the air-bone gap. Studebaker's method for selection of appropriate masking levels can be summarized in the following equation:

$$dB\ EM = PL_T + (AB\ Gap_{NT} - AB\ Gap_T)\ /\ 2$$

where dB EM is the effective masking level defined relative to a 50 percent response criterion, PL_T is the presentation level of the speech signal at the test ear, AB Gap_{NT} is the air-bone gap in the nontest ear, and AB Gap_T is the air-bone gap in the test ear. Studebaker (1979) recommended that these calculations be based on "on the average of the two largest of the air-bone gaps at those pure tone frequencies that correlate best with performance on the particular speech test being used" (p. 93). A more conservative approach would involve adjusting for the largest air-bone gap at frequencies from 250 to 4000 Hz in each ear.

It should be noted that effective masking level is equal to the presentation level of the test signal (PL_T) in those cases in which there are no air-bone gaps in either ear or where there are equal air-bone gaps in both ears. Consequently, very high levels of maskings can result, particularly during suprathreshold speech recognition testing. Studebaker (1979) states that it is possible to significantly reduce the intensity level of the masker below the presentation level of the signal (PL_T). Specifically, the effective masking level can be reduced by the smallest expected interaural attenuation value; a value of 20 dB is subsequently added to the effective masking level as a safety factor. (*Note:* If an air-bone gap exists in the nontest ear, the effective masking level must also be increased by an amount equal to the air-bone gap.)

Studebaker's method for selection of appropriate masking levels *in those cases in which there are no air-bone gaps in the nontest ear* can be restated in the following equation:

$$dB\ EM = PL_T - IA + 20\ dB\ safety\ factor$$

Studebaker indicates that application of this procedure will provide the amount by which the masker can be decreased below the presentation level of the speech signal while maintaining an effective masking level at least 10 dB above the required minimum. In practice, it is permissible to reduce the effective masking level from the presentation level of the speech signal (PL_T) by 15 to 25 dB, assuming that there is not a conductive hearing loss in the nontest ear.

In summary, the optimal masking level during speech audiometry is one that falls above the minimum effective masking and below the maximum permissible masking levels. Specifically, the goal is to select a masker level that falls at the middle of the masking plateau. Two approaches to the selection of appropriate masking levels have been discussed. The first method involves directly calculating mid-masking level based upon information on the minimum and maximum masking levels. The second method, proposed by Studebaker (1979) and endorsed by Konkle and Berry (1983), involves presenting the masker at an effective level equal to the presentation level of the speech signal in the test ear, adjusted for the difference in the air-bone gaps exhibited in the two ears. Although the method proposed by Studebaker typically will result in the selection of an appropriate masker level, it does not alert the clinician to the possibility of overmasking. Masker levels can be selected that theoretically can exceed maximum masking levels, particularly during the assessment of suprathreshold speech recognition in cases of conductive hearing impairment or when presenting speech at high intensity levels (e.g., constructing a performance-intensity function). The direct calculation of mid-masking level is generally recommended because it provides the clinician with quantitative information about the width of the masking plateau, as well as with estimated minimum and maximum masking levels. In cases in which the masking plateau is very narrow or nonexistent, knowledge about the minimum and maximum masking levels will permit the audiologist to make a judicious decision when selecting an appropriate masking level.

A simplified approach, based on the underlying concepts of both the *mid-plateau* and *Studebaker* acoustic procedures, can be derived when selecting contralateral masking levels during assessment of suprathreshold speech recognition. Stated simply, the effective masking level is equal to the presentation level of the speech signal at the test ear (PL_T) minus 20 dB:

$$dB\ EM = PL_T - 20\ dB$$

It should be apparent that this "short-cut" approach to selecting an appropriate level of masking is basically a modification of Studebaker's (1979) original equation:

$$dB\ EM = PL_T - IA + 20\ dB\ safety\ factor$$

If we assume that interaural attenuation for speech is approximately equal to 40 dB, then Studebaker's equation can be simplified as follows:

$$\begin{aligned} dB\ EM &= PL_T - IA + 20\ dB\ safety\ factor \\ &= PL_T - 40\ dB + 20\ dB\ safety\ factor \\ &= PL_T - 20\ dB \end{aligned}$$

This "short-cut" procedure proves very effective *given the following two conditions*:

1. There are no *significant* air-bone gaps in either ear.
2. Suprathreshold speech recognition is being evaluated at a *moderate* sensation level (i.e., approximately 40 dB SL). Given these two prerequisites, the selected masking level will occur approximately at midplateau. The use of the short-cut procedure is not recommended when assessing suprathreshold speech recognition at higher sensation levels (i.e., greater than approximately 50 dB SL) because of the increased likelihood of overmasking.

Reconsider the example presented in Figure 6-3. Recall that contralateral masking was required when evaluating suprathreshold speech recognition in the left ear. The short-cut acoustic procedure for selecting the effective masking level should prove efficient in this case because both prerequisites have been met: There are no significant air-bone gaps in either ear and suprathreshold speech recognition is evaluated at a moderate sensation level (i.e., 40 dB SL). Effective masking level is calculated as follows:

$$\begin{aligned} dB\ EM &= PL_T - 20\ dB \\ &= (40\ dB\ HL + 40\ dB\ SL) - 20\ dB \\ &= 80\ dB\ HL - 20\ dB \\ &= 60\ dB\ EM \end{aligned}$$

It should be noted that the effective masking level of 60 dB EM calculated using the short-cut approach is the same as that determined using the midplateau procedure. It is very important to remember, however, that both conditions must be met in order to use the short-cut masking procedure with confidence. The presence of a conductive component in either ear or the use of high sensation levels (e.g., constructing a performance-intensity function) can result in calculated effective masking levels that produce undermasking or overmasking. In addition, audiometric configuration may have an influence on the effectiveness of the short-cut approach. For example, the procedure may prove most effective when the audiometric configuration in the test ear is flat rather than rising or sloping (or more generally when the SRT correlates with the best pure-tone thresholds from 250 through 4000 Hz). The use of the short-cut masking procedure *when appropriate* can significantly simplify the calculations required for the determination of mid-masking level. However, it should *always* be used with caution.

Psychoacoustic Masking Procedures

When measuring masked speech thresholds (i.e., SRT or SDT), either acoustic or psychoacoustic masking procedures can be used. Recall that psychoacoustic procedures rely on observations of measured threshold shifts in the test ear as a function of masker effective levels in the nontest ear. Therefore, threshold shift masking procedures will prove effective for measuring any type of *threshold* response (i.e., pure-tone and speech).

The plateau procedure, as originally described by Hood (1960) for use during bone-conduction audiometry, can be applied during measurement of speech thresholds (Konkle & Berry, 1983; Martin, 1994; Studebaker, 1979). A major advantage of the plateau procedure is that information about bone-conduction sensitivity in each ear is not required when selecting appropriate masking levels. The following procedure for assessing the masked SRT incorporates the original concept of the masking plateau. Very simply, speech threshold is re-established for a series of 10-dB increments in masker level.

1. An unmasked SRT is initially obtained in the test ear.

2. Masking noise is introduced at an effective level 10 dB above the SRT of the nontest ear (i.e., initial minimum masking level):

$$M_{min} = SRT_{NT} + 10 \text{ dB safety factor)}$$

3. The SRT is re-established in the presence of masking in the nontest ear.

4. If the initial level of effective masking does not shift the SRT by more than 5 dB from the unmasked condition (i.e., the effect of central masking), the response is recorded as the true threshold of the test ear.

5. If there is an increase in the SRT from the unmasked condition, the masker level is increased by 10 dB and the speech threshold is re-established. Specifically, if fewer than three out of six words are repeated correctly, the signal level is increased by 5 dB; if three correct responses are obtained, the masker level is increased by 10 dB. The true threshold of the test ear is reached when the masker level can be increased over a range of 20 to 30 dB (i.e., two to three successive 10-dB steps) without a change in measured threshold.

The clinician is again cautioned about using only one masking level (i.e., initial minimum masking level) when establishing threshold using the psychoacoustic procedure. When low effective masking levels are used, under-masking can result in a small percentage of individual cases because of intersubject variability of effective masking level. If the SRT is not shifted by more than 5 dB with the introduction of initial masking (see Step 4 above), an additional 10-dB masking increment should be used to ensure that the initial masking level was sufficient.

The threshold shift procedure often requires that several speech recognition thresholds be measured before establishing a masking plateau. Thus, the procedure can prove very time-consuming. Although either acoustic or psychoacoustic masking procedures are effective when assessing speech recognition threshold, the acoustic method proves to be the method of choice because of its greater time efficiency (Konkle & Berry, 1983; Studebaker, 1979).

The threshold shift procedure proves to be efficient during measurement of speech detection threshold because of the nature of the response task (i.e., detection rather than recognition). A small modification of the plateau procedure is required, however, when establishing the SDT. Recall that when establishing a masked SRT, masking noise is initially introduced at an effective level 10 dB above the SRT of the nontest ear (i.e., $M_{min} = SRT_{NT} + 10$ dB safety factor). Because the effective masking level for speech typically is referenced to the SRT (i.e., the effective masking for speech refers to the dB HL to which the speech recognition threshold is shifted by a given level of noise), an adjustment in masker level is required when determining the initial masking during assessment of the speech detection threshold. Recall that speech can be detected at a lower intensity than that required to reach the SRT; this difference between speech thresholds averages about 8 to 9 dB (e.g., Beattie et al., 1978). Therefore, it will be necessary to use at least an 8 to 9 dB greater level of noise during assessment of the SDT when the masker level is referenced to the SRT. Although a given level of noise may prove sufficient to just mask the SRT in the nontest ear, a detection response to speech theoretically can still occur. Given these assumptions, the initial masking level must be increased by an additional 10 dB when measuring a masked SDT using the threshold shift procedure in order to eliminate a detection response from the nontest ear:

$$M_{min} = SRT_{NT} + 10 \text{ dB correction factor} + 10 \text{ dB safety factor}$$
$$= SRT_{NT} + 20 \text{ dB (correction + safety factors)}$$

In summary, both acoustic and psychoacoustic masking procedures can be used during speech audiometry. While acoustic procedures are most appropriate for suprathreshold speech recognition tests, either masking method is applicable during measurement of speech thresholds.

Summary

While the psychoacoustic masking approach proved efficient for pure-tone threshold measurement, acoustic masking procedures will be required during speech audiometry, particularly during assessment of suprathreshold speech recognition. One of the goals of the acoustic or formula method is to use rules that will place the selected masking level at approximately the middle of the range of correct values (i.e., midplateau). The optimal masking level during speech audiometry is one that falls above the minimum effective masking and below the maximum permissible masking levels.

Three factors influence minimum masking levels during speech audiometry: (1) Presentation level of the test signal; (2) interaural attenuation; and (3) the presence of an air-bone gap in the nontest ear. The formula for calculating minimum masking level (M_{min}) is as follows:

$$M_{min} = PL_T - IA + \text{Max AB gap}_{NT}$$

where PL_T is the presentation level of the speech signal in dB HL at the test ear, IA is the interaural attenuation value for the particular speech measurement, and Max AB Gap_{NT} is the maximum air-bone gap in the nontest ear in the frequency range from 250 to 4000 Hz.

Two factors influence the maximum masking level during speech audiometry: (1) The bone-conduction hearing sensitivity of the test ear and (2) interaural attenuation. The formula for calculating maximum masking level (M_{max}) is as follows:

$$M_{max} = Best\ BC_T + IA - 5\ dB$$

where Best BC_T is equal to the best bone-conduction threshold in the test ear in the frequency range from 250 to 4000 Hz and IA is equal to interaural attenuation for the particular speech measurement.

Given that minimum and maximum masking levels respectively represent the lower and upper limits of the masking plateau, our goal clinically is to select a masker level that occurs at the middle of the range (i.e., midplateau). A direct approach to calculating the mid-masking level (M_{mid}) involves determining the average of the minimum and maximum masking levels:

$$M_{mid} = (M_{max} + M_{min})\ /\ 2$$

Studebaker (1979) has described an alternate acoustic masking procedure for use during speech audiometry that is consistent with the goal of selecting a masker level that occurs at midplateau. Specifically, he states that the recommended effective masking level is equal to the level of the speech signal in the test ear (PL_T), adjusted for the difference in the air-bone gaps exhibited in the test (AB Gap_T) and nontest (AB Gap_{NT}) ears. Studebaker's method for selection of the appropriate masking levels can be summarized as follows:

$$dB\ EM = PL_T + (AB\ Gap_{NT} - AB\ Gap_T)\ /\ 2$$

A conservative approach would involve adjusting for the largest air-bone gap at frequencies from 250 to 4000 Hz in each ear.

Studebaker (1979) states that it is possible to reduce the intensity level of the masker below the presentation level of the signal in some situations. Studebaker's method for selecting appropriate masking levels in those cases in which there are no air-bone gaps in the nontest ear can be restated in the following equation:

$$dB\ EM = PL_T - IA + 20\ dB\ safety\ factor$$

The direct calculation of the mid-masking level is generally recommended because it provides the clinician with quantitative information about the width of the masking plateau as well as with the estimated minimum and maximum masking levels. A simplified approach, based on the underlying concepts of both the midplateau and Studebaker acoustic procedures, can be used when selecting appropriate levels of contralateral masking during measurement of suprathreshold speech recognition. Specifically, effective masking level is equal to the presentation level of the speech signal at the test ear (PL_T) minus 20 dB:

$$dB\ EM = PL_T - 20\ dB$$

This short-cut masking procedure proves very effective *given the following two conditions*:

1. There are *significant* no air-bone gaps in either ear.
2. Suprathreshold speech recognition is evaluated at moderate sensation levels (i.e., approximately 40 dB).

Given these two prerequisites, the selected masking level will occur approximately at midplateau.

Either acoustic or psychoacoustic masking procedures can be used when measuring masked speech thresholds. The plateau procedure can be applied during measurement of both speech detection and recognition thresholds. An advantage of the plateau procedure is that information about bone-conduction sensitivity in each ear is not required when selecting appropriate masking levels. The acoustic method generally proves to be the method of choice because of greater time efficiency, particularly during measurement of speech recognition threshold.

Study Questions

1. What are the three factors that influence the minimum masking level during air-conduction speech audiometry?
2. State the equation for calculating minimum masking level.
3. Explain why the largest air-bone gap in the nontest ear must be compensated for when calculating minimum masking level during speech audiometry.
4. The frequency range from 250 to 4000 Hz is considered when determining the minimum masking level for speech. Briefly discuss.
5. What are the two factors that influence maximum masking level during speech audiometry?
6. State the equation for calculating maximum masking level.
7. What is considered an optimal masking level during speech audiometry? Stated differently, what is our goal when selecting an appropriate masking level?
8. How does the mid-masking level relate to minimum and maximum masking levels? State the equation for calculating mid-masking level.
9. Briefly discuss the two advantages of the midplateau masking procedure.
10. Studebaker (1979) has described an alternate acoustic masking procedure for use during speech audiometry. What three factors are accounted for when selecting an appropriate masking level? State the equation for selecting the effective masking level.
11. There are two major approaches to selecting appropriate masking levels during speech audiometry. Briefly discuss the advantages and disadvantages of each.
12. Discuss the short-cut acoustic approach to selecting appropriate levels of masking during speech audiometry. State the equation for calculating effective masking level. What two conditions must be met to use this simplified procedure?

13. Psychoacoustic masking procedures can be used when measuring speech thresholds. Briefly describe the plateau procedure for measuring masked speech detection and recognition thresholds. What are the advantages and disadvantages of the plateau procedure for measuring speech thresholds?

7

Clinical Masking Procedures: Suprathreshold Pure-Tone Audiometry

Our discussion so far has focused on the use of contralateral masking during the basic audiological evaluation. Specifically, the principles and clinical applications of masking during threshold pure-tone audiometry and threshold and suprathreshold speech audiometry have been reviewed. Suprathreshold pure-tone tests, although not a component of the basic audiological evaluation, historically have played an important role in the classic behavioral site-of-lesion test battery. Contralateral masking is sometimes required during the administration of such diagnostic tests.

Site-of-lesion assessment typically refers to the differentiation of cochlear versus eighth-nerve pathology. The classic site-of-lesion tests are related to assessment of one of three auditory phenomena: (1) Abnormal growth of loudness (e.g., alternate binaural loudness balance, ABLB), (2) auditory adaptation (e.g., tone decay tests, Bekésy audiometry), and (3) differential threshold for intensity (e.g., short increment sensitivity index, SISI) (see Hall, 1991, for an excellent historical and critical review of the classic site-of-lesion test battery).

Over approximately the past fifteen years, the use of the traditional site-of-lesion test battery, which requires *behavioral* responses from the patient, has declined significantly. Conversely, the use of *physiological* tests (e.g., acoustic immittance measures, auditory brain stem response, ABR) for differential diagnosis of cochlear versus eighth-nerve pathology has increased dramatically (Hall, 1991; Martin et al., 1994; Martin & Morris, 1989). Since the early 1970s, Frederick Martin has conducted a series of surveys of audiologic practices in the United States (Martin et al., 1994; Martin & Forbis, 1978; Martin & Morris, 1989; Martin & Pennington, 1971; Martin & Sides, 1985; Pennington & Martin, 1972). In the most recent survey (conducted in 1992), Martin reported a significant decrease since 1972 in the use of behavioral tests for site of lesion (Martin et al., 1994). For example, the routine use of Bekésy audiometry by surveyed audiologists has decreased from 71 percent in 1972 to approximately 10 percent in 1992. Only one behavioral test for site of lesion appears to have remained relatively popular over the years. As of 1992, 72 percent of surveyed audiologists reported the routine use tone decay tests (Martin et al., 1994).

During the same period of time that there was a decrease in the routine use of behavioral tests, there was extraordinary growth in the use of acoustic immittance measures and electrophysiological tests. As of 1992, 96 percent of surveyed audiologists used acoustic immittance measures (including acoustic reflex measurement) on a routine basis; auditory brain stem response measurement (ABR), the most popular electrophysiological procedure, was used by 65 percent of audiologists in clinical practice. In fact, the majority of audiologists who measure auditory evoked potentials typically use them for site-of-lesion testing (Martin et al., 1994). Hall (1991) suggests that the current clinical popularity of acoustic reflex measurements (i.e., threshold and decay) and ABR and the "demise" of the traditional behavioral test battery are partly the consequence of strong empirical evidence of the former's superior accuracy in differentiating cochlear versus eighth-nerve pathology.

It is beyond the scope of this book to discuss the use of contralateral masking during administration of all site-of-lesion behavioral pure-tone tests.[1] Generally, these tests are presented at suprathreshold levels. And thus the same principles of contralateral masking can be applied. Because the tone decay tests continue to be used with some frequency (Martin et al., 1994), they will be used as examples when discussing the principles of contralateral masking for suprathreshold pure-tone tests.

Auditory adaptation is defined as the temporary decrease in auditory sensitivity that results from sustained (i.e., continuous) acoustic stimulation at *suprathreshold* intensity. Individuals with normal hearing or *cochlear* hearing impairment typically exhibit no greater than minimal adaptation. Conversely, subjects with eighth-nerve pathology experience excessive (i.e., abnormal) adaptation (Konkle & Orchik, 1979). The assessment of auditory adaptation historically has played an important role in differentiating cochlear versus eighth-nerve pathology (Hall, 1991; Konkle & Orchik, 1979).

There are different manual pure-tone techniques for assessing auditory adaptation or tone decay (e.g., Carhart, 1957; Hood, 1955; Jerger & Jerger, 1975; Olsen & Noffsinger, 1974; Rosenberg, 1958).[2] All procedures involve presenting a continuous pure-tone stimulus and determining whether auditory sensitivity decreases over time. An important variable in the assessment of tone decay is the initial presentation level of the test tone. According to the most recent survey of audiologic practices conducted by Martin (Martin et al., 1994), the most frequently used initial level continues to be 20 dB SL. This is the initial presentation level recommended by Olsen and Noffsinger (1974) in their modification of the classic Carhart (1957) tone decay procedure.

The basic features of the Olsen and Noffsinger (1974) modification of the Carhart threshold tone decay test can be summarized as follows:

1. A pure-tone stimulus is presented *continuously* at 20 dB SL relative to the patient's threshold.

2. The patient is instructed to respond (e.g., press response button, raise hand) as soon as the tone is perceived and to continue responding for as long as the tone is audible. Using a stopwatch, a timing period is initiated.

3. If the patient can perceive the tone for 60 seconds, the test is terminated. If the patient stops responding during the 60-second interval, the tone is raised (*without interruption*) in 5-dB steps until the patient responds again. A new minute of timing is initiated. This procedure is continued until the patient can perceive the tone for the 60-second response criterion.

4. The magnitude of tone decay is calculated by subtracting the patient's pure-tone threshold from the level at which the tone is perceived for the 60-

second time period (i.e., the level at which the test is terminated). For example, if pure-tone threshold is 30 dB HL and the level at which the patient can perceive the tone for 60 seconds is 70 dB HL, then tone decay is calculated as 40 dB.

The Olsen-Noffsinger (1974) tone decay test follows the original guidelines of the Carhart (1957) threshold tone decay test with the exception that the tone is initially presented at 20 dB SL rather than at threshold. An initial presentation level of 20 dB SL was recommended for two reasons. First, a tone of 20 dB SL is clearly audible, resulting in an easier listening task at the beginning of the test. Second, a presentation level of 20 dB SL will effectively screen out individuals with lesions peripheral to the eighth nerve (i.e., measured tone decay ≤ 20 dB), yet still permit measurement of excess tone decay (i.e., ≥ 35 dB) in cases of eighth-nerve pathology. Olsen and Noffsinger reported that 95 percent of cases of confirmed eighth-nerve tumor exhibited excess tone decay measured with either the Carhart or 20 dB SL procedure. Because the Olsen-Noffsinger modification of the Carhart tone decay test is the most frequently used behavioral procedure for measuring auditory adaptation (Martin et al., 1994), it will be used in the examples to facilitate an understanding of contralateral masking during suprathreshold pure-tone tests.

Consider the audiogram presented in Figure 7-1. Pure-tone testing reveals normal hearing sensitivity in the right ear. There is a mild-to-moderate sensorineural hearing loss of sloping configuration in the left ear. Tone decay will be measured at one low frequency, 500 Hz, and one high frequency, 4000 Hz, using the 20 dB SL procedure. We will use this example in our discussion of when and how to mask during suprathreshold pure-tone tests.

When to Mask

Recall from Chapter 3 that there are three factors to consider when determining the need for masking during air-conduction threshold audiometry:

1. Intensity level of the signal at the test ear (AC_T)
2. Interaural attenuation (IA)
3. Bone-conduction hearing sensitivity in the nontest ear (BC_{NT})

The equation for when to mask during air-conduction threshold audiometry was stated as follows:

$$AC_T - BC_{NT} \geq IA$$

or

$$AC_T - IA \geq BC_{NT}$$

The same rule will be used when making a decision on the need for masking during suprathreshold pure-tone audiometry. We again will use 40 dB as the conservative estimate of interaural attenuation. During suprathreshold pure-tone audiometry, AC_T refers to the intensity or presentation level of the test tone (Presentation level$_T$) rather than air-conduction threshold as is the case of threshold audiometry. We can restate our rule for when to mask during suprathreshold pure-tone tests as follows:

FIGURE 7–1   Audiogram presenting normal hearing in the right ear and a mild-to-moderate sensorineural hearing loss of sloping configuration in the left ear. Tone decay will be measured at 500 and 4000 Hz using an initial level of 20 dB SL (Olsen & Noffsinger, 1974). Contralateral masking will be required when assessing tone decay in the left ear at both 500 and 4000 Hz.

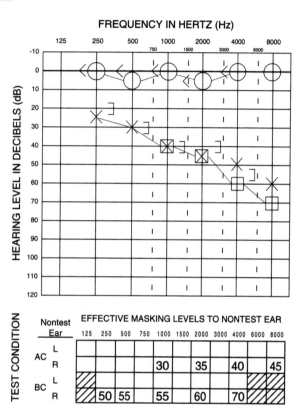

$$\text{Presentation level}_T - BC_{NT} \geq IA$$

or

$$\text{Presentation level}_T - IA \geq BC_{NT}$$

500 Hz: Is contralateral masking required when measuring tone decay at 500 Hz in the left ear? Pure-tone threshold is 30 dB HL; assessment of tone decay will be initiated at 20 dB SL, that is 50 dB HL. Although masking was not needed when measuring pure-tone threshold in the left ear, contralateral masking will be required when assessing tone decay. The presentation level of the test tone (i.e., 50 dB HL) equals or exceeds bone-conduction threshold in the nontest ear (i.e., 0 dB HL) by the amount of interaural attenuation (i.e., 40 dB):

$$\text{Presentation level}_T - IA \geq BC_{NT}$$
$$50 \text{ dB HL} - 40 \text{ dB} \geq 0 \text{ dB HL?}$$
$$10 \text{ dB HL} \geq 0 \text{ dB HL?} \qquad Yes$$

4000 Hz: Is contralateral masking required when measuring tone decay at 4000 Hz in the left ear? Masked pure-tone threshold is 60 dB HL; assessment of tone decay will be initiated at 20 dB SL, that is, 80 dB HL. Therefore, contralateral masking will be required when measuring tone decay at 4000 Hz in the left ear. The presentation level of the test tone (i.e., 80 dB HL) equals or exceeds bone-conduction threshold in the nontest ear (i.e., 0 dB HL) by the amount of interaural attenuation (i.e., 40 dB):

$$\text{Presentation level}_T - IA \geq BC_{NT}$$
$$80 \text{ dB HL} - 40 \text{ dB} \geq 0 \text{ dB HL?}$$
$$40 \text{ dB HL} \geq 0 \text{ dB HL?} \qquad \textit{Yes}$$

Because contralateral masking was required earlier during air-conduction *threshold* measurement, it follows that masking will also be required during any *suprathreshold* pure-tone test.

Selection of Appropriate Masking Levels

How much masking is required when assessing tone decay at 500 and 4000 Hz in the left ear? Just as during pure-tone threshold audiometry, a decision about how much masking to use will involve estimating the minimum and maximum masking levels.

Recall from Chapter 5 the formulas for estimating the minimum and maximum masking levels:

$$M_{min} = AC_T - IA + AB\ Gap_{NT}$$
$$M_{max} = BC_T + IA - 5 \text{ dB}$$

Remember that during suprathreshold pure-tone audiometry, AC_T refers to the *presentation level* of the test tone (Presentation level$_T$). We can restate our equation for minimum masking level as follows:

$$M_{min} = \text{Presentation level}_T - IA + AB\ Gap_{NT}$$

It is important to note that we are using the "formula" approach for calculating minimum masking level. This is an "acoustic" masking approach that proves necessary during any *suprathreshold* auditory test. Martin's simplified approach for determining the initial minimum masking level (i.e., $M_{min} = AC_{NT}$) is appropriate *only* when using a psychoacoustic masking approach *during threshold auditory tests*. Consequently, it cannot be used when determining the minimum masking level needed during measurement of tone decay, a suprathreshold test.

500 Hz: Recall that the test tone will be presented *initially* at 50 dB HL (i.e., 20 dB SL). We will first determine M_{min}, the minimum level of noise needed to just mask a cross-hearing signal in the nontest ear (i.e., right ear). Because a difference of 40 dB or greater did not exist between the unmasked air-conduction threshold in the test ear (i.e., left ear) and the bone-conduction threshold in the nontest ear (i.e., right ear), there was no need to obtain a masked pure-tone threshold at 500 Hz. It will be necessary, then, to assume that interaural attenuation can be as small as 40 dB: We do not have a better estimate of IA for this patient.

$$M_{min} = \text{Presentation level}_T - IA + AB\ Gap_{NT}$$
$$= 50 \text{ dB HL} - 40 \text{ dB} + 5 \text{ dB}$$
$$= 15 \text{ dB EM}$$

Next, we will estimate M_{max}, the maximum masking level that will not result in overmasking. It is important to note that M_{max} is calculated in the same way for both threshold and suprathreshold pure-tone tests.

$$M_{max} = BC_T + IA - 5 \text{ dB}$$
$$= 30 \text{ dB HL} + 40 \text{ dB} - 5 \text{ dB}$$
$$= 65 \text{ dB EM}$$

In this particular example, when tone decay is assessed at an initial presentation level of 50 dB HL, the range of acceptable masking levels is 15 dB EM to 65 dB EM.

4000 Hz: The test tone will be presented *initially* to the left ear at 80 dB HL (i.e., 20 dB SL). Because a difference of 40 dB or greater did exist between the unmasked air-conduction threshold in the test ear (i.e., left ear) and the bone-conduction threshold in the nontest ear (i.e., right ear) at 4000 Hz, a masked pure-tone threshold was required. Therefore, we can use a more accurate estimate of interaural attenuation in our equations for calculation of both M_{min} and M_{max}. In this particular example, the difference between the unmasked air-conduction threshold in the left ear (i.e., 50 dB HL) and the bone-conduction threshold in the nontest ear (i.e., 0 dB) is 50 dB. Thus, interaural attenuation is at least 50 dB. The use of the greater and more accurate estimate of interaural attenuation will reduce M_{min} by 10 dB and increase M_{max} by 10 dB, thereby increasing the permissible range of masking by 20 dB.

$$M_{min} = \text{Presentation level}_T - IA + AB \text{ Gap}_{NT}$$
$$= 80 \text{ dB HL} - 50 \text{ dB} + 0 \text{ dB}$$
$$= 30 \text{ dB EM}$$
$$M_{max} = BC_T + IA - 5 \text{ dB}$$
$$= 55 \text{ dB HL} + 50 \text{ dB} - 5 \text{ dB}$$
$$= 100 \text{ dB EM}$$

In this particular example, when tone decay is assessed at an initial presentation level of 80 dB HL, the range of acceptable masking levels is 30 dB EM to 100 dB EM.

Clinical Masking Procedures

Remember that a psychoacoustic masking procedure, specifically the plateau method, was used during the establishment of masked pure-tone thresholds. Masking during suprathreshold pure-tone tests, however, will require the use of an acoustic procedure. Specifically, the required masking level will be derived by calculating the estimated acoustic levels of the test and the masker signals in the test and nontest ears.

The optimal masking level during a suprathreshold pure-tone test is one that falls above the minimum effective masking and does not exceed the maximum permissible masking level. During speech audiometry, a midplateau masking method was recommended. The minimum and maximum masking levels respectively represent the lower and upper limits of the masking plateau. Therefore, the goal when using a midplateau method was to select a masker level that occurred approximately at the middle of the range (i.e., midplateau).

The midplateau masking procedure proves very efficient during suprathreshold speech and pure-tone tests whenever there is minimal or no variation in the presentation level of the test signal during the course of the test. However, it often is necessary to significantly increase the presentation level of the test signal during assessment of tone decay. Consequently, it will be necessary to reassess the required minimum masking level as the intensity level of the tone is increased. The use of a midplateau masking procedure during measurement of tone decay may prove inefficient whenever the intensity level of the test signal must be increased in order for the patient to maintain audibility. Starting at a mid-masking level can significantly limit the range of masking levels available should it prove necessary to progressively increase the level of the test tone.

Whenever there exists the possibility that the test signal will be increased systematically during a suprathreshold pure-tone test (e.g., a tone decay procedure), it is recommended that the initial masking level be introduced as close as possible to the minimum required. This will permit the level of the masking noise to be increased systematically as the level of the tone is increased. Rather than using the midplateau masking method during suprathreshold pure-tone tests, a minimum noise method is recommended. Specifically, the minimum amount of noise required to mask the cross-hearing signal is introduced to the nontest ear. By introducing the masking noise at a level slightly greater than the minimum required, the audiologist can take advantage of a wider range of acceptable levels of masking *without overmasking*.

Consider again the audiogram presented in Figure 7-1. We already have decided that contralateral masking will be required when assessing tone decay at 500 and 4000 Hz in the left ear when using the 20 dB SL procedure.

500 Hz: Recall that the tone decay test will be initiated at 50 dB HL (i.e., pure-tone threshold of 30 dB HL + 20 dB SL = 50 dB HL presentation level). When using the minimum noise method, we first need to determine the acceptable range of masking levels. Specifically, we need to estimate minimum (i.e., M_{min}) and maximum (M_{max}) masking levels. Recall from our previous calculations that M_{min} and M_{max} are equal to 15 dB EM and 65 dB EM, respectively. If we begin our assessment of tone decay at 50 dB HL, we will need an initial masking level of at least 15 dB EM. Because calibration of effective masking level is based on the averaged responses of a group of normal-hearing subjects, a given effective making level will not prove equally effective for all subjects. A safety factor of not less than 10 dB (usually 10 to 15 dB) should be added to the initial minimum masking level to ensure adequate masking for all subjects. In this particular example, a beginning masking level of 25 to 30 dB EM (i.e., M_{min} of 15 dB EM plus a safety factor of 10 to 15 dB) is recommended. If it is necessary to increase the level of the signal during the course of the tone decay procedure, the masking level should be increased proportionally. In order to avoid the possibility of overmasking, the masking level should not exceed M_{max}. In this particular example, masking should be restricted to levels not exceeding 65 dB EM.

4000 Hz: Contralateral masking is also required when assessing tone decay at 4000 Hz in the left ear. The test tone will be presented *initially* to the left ear at 80 dB HL (i.e., 20 dB SL). Again when using the minimum noise method, we need to determine the acceptable range of masking levels (i.e., the lower and upper limits of the masking plateau). Recall from our previous calculations that M_{min} and M_{max} are equal to 30 dB EM and 100 dB EM, respectively. An appropriate starting level for the 20 dB SL tone decay procedure at 4000 Hz would be 40 to 45 dB EM (i.e., M_{min} of 30 dB EM plus a 10 to 15 dB safety factor). If it is necessary to increase the level of the tone during the course of the test, theoretically the masking level can be increased to 100 dB EM (i.e., M_{max}) without risk of overmasking.

The masker level can be increased using either a *manual* or *automatic* procedure. When using the manual procedure, it is necessary for the audiologist to increase the level of the masker by a proportional amount each time that the tone is increased by 5 or 10 dB. This will take some practice for the beginning audiologist: Two attenuators that independently control the levels of the tone and masker *and* a stopwatch must be manipulated almost simultaneously. Remember that each time the level of the tone is increased, the masker level must be increased proportionally as well. In addition, when the patient responds again to the tone after loss of audibility, it will be necessary to reset the stopwatch for a 60-second time period.

The automatic procedure greatly simplifies the audiologist's task. Some current two-channel audiometers provide a "tracking" option. When the tracking mode is selected, any decibel change to the Channel 1 attenuator (i.e., the dB HL control for the test tone) will automatically change the decibel output for the Channel 2 attenuator (i.e., dB level control for the masker) by the same amount. Once the audiologist sets the masker level for the tone's initial presentation level, the audiometer will automatically increase the masker level by 5 dB each time that the tone is increased by 5 dB. The audiologist only needs to control the level of the test tone once the initial masking level is selected.

Summary

There are three factors that must be considered when determining the need for contralateral making during suprathreshold pure-tone audiometry:

1. Intensity level of the signal at the test ear (Presentation level$_T$)
2. Interaural attenuation (IA)
3. Bone-conduction hearing sensitivity in the nontest ear (BC_{NT})

The equation for when to mask during suprathreshold pure-tone audiometry can be stated as follows:

$$\text{Presentation level}_T - BC_{NT} \geq IA$$

or

$$\text{Presentation level}_T - IA \geq BC_{NT}$$

A decision about how much masking to use will involve estimating the minimum and maximum masking levels. The equations for estimating minimum and maximum masking levels during suprathreshold pure-tone audiometry can be summarized as follows:

$$M_{min} = \text{Presentation level}_T - IA + AB\ Gap_{NT}$$
$$M_{max} = BC_T + IA - 5\ dB$$

The optimal masking level during a suprathreshold pure-tone test is one that falls above the minimum effective masking, yet does not exceed the maximum permissible masking level. The midplateau masking procedure proves very efficient during suprathreshold pure-tone tests whenever there is minimal or no variation in the presentation level of the test signal during the course of the test. Whenever it is anticipated that the test signal will be increased systematically during a suprathreshold pure-tone test, it is recommended that the initial masking level be introduced as close as possible to the minimum required. Rather than using the midplateau masking method during suprathreshold pure-tone tests, a minimum noise method can be employed. Specifically, the minimum amount of noise required to mask the cross-hearing signal (i.e., M_{min} + 10 or 15 dB safety factor) is introduced to the nontest ear. By introducing the masking noise at a level slightly greater than the minimum required, the audiologist can take advantage of a wider range of acceptable levels of masking during the course of the test.

Study Questions

1. What three factors must be considered when determining the need for masking during suprathreshold pure-tone audiometry?

2. State the equation for when to mask during suprathreshold pure-tone audiometry.

3. What two factors must be considered when deciding how much masking to use during suprathreshold pure-tone audiometry?

4. State the formulas for estimating the minimum and maximum masking levels during suprathreshold pure-tone audiometry.

5. Briefly describe the minimum noise method of masking. When is the minimum noise method more appropriate than the midplateau procedure when selecting an appropriate masking level during suprathreshold pure-tone audiometry?

Endnotes

1. Because this book focuses on the principles and clinical applications of masking during *behavioral* auditory assessment, the use of contralateral masking during ABR measurements, an electrophysiological test, will not be discussed here. The concepts necessary for understanding contralateral masking and behavioral auditory tests, however, will facilitate an understanding of masking during auditory evoked response (AER) measurement. Hall (1992) provides an excellent discussion of contralateral masking during AER measurement in his comprehensive text *Handbook of Auditory Evoked Responses* (pp. 170–175).

2. Hall (1991), Konkle and Orchik (1979), and Silman and Silverman (1991) provide excellent critical reviews of behavioral tests of auditory adaptation.

8

The Use of Insert Earphones

There are three major types of earphones currently used in audiological testing: supra-aural, circumaural, and insert. Supra-aural earphones use cushions that are pressed against the pinna. Circumaural earphones use cushions that encircle or surround the pinna. Insert earphones are coupled to the ear by insertion into the ear canal. (See Killion & Villchur, 1989, and Zwislocki et al., 1988, for a review of advantages and disadvantages of earphones in audiometry.)

Supra-aural earphones currently are the standard configuration used in audiometric testing. The most common supra-aural earphones supplied with audiometers are the Telephonics TDH-39, TDH-49, TDH-50, or Telex 1470A earphones, encased in either an MX-41/AR or Telephonics Model 51 rubber cushion.[1] However, several limitations of the traditional supra-aural earphone have been reported and are listed below.

1. There is often reduced reliability at low frequencies because of variable and sometimes inadequate coupling between the earphone cushion and the pinna (Clemis, Ballad, & Killion, 1986; Killion, 1984; Zwislocki et al., 1988).

2. There is limited attenuation of ambient noise (i.e., real ear attenuation), particularly in the low frequencies (Berger & Kerivan, 1983; Berger & Killion, 1989; Clark & Roeser, 1988; Clemis et al., 1986; Franks, Engel, & Themann, 1992; Killion, 1984; Wright & Frank, 1992). This is an important consideration when testing is conducted in an environment other than a sound-treated booth (e.g., hearing screening in schools, testing at bedside in hospitals).

3. There is a required headband force that can make the headphones uncomfortable to wear for prolonged periods of time (Killion, 1984).

4. Because supra-aural earphone cushions exert pressure *against* the pinna, they sometimes can result in collapse of the external ear canal (Ventry et al., 1961; Hildyard & Valentine, 1962), particularly in the elderly population (e.g., Schow & Goldbaum, 1980). The consequence is often poorer air-conduction thresholds, usually in the higher frequencies (Chaiklin & McClellan, 1971).

5. Because of close proximity between the earphone and recording electrodes during auditory brain stem response (ABR) measurements, large stimulus artifacts can result in the averaged ABR response (Beauchaine et al., 1987; Killion, 1984).

6. The limited high-frequency response of supra-aural earphones can contribute to unreliable responses during high-frequency audiometry (Killion, 1984).

7. Measurements made with standard earphones are difficult to relate to hearing aid data (Clemis et al., 1986). Specifically, the ability to convert audiometric data to relevant hearing aid characteristics is limited because the supra-aural earphone and hearing aid are not calibrated with the same acoustic coupler (Mueller & Bright, 1994).

8. Limited interaural attenuation (IA) of supra-aural earphones often necessitates masking in the nontest ear (Clemis et al., 1986; Killion, 1984; Killion et al., 1985).

Over forty-five years ago, Bekésy (1948) first demonstrated that an insert earphone could be used to increase both interaural attenuation and background noise attenuation when compared to the supra-aural earphone. Bekésy constructed an insert earphone using a hearing aid receiver coupled to the ear using a plastic tube and perforated earplug. Using a similar (yet greatly improved) design, Killion (1984) described new insert earphones for audiometry—Etymotic Research "tubephones." There are different models of the Etymotic Research insert earphone available, each differing in electroacoustic characteristics. The Etymotic Research ER-3A, however, is currently the most commonly used clinical audiometric insert earphone (Killion & Villchur, 1989) and has been researched extensively since its development.

The 3A tubephones are presented in Figure 8-1*A*. The *transducers* are contained within rectangular cases that are shoulder-mounted on each side of the neck. The transducers can be clipped to the patient's clothing or placed there using a Velcro strap neck loop. Each transducer is coupled to the ear canal using a *sound tube* of precisely defined dimensions (278-mm length of #16 tubing) and a *modified* E-A-R™ foam earplug (Cabot Safety Corporation). The foam eartips, which are disposable, are available in three sizes. The Etymotic Research ER3-14 eartip is designed for use by individuals with normal-size ear canals. The ER3-14B is designed for individuals with small ear canals while the ER3-14C is intended for patients with very large ear canals.

More recently, the Auditory Systems Division of Cabot Safety Corporation (1990) manufactured an insert earphone known as the E-A-RTONE™ 3A. The Etymotic Research ER-3A and the E-A-RTONE 3A insert earphones are functionally equivalent because they are built to identical specifications (Frank & Vavrek, 1992). The E-A-RTONE 3A insert earphone uses foam eartips known as E-A-RLINKs, which are available in three sizes: 3A, 3B, and 3C. The E-A-RLINK 3A, 3B, and 3C eartips are functionally equivalent to the Etymotic Research ER3-14, ER3-14B, and ER3-14C eartips, respectively (Frank & Vavrek, 1992).

The Etymotic Research ER-3A insert earphone was designed to simulate the frequency response of the TDH-39 supra-aural earphone at the tympanic membrane so that the two transducers could be used interchangeably (Killion & Villchur, 1989). In fact, the 3A insert earphone can directly replace the Telephonics TDH-39, TDH-49, TDH-50, or Telex 1470A supra-aural earphones without need for recalibrating the audiometer. In other words, the 3A insert earphone can be used as a "plug-in" substitute for the traditional supra-aural earphone. In fact, when the 3A insert earphone is plugged into an audiometer calibrated for the traditional supra-aural earphone, only small correction factors are required (typically at the low and high frequencies). The manufacturers of these devices (Etymotic Research and Cabot Safety Corporation) have provided recommended correction factors when the 3A insert earphone is used as a complement to the traditional supra-aural earphones (i.e., the supra-aural earphone serves as the primary air-conduction transducer). These correction factors are

FIGURE 8–1 Two types of insert earphones. (A) The 3A Tubephone (Etymotic Research ER-3A and E-A-RTONE™ 3A) with foam eartips and (B) the standard "button" transducer (Grason-Stadler).

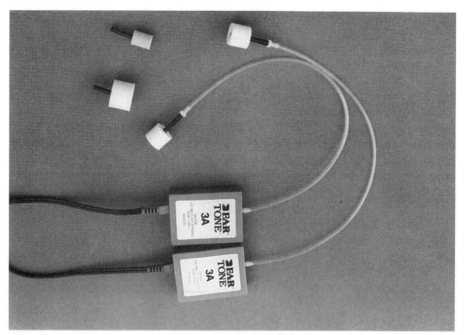

A

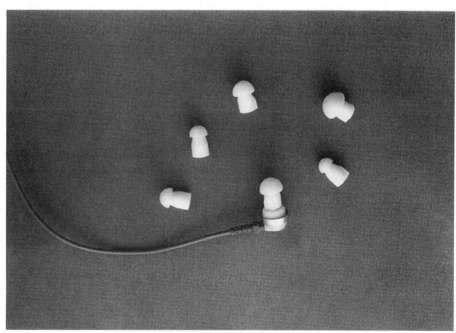

B

provided in Table 8-1. When the Etymotic Research ER-3A or E-A-RTONE 3A insert earphone is used as the primary transducer, however, the audiometer should be calibrated using the interim reference threshold levels specified in the American National Standard *Specification for Audiometers* (ANSI S3.6-1989, Appendix G). Consequently, correction factors would not be required.

When the 3A insert is used as a plug-in substitute for a supra-aural earphone during speech audiometry, a correction factor typically is not required. The standard reference sound pressure level for speech is always *12.5 dB above the 1000 Hz standard reference sound pressure level threshold* for a particular earphone as specified in ANSI S3.6-1989. For example, the standard reference threshold sound pressure level for a Telephonics TDH-49 supra-aural earphone at 1000 Hz is 7.5 dB. Consequently, the standard reference level for speech is 20 dB SPL for that particular earphone (calibrated in a standard 6-cc, NBS 9-A coupler). When using the 3A insert earphone, the interim standard reference equivalent threshold sound pressure level at 1000 Hz is 3.5 dB (calibrated in a standard 2-cc, HA-1 coupler). Therefore, the standard reference level for speech will be 16 dB SPL when using the 3A insert earphone. Because the manufacturers of the 3A insert earphone recommend a plug-in correction factor of 0 dB at 1000 Hz (see Table 8-1), a correction factor for speech will not be necessary when the insert is used as a plug-in substitute for a calibrated supra-aural earphone.

The manufacturer of the E-A-RTONE 3A insert earphone cautions that the provided correction factors assume that the integrity of the original earphones remains undisturbed (see Lilly & Purdy, 1993, for a review of potential problems with the Tubephone insert earphones). If the audiologist is using the Tubephone insert earphone as a plug-in substitute for the supra-aural earphone, *verification of the appropriateness of the provided correction factors is recommended each time that the audiometer is calibrated*. The manufacturer of the E-A-RTONE 3A insert earphone (Cabot Safety Corporation, Auditory Systems Division, 1990) recommends the following calibration procedure when determining *individual correction factors* for 3A insert earphones:

1. Calibrate the audiometer for the primary transducer (i.e., supra-aural earphone) using the appropriate standard (i.e., ANSI S3.6-1989).

2. Unplug the supra-aural earphones and connect the 3A insert earphones to the audiometer.

TABLE 8–1 Plug-in correction factors (dB HL) for the Etymotic Research ER-3A and E-A-RTONE™ 3A insert earphones when used as a complement to the Telephonics TDH-39, 49, or 50 earphones or the Telex 1470A earphone.

Transducer	Frequency (in Hz)										
	125	*250*	*500*	*750*	*1000*	*1500*	*2000*	*3000*	*4000*	*6000*	*8000*
TDH-39, 49, 50	15	5	0	–5	0	0	0	0	0	–10	–10
1470A	15	5	0	–5	0	0	0	–5	0	–10	–15
	Decibel (dB) value to be added to dB HL dial setting.										

From *Instructions for Use of E-A-RTONE™ 3A Insert Earphones* by Cabot Safety Corporation, Auditory Systems Division, 1990, Indianapolis, Indiana and *ER-3A Tubephone™ Insert Earphone*, Etymotic Research, 1991, Elk Grove Village, Illinois. Reprinted by permission.

3. Measure the SPL output in a 2-cc coupler and compare to the interim reference threshold levels for insert earphones provided in ANSI S3.6-1989 (or the instructions manual for the 3A insert earphone).

4. Tabulate the difference between the actual (i.e., measured) and the target (i.e., interim reference threshold levels for insert earphones) sound pressure levels at each frequency.

5. This table comprises the appropriate correction factors (rounded to the nearest 5 dB) for your 3A insert earphone when used as a plug-in substitute for the supra-aural earphone. (For example, if the target SPL at 250 Hz is 84.0 dB and the measured SPL is 89.0 dB, then the rounded correction factor is +5 dB.)

There currently is considerable empirical evidence suggesting that the Etymotic Research ER-3A or E-A-RTONE 3A insert earphones offer a valid alternative in many audiometric applications because they solve several of the problems associated with conventional supra-aural earphones (Beauchaine et al., 1987; Berger & Killion, 1989; Borton, Nolen, Luks, & Meline, 1989; Clark & Roeser, 1988; Clemis et al., 1986; Frank & Wright, 1990; Hosford-Dunn, Kuklinski, Raggio, & Haggerty, 1986; Killion, 1984; Killion et al., 1985; Lindgren, 1990; Martin, Severance, & Thibodeau, 1991; Mueller & Bright, 1994; Sklare & Denenberg, 1987; Stuart, Stenstrom, Tompkins, & Vandenhoff, 1991; Valente, Valente, & Goebel, 1992; Wright & Frank, 1992). A major advantage of the 3A insert earphone compared to the conventional supra-aural earphone is *increased interaural attenuation* for air-conducted sound, particularly in the lower frequencies (e.g., Hosford-Dunn et al., 1986; Killion et al., 1985; Sklare & Denenberg, 1987; Van Campen et al., 1990). This is clearly illustrated in the results of a study by Killion and colleagues (1985) (see Figure 8-2). Increased interaural attenuation with insert earphones appears to be partly the result of the reduced contact area of the earphone with the skull.

Zwislocki (1953) evaluated interaural attenuation using three types of earphones: circumaural, supra-aural ("small rubber cushion"), and insert ("perforated ear plug"). Results suggested that interaural attenuation for air-conducted sound increased as the contact area of the earphone with the skull decreased: Interaural attenuation was greatest for the insert earphone and smallest for the receiver encased in a circumaural cushion. When an acoustic signal is delivered to the ear through an earphone, the resultant sound pressure acts over a surface area of the skull determined by the earphone cushion. The acoustic force applied to the head at a specific sound pressure level is assumed to be proportional to the contact area of the earphone cushion with the skull. The surface area under the smaller cushion of an insert earphone will result in a smaller applied force to the skull, resulting in reduced bone-conduction transmission.

Chaiklin (1967) has also suggested that interaural attenuation may be increased in the low frequencies with a *deep* insert because of a reduction of the occlusion effect. There is considerable evidence that the occlusion effect influences the measured interaural attenuation for air-conducted sound (e.g., Berrett, 1973; Chaiklin, 1967; Killion et al., 1985). In fact, there is an inverse relationship between magnitude of the occlusion effect and the measured interaural attenuation in the low frequencies: An earphone that reduces the occlusion effect will exhibit increased interaural attenuation for air-conducted sound. If the opposite ear is occluded and exhibits a normal occlusion effect, then interaural attenuation will be increased in magnitude by the size of the occlusion effect (Berrett, 1973). It is probable that the increased interaural attenuation for air-conducted

FIGURE 8–2   Average and range of interaural attenuation values obtained on six subjects using two earphones: TDH-39 encased in MX-41/AR supra-aural cushion (●) and ER-3A insert earphone with deeply inserted plugs (■). NOTE: From "Insert earphones for more interaural attenuation" by M.C. Killion, L.A. Wilber, and G.I. Gudmundsen, 1985, *Hearing Instruments, 36*, 34, 36. Reprinted by permission.

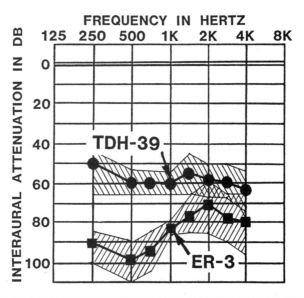

sound observed in the low frequencies when using 3A insert earphones (with deeply inserted earplugs) is primarily related to a significant reduction (or elimination) of the occlusion effect. (Refer to the section The Occlusion Effect and Air Conduction in Chapter 5 for further discussion of the occlusion effect and interaural attenuation for air-conducted sound.)

The use of insert earphones to increase interaural attenuation has been recommended for many years (Coles & Priede, 1970; Feldman, 1963; Hood, 1960; Littler, Knight, & Strange, 1952; Studebaker, 1962; Zwislocki, 1953). The use of a transducer that yields increased interaural attenuation for air-conducted sound provides two major advantages. First, the need for contralateral masking is significantly reduced during air-conduction audiometry. Second, the range between minimum and maximum masking levels is increased, thereby increasing the width of the masking plateau and the range of permissible masking (Studebaker, 1962) during both air- and bone-conduction audiometry. Thus, the risk of overmasking is significantly reduced. In fact, the use of an insert earphone can often solve the audiometric "masking dilemma" (Clemis et al., 1986; Hosford-Dunn et al., 1986; Killion et al., 1985; Sklare & Denenberg, 1987).

Some two-channel diagnostic audiometers now come equipped with a single insert earphone, typically the standard "button" transducer. If increased interaural attenuation is the primary goal in the selection of an insert earphone, however, then the Etymotic Research ER-3A or E-A-RTONE 3A is clearly the transducer of choice. Evidence suggests that the ER-3A insert provides significantly greater interaural attenuation than the standard button transducer (Blackwell, Oyler, & Seyfried, 1991; Hosford-Dunn et al., 1986). Blackwell and colleagues (1991) compared the interaural attenuation obtained with a Grason-

Stadler (GS) insert earphone and a standard TDH-50P supra-aural earphone. The GS insert is a button transducer fitted with standard immittance probe cuffs (see Figure 8-1*B*). Although Blackwell and colleagues observed greater interaural attenuation with the GS insert, the difference between the insert and standard earphones did not exceed 10 dB at any frequency. Figure 8-3 compares average interaural attenuation values obtained with standard supra-aural earphones (Blackwell et al., 1991), the GS insert earphone (Blackwell et al., 1991), and the Etymotic Research ER-3A insert using deeply inserted foam plugs (Killion et al., 1985). It is evident that the ER-3A provides significantly greater average interaural attenuation than does the GS insert, particularly in the lower frequencies (approximately 20 to 30 dB greater interaural attenuation). Hosford-Dunn and colleagues (1986) suggest that the ER-3A insert earphone provides superior interaural attenuation because of the large distance (i.e., 278-mm length of plastic tubing) between the transducer and the ear insert, thereby reducing the vibrating surface for bone conduction. The GS insert has a greater vibrating surface because the transducer is coupled directly to the immittance probe cuff inserted into the ear canal.

It is also probable that the 3A insert exhibits superior interaural attenuation in the low frequencies because of a significantly reduced occlusion effect. There is evidence that the occlusion effect is negligible when using either *deeply or intermediately inserted* insert earphones. In fact, the advantage of a greatly reduced occlusion effect is lost when a shallow insertion is used (Berger & Kerivan, 1983). Because of its relatively shallow insertion, the GS insert may exhibit an occlusion effect that is more similar to that achieved with conventional supra-aural ear-

FIGURE 8–3 Average interaural attenuation values obtained with three earphones. TDH-50P standard supra-aural earphones (ɔ) (Blackwell, Oyler, & Seyfried, 1991); Grason-Stadler (GS) insert earphone (h) Blackwell, Oyler, & Seyfried, 1991); and ER-3A insert earphone with deeply inserted foam plugs (■) (Killion, Wilber, & Gudmundsen, 1985).

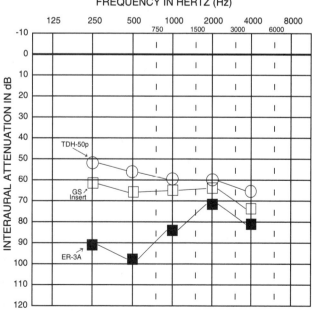

phones. Thus, the GS insert and supra-aural earphones will also yield more similar values of interaural attenuation in the low frequencies.

Our discussion of the use of insert earphones during clinical masking procedures will focus on the ER-3A for two reasons. First, the ER-3A currently appears be the most commonly used insert earphone for clinical audiometric applications (Killion & Villchur, 1989). Second, the ER-3A provides the greatest interaural attenuation for air-conducted sound when compared to other commercially available insert earphones (e.g., Blackwell et al., 1991; Hosford-Dunn et al., 1986; Killion et al., 1985; Sklare & Denenberg, 1987; Van Campen et al., 1990).[2]

The same basic principles will be applied when using either the conventional supra-aural earphone or the ER-3A insert earphone during clinical masking procedures. Therefore, a significant portion of the following discussion of the use of insert earphones will simply reinforce what you already know about clinical masking procedures.

Pure-Tone Air-Conduction Audiometry

When to Mask

Recall from our discussion in Chapter 3 that three factors must be considered when making a decision about the need for masking during pure-tone air-conduction testing:

1. Unmasked air-conduction threshold in the test ear (AC_T)
2. Interaural attenuation (IA)
3. Bone-conduction hearing sensitivity in the nontest ear (BC_{NT})

When supra-aural earphones were used, the rule for when to mask was stated as follows:

$$AC_T - BC_{NT} \text{ (or } AC_{NT}) \geq 40 \text{ dB}$$

or

$$AC_T - 40 \text{ dB} \geq BC_{NT} \text{ (or } AC_{NT})$$

We essentially can employ the same masking rule when using the ER-3A insert earphone. The only modification required is the use of a larger value of interaural attenuation than 40 dB.

Table 8-2 presents interaural attenuation values for pure-tone air-conducted signals using Etymotic Research ER-3A insert earphones with foam earplugs. As was noted with supra-aural earphones, interaural attenuation values vary across frequency and subject, ranging from 50 to 110 dB. Following Studebaker's (1967a) recommendation, we again will use the smallest interaural attenuation value reported when making a decision about the need for masking. However, to take advantage of the significantly increased interaural attenuation provided by the ER-3A earphone in the low frequencies, a single value of interaural attenuation value will not be employed across the frequency range. Rather, a different value of interaural attenuation will be used for the low and high frequencies when making a decision about the need for masking. *Based on currently available data, conservative estimates of interaural attenuation for the ER-3A insert earphone are 75 dB at 1000 Hz and below and 50 dB at frequencies above 1000 Hz.* The rules for when to mask during pure-tone air-conduction audiometry when using 3A insert earphones with foam plugs can be summarized as follows:

TABLE 8-2 Range of interaural attenuation values (in dB) for pure-tone air-conducted signals using Etymotic Research ER-3A insert earphones with foam earplugs.

			Frequency (Hz)											
Study	Insertion Depth	Number of Subjects	125	250	500	750	1000	1500	2000	3000	4000	6000	8000
Killion, Wilber, & Gudmundsen (1985)	Deep	N = 6	—	85 – 100	90 – 110	85 – 105	78 – 85	65 – 85	60 – 85	65 – 90	65 – 95	—	—
Sklare & Denenberg (1987)	Deep	N = 7	—	75$^+$ – 100$^+$	85 – 105	80 – 100	75 – 90	65 – 85	55 – 90	50 – 80	60 – 85	60$^+$ – 95	—
Van Campen, Sammeth, & Peek (1990)	Intermediate	N = 2	—	85 – 90	85 – 90	—	80 – 85	—	65 – 80	—	75 – 85	—	75$^+$ – 80

$$AC_T - BC_{NT} \text{ (or } AC_{NT}) \geq IA$$

or

$$AC_T - IA \geq BC_{NT} \text{ (or } AC_{NT})$$

where interaural attenuation is equal to

75 dB at frequencies $\leq$ 1000 Hz

50 dB at frequencies > 1000 Hz

It should be apparent that because of the greater interaural attenuation provided by the ER-3A insert earphone, the need for masking will be reduced, particularly in the lower frequencies.

The interaural attenuation values recommended clinically for ER-3A earphones assume that *deeply inserted* foam eartips are used. It is very important to note that maximum interaural attenuation for the ER-3A insert earphone is achieved in the low frequencies when a deep earplug insertion is used (Killion et al., 1985). Because the eartips are 12 mm in length, the correct insertion depth is achieved when the outer edge of the earplug is 2 to 3 mm *inside* the entrance of the ear canal (Cabot Safety Corporation, 1990). Conversely, a shallow insertion is obtained when the outer edge of the earplug protrudes from the entrance of the ear canal. An intermediate insertion is achieved when the outer edge of the earplug is flush with the opening of the ear canal (Van Campen et al., 1990). Figure 8-4 presents a schematic diagram of deep and shallow insertions.

Killion and co-workers (1985) evaluated interaural attenuation in a single subject using deep and shallow earplug insertion in both ears. They stated that the soft cartilage of the ear canal is exposed in the shallow insertion; conversely, the soft cartilage is essentially covered with a deep insertion. Their data suggested that an additional 15 to 20 dB of interaural attenuation could be achieved in the low frequencies *for each ear* in which the earplug was deeply inserted (i.e., total interaural attenuation of 30 to 40 dB). It should be noted, however, that there is limited data suggesting that interaural attenuation is similar for either *intermediate* or *deep* insertion of the foam plug; a shallow insertion appears to significantly reduce interaural attenuation (Killion et al., 1985; Sklare & Denenberg, 1987; Van Campen et al., 1990).

Consider the unmasked audiogram presented in Figure 8-5*A*. Air-conduction thresholds have been obtained using ER-3A insert earphones. Is masking required in either ear during air-conduction testing? Remember that we will consider the unmasked bone-conduction responses as possible thresholds for either ear. We will use the following equation when making a decision about the need for masking:

$$AC_T - IA \geq BC_{NT}$$

Right Ear (Test Ear)		Masking Needed?
250 Hz	$5 - 75 \geq 5$?	No
500 Hz	$5 - 75 \geq 5$?	No
1000 Hz	$10 - 75 \geq 5$?	No
2000 Hz	$5 - 50 \geq 5$?	No
4000 Hz	$5 - 50 \geq 5$?	No
8000 Hz	$10 - 50 \geq 10^*$?	No

*Estimated bone-conduction threshold

FIGURE 8–4   A schematic diagram of shallow (A) and deep (B) insertion of foam earplugs used with 3A insert earphones. From "Insert earphones for more interaural attenuation" by M.C. Killion, LA. Wilber, and G.I. Gudmundsen, 1985, *Hearing Instruments, 36*, 34, 36. Reprinted by permission.

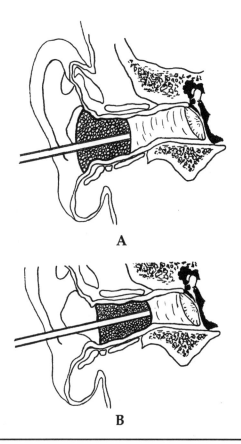

A

B

Contralateral masking is not required when obtaining air-conduction thresholds at any frequency in the right ear. The estimated level of the cross hearing signal (i.e., $AC_T - IA$) does not equal or exceed the apparent bone-conduction threshold in the nontest ear. Because bone-conduction threshold cannot be measured at 8000 Hz, it was necessary to predict a possible unmasked bone-conduction response. Given that unmasked bone-conduction responses interweave with air-conduction thresholds in the right ear at octave frequencies from 250 through 4000 Hz, it is reasonable to assume that a similar relationship would also occur at 8000 Hz (i.e., the bone-conduction threshold is essentially the same as that obtained by air conduction).

It should be apparent that whenever the obtained air-conduction threshold is significantly less than the estimate of interaural attenuation, contralateral masking typically will not be needed. This would require bone-conduction threshold responses at *negative* decibel values. For example, a bone-conduction threshold would be required at –65 dB HL at 1000 Hz (i.e., AC_T of 10 dB HL – IA of 75 dB = –65 dB HL) in order for the left ear to perceive a cross-hearing signal from the right ear! With clinical experience, it will become evident that it is not necessary to evaluate the need for contralateral masking during air-conduction threshold audiometry whenever the test ear exhibits normal hearing.

Contralateral masking will be required, however, when measuring air-conduction thresholds in the left ear.

FIGURE 8–5   Audiogram A presents unmasked air- and bone-conduction thresholds. Air-conduction thresholds were measured using 3A insert earphones with foam earplugs. Contralateral masking is needed when measuring air-conduction thresholds at 2000, 4000, and 8000 Hz in the left ear. After masked air-conduction thresholds are obtained in the left ear (Audiogram B), it also will be necessary to measure masked bone-conduction thresholds in the left ear at all frequencies (i.e., octave frequencies from 250 to 4000 Hz).

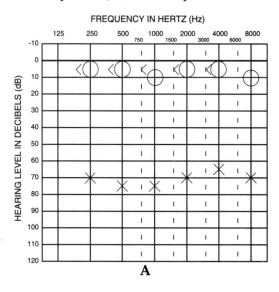

A

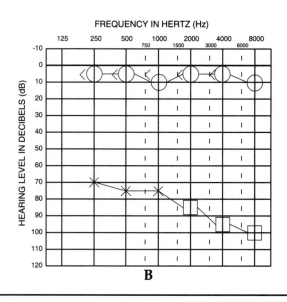

B

$$AC_T - IA \geq BC_{NT}$$

Left Ear (Test Ear)		Masking Needed?
250 Hz	$70 - 75 \geq 5$?	No
500 Hz	$75 - 75 \geq 5$?	No
1000 Hz	$75 - 75 \geq 5$?	No
2000 Hz	$70 - 50 \geq 5$?	Yes
4000 Hz	$65 - 50 \geq 5$?	Yes
8000 Hz	$70 - 50 \geq 10^*$?	Yes

*Estimated bone-conduction threshold

It is necessary to obtained masked air-conduction thresholds at 2000, 4000, and 8000 Hz because the estimated level of the cross-hearing signal equals or exceeds the apparent bone-conduction threshold in the nontest ear. It should be noted that contralateral masking also would have been required at 250, 500, and 1000 Hz *if supra-aural earphones had been used*: AC_T exceeds BC_{NT} by at least 40 dB (i.e., IA for supra-aural earphones). In this particular case, the use of ER-3A insert earphones eliminated the need for contralateral masking in the lower frequencies.

Selection of Appropriate Masking Levels

Our next step will be to determine the appropriate masking levels during measurement of pure tone air-conduction thresholds. We will continue to use the audiogram presented in Figure 8-5*A* to illustrate the selection of masking levels. We already have decided that contralateral masking is required when measuring air-conduction thresholds at 2000, 4000, and 8000 Hz in the left ear. Recall from our discussion in Chapter 5 the formulas for determining minimum (M_{min}) and maximum (M_{max}) masking levels:

$$M_{min} = AC_{NT} + 10 \text{ dB safety factor}$$
$$M_{max} = B_T + IA - 5 \text{ dB}$$

Regardless of the transducer type used to deliver the contralateral masking, M_{min} is always equal to the air-conduction threshold of the nontest ear. No modification is required when using an insert earphone.

$$M_{min} = AC_{NT} + 10 \text{ dB safety factor}$$

2000 Hz	$M_{min} = 5 \text{ dB HL} + 10 \text{ dB} = 15 \text{ dB EM}$
4000 Hz	$M_{min} = 5 \text{ dB HL} + 10 \text{ dB} = 15 \text{ dB EM}$
8000 Hz	$M_{min} = 10 \text{ dB HL} + 10 \text{ dB} = 20 \text{ dB EM}$

Although M_{max} is calculated in the same way when using an insert earphone, the estimated value theoretically should be greater because of the increased interaural attenuation.

$$M_{max} = B_T + IA - 5 \text{ dB}$$

2000 Hz	$M_{max} = 5 \text{ dB HL} + 65 \text{ dB} - 5 \text{ dB} = 65 \text{ dB EM}$
4000 Hz	$M_{max} = 5 \text{ dB HL} + 60 \text{ dB} - 5 \text{ dB} = 60 \text{ dB EM}$
8000 Hz	$M_{max} = 10 \text{ dB HL} + 60 \text{ dB} - 5 \text{ dB} = 65 \text{ dB EM}$

Two points should be noted in the above calculations. First, remember that our estimate of M_{max} is typically *very* conservative if we use the unmasked bone-conduction thresholds (i.e., 5 dB HL at 2000 and 4000 Hz, and the predicted 10 dB HL at 8000 Hz) as our estimate of BC_T. Consequently, M_{max} will be considerably greater if there is a sensorineural hearing loss in the test ear. Second, we have used the more accurate estimates of interaural attenuation (i.e., 65 dB at 2000 Hz and 60 dB at 4000 and 8000 Hz) when calculating M_{max} rather than the more conservative estimate of 50 dB. (Interaural attenuation was estimated by comparing the unmasked bone-conduction threshold to the unmasked air-conduction threshold at each frequency.) The important point to remember here is that M_{max} should be increased significantly when using the ER-3A insert earphone because of greater interaural attenuation. Therefore, greater levels of masking can be used without overmasking.

Pure-Tone Bone-Conduction Audiometry

When to Mask

Recall the rule for when to mask during bone-conduction audiometry:

The use of masking is indicated when there exists a potential air-bone gap (AB Gap_T) of 15 dB or greater in the test ear.

$$AB\ Gap_T \geq 15\ dB$$

A decision about when to mask during bone-conduction audiometry is not affected by the transducer type used to deliver contralateral masking.

Consider the pure-tone audiogram presented in Figure 8-5*B*. This is the same audiogram presented in Figure 8-5*A*; however, masked air-conduction thresholds at 2000, 4000, and 8000 Hz in the left ear are now included. When we compare the unmasked bone-conduction thresholds to the air-conduction thresholds in the right ear, there is no evidence of a significant air-bone gap at any frequency (i.e., no air-bone gap $\geq$ 15 dB). However, there are potentially significant air-bone gaps in the left ear (i.e., 65 dB at 250 Hz, 70 dB at 500 Hz, 70 dB at 1000 Hz, 80 dB at 2000 Hz, and 90 dB at 4000 Hz). Thus, contralateral masking is required when measuring bone-conduction thresholds at all frequencies in the left ear. Remember that there is no need to consider the transducer used for delivering contralateral masking (i.e., supra-aural versus insert) when making a decision about when to mask during bone-conduction audiometry.

Selection of Appropriate Masking Levels

Recall from our discussion in Chapter 5 the formulas for determining minimum (M_{min}) and maximum (M_{max}) masking levels during bone-conduction audiometry:

$$M_{min} = AC_{NT} + OE + 10\ dB\ safety\ factor$$
$$M_{max} = B_T + IA - 5\ dB$$

Although the transducer type for delivering masking did not affect our decision about the need to mask, it will affect the estimated minimum and maximum masking levels.

Recall that calculation of M_{min} includes a correction for the occlusion effect in the lower frequencies. There is evidence, however, that the occlusion effect is negligible when using deeply inserted insert earphones (Berger & Kerivan, 1983; Chaiklin, 1967). Berger and Kerivan (1983) studied the magnitude of the occlusion effect in normal-hearing subjects for different occluding devices, including E-A-R plugs, the foam insert used with the ER-3A and E-A-RTONE 3A insert earphones. Their results for four occluding devices are presented in Table 8-3. Three of their findings have importance when using air-conduction transducers to deliver contralateral ear masking during bone-conduction audiometry. First, the average occlusion effect is negligible when occluding the ear using an E-A-R foam plug with either deep or standard (i.e., intermediate) insertion. In fact, a significant occlusion effect is observed only at 250 Hz. Second, the advantage of a greatly reduced occlusion effect for the E-A-R foam plug is lost when a partial or shallow insertion is used. Third, partial insertion of an E-A-R foam plug yields occlusion effects that are similar to those achieved with the conventional air-conduction transducer (i.e., TDH-50 earphone encased in MX-41/AR cushion).

Different theories have been proposed to explain the reduced occlusion effect as an insert device occupies a greater volume of the ear canal (Berger & Kerivan, 1983; Tonndorf, 1972).

1. The "tuning" or resonance of the entrapped air within the ear canal is shifted to higher frequencies as the occlusion occurs more deeply (i.e., the unoccluded ear canal becomes progressively shorter). Consequently, there is reduced responsiveness in the lower frequencies at which the occlusion effect is demonstrated (Tonndorf, 1972).

2. The surface area of the ear canal is reduced as an occlusion occurs more deeply. Because less of the canal wall is exposed, there is less sound energy radiated into the canal (Tonndorf, 1972).

TABLE 8–3   Mean occlusion effects in dB (and standard deviations) for six normal-hearing subjects using four occluding devices: E-A-R Plug with deep, standard, and partial insertions and TDH-50 earphone encased in MX-41/AR supra-aural cushion. The approximate occluded volume (in cc) for each device is also reported.

Device	Approximate occluded volume (in cc)	250	500	1000	2000
E-A-R Plug, deep insertion	0.2	3.4 (4.3)	–5.1 (4.6)	0.3 (2.9)	0.3 (3.9)
E-A-R Plug, standard insertion	0.5	6.9 (4.3)	–0.7 (7.1)	0.9 (3.0)	–1.1 (2.4)
E-A-R Plug, partial insertion	0.8	21.2 (4.9)	15.5 (5.3)	9.9 (6.1)	–1.6 (5.1)
TDH-50, MX-41/AR	6.0	20.3 (7.2)	21.6 (6.3)	7.5 (3.0)	–1.3 (5.1)

Occlusion Effect (in dB), Frequency in Hz.

From "Comparison of the noise attenuation of three audiometric earphones, with additional data on masking new threshold," by E.H. Berger and M.C. Killion, 1989. *Journal of the Aconstical Society of America, 86,* 84, 89, 1989. Reprinted with permission.

3. Because the medial portion of the ear canal is osseous, it may be stiffer than the lateral portion, which is cartilaginous. As an occlusion occurs more deeply, the exposed ear canal that is osseous may radiate less low-frequency sound than the covered, cartilaginous portion (Berger & Kerivan, 1983).

4. The stiffness of the entrapped air within the ear canal increases as the occlusion occurs more deeply. The tympanic membrane eventually becomes "immobilized," consequently impairing sound transmission through the middle ear (Tonndorf, 1972).

5. When the ear canal is occluded more deeply, a reduced length of the ear canal is unsupported. A more rigid structure may be more difficult to set into vibration (Berger & Kerivan, 1983).

Although the occlusion effect is negligible when using the E-A-R foam plug with either the ER-3A and E-A-RTONE 3A insert earphones with either deep or intermediate insertion, a small correction factor typically will need to be added to M_{min} at 250 Hz. Recall from Chapter 5 that there are two approaches to correcting for the occlusion effect: The clinician can use either *average* or *individual* occlusion effect values. Unfortunately, there is very limited research available on the occlusion effect produced by the E-A-R foam plug. Based on the average occlusion effects reported in the research conducted by Berger and Kerivan (1983), the following values are recommended for clinical use: 10 dB at 250 Hz and 0 dB at frequencies of 500 Hz and higher. It is important to remember that these corrections are appropriate *only when using E-A-R foam plugs with either intermediate or deep insertion.*

It should be noted that the depth of the foam earplug's insertion is related to both interaural attenuation and the occlusion effect. Limited empirical data suggest that interaural attenuation is similar for either intermediate or deep insertion of the foam plug; a shallow insertion significantly decreases interaural attenuation (Killion et al., 1985; Sklare & Denenberg, 1987; Van Campen et al., 1990). Similarly, the magnitude of the occlusion effect is equivalent for both intermediate and deep insertions of the foam plug (Berger & Kerivan, 1983). A shallowly inserted foam plug, however, will increase the occlusion effect and decrease interaural attenuation. Although a deeply inserted foam plug is desirable, there is limited evidence to suggest that an intermediate insertion will prove clinically acceptable in most instances.

Consider again the audiogram presented in Figure 8-5B. We already have decided that masked bone-conduction thresholds are required at all frequencies when testing the left ear: Unmasked bone-conduction thresholds suggest potential air-bone gaps of 15 dB or greater. Calculate M_{min} using the following equation:

$$M_{min} = AC_{NT} + OE + 10\ dB\ (safety\ factor)$$

250 Hz	$M_{min} = 5\ dB\ HL + 10\ dB + 10\ dB = 25\ dB\ EM$
500 Hz	$M_{min} = 5\ dB\ HL + 0\ dB + 10\ dB = 15\ dB\ EM$
1000 Hz	$M_{min} = 10\ dB\ HL + 0\ dB + 10\ dB = 20\ dB\ EM$
2000 Hz	$M_{min} = 5\ dB\ HL + 0\ dB + 10\ dB = 15\ dB\ EM$
4000 Hz	$M_{min} = 5\ dB\ HL + 0\ dB + 10\ dB = 15\ dB\ EM$

Rather than using average occlusion effect values, the audiologist also can use individually measured occlusion effects when determining required masking levels (Martin et al., 1974). Remember that the occlusion effect is added to M_{min} only when there is no evidence of a significant conductive component in the nontest (i.e., masked) ear.

Although M_{max} is calculated in the same way when using an insert earphone, remember that theoretically the estimated value should be greater because of increased interaural attenuation. We again will use the estimated interaural attenuation values of 65 dB at 2000 Hz and 60 dB at 4000 Hz when calculating M_{max} (i.e., unmasked air-conduction threshold in the left ear minus unmasked bone-conduction threshold). Standard interaural attenuation values of 75 dB are used at 1000 HZ and below.

$$M_{max} = B_T + IA - 5 \text{ dB}$$

250 Hz	M_{max} = 5 dB HL + 75 dB − 5 dB = 75 dB EM
500 Hz	M_{max} = 5 dB HL + 75 dB − 5 dB = 75 dB EM
1000 Hz	M_{max} = 5 dB HL + 75 dB − 5 dB = 75 dB EM
2000 Hz	M_{max} = 5 dB HL + 65 dB − 5 dB = 65 dB EM
4000 Hz	M_{max} = 5 dB HL + 60 dB − 5 dB = 60 dB EM

Because we used the unmasked bone-conduction thresholds as estimates of BC_T, our estimates of M_{max} are very conservative. In fact, M_{max} is very likely greater than the values estimated using unmasked bone-conduction thresholds. The maximum conductive hearing loss is approximately 60 dB. Because the potential air-bone gaps exceed 60 dB in the left ear, it is probable that the unmasked bone-conduction thresholds reflect hearing in the right ear. If there is a sensorineural hearing loss in the left ear, the actual values of M_{max} will be greatly increased. Recall from our discussion in Chapter 5 that estimates of M_{max} are typically very conservative. These estimates simply alert the audiologist to the possibility of overmasking *if the unmasked bone-conduction thresholds reflect hearing in the test ear*.

Speech Audiometry

When to Mask

Recall from Chapter 4 that contralateral masking is indicated during speech audiometry whenever the presentation level of the signal at the test ear (Presentation level$_T$) equals or exceeds the best pure-tone bone-conduction threshold (from 250 to 4000 Hz) in the nontest ear (Best BC_{NT}) by the amount of interaural attenuation (IA):

$$\text{Presentation level}_T - IA \geq \text{Best } BC_{NT}$$

Unfortunately, there is only limited data available about interaural attenuation for speech using insert earphones. Sklare and Denenberg (1987) reported interaural attenuation for speech (i.e., SRT using spondaic words) in seven adult subjects with unilateral, profound sensorineural hearing loss using Etymotic Research 3A insert earphones with foam plugs. Interaural attenuation values ranged from 68 to 84 dB. Remember that a single value defining the lower limit of interaural attenuation will be most useful when making a decision about the need for contralateral masking (Studebaker, 1967a). A conservative estimate of interaural attenuation for spondees using 3A insert earphones, therefore, is 68 dB. It should be noted that the smallest reported value of interaural attenuation for spondaic words is exactly 20 dB greater when using 3A insert earphones with foam plugs (i.e., IA = 68 dB) than when using traditional supra-aural earphones (i.e., IA = 48 dB). This will make it very convenient to modify our rules for when to mask during speech audiometry using the traditional supra-aural earphones that were first discussed in Chapter 4: We only need to apply a 20-dB correction factor.

Recall from Chapter 4 that there are two basic approaches to making a decision about the need for contralateral masking during speech audiometry using supra-aural earphones:

1. The use of a single interaural attenuation value (i.e., IA = 40 dB) for *all* threshold and suprathreshold speech measurements;

2. The use of different interaural attenuation values for each test of the speech audiometric test battery (i.e., IA = 45 dB for SRT, IA = 35 dB for SDT and suprathreshold speech recognition).

Regardless of the selected approach, it is necessary to add a correction factor of 20 dB to the interaural attenuation value used with supra-aural earphones. That is, the audiologist can use either a single value of interaural attenuation (i.e., IA = 60 dB) for all speech audiometric measurements or different interaural attenuation values for each component of the test battery (i.e., IA = 65 dB for SRT, IA = 55 dB for SDT and suprathreshold speech recognition). The rules for when to mask during speech audiometry using 3A insert earphones are summarized as follows:

$$\text{Presentation level}_T - \text{IA} \geq \text{Best BC}_{NT}$$

or

$$\text{Presentation level}_T - \text{Best BC}_{NT} \geq \text{IA}$$

where interaural attenuation values for speech are equal to

65 dB	Speech recognition threshold
55 dB	Speech detection threshold
55 dB	Suprathreshold speech recognition

or

60 dB	All speech audiometric measurements

Consider the audiogram presented in Figure 8-6. Pure-tone testing reveals normal hearing in the left ear and a moderate, sensorineural hearing loss of flat configuration in the right ear. In this example, we will use the same value of interaural attenuation (i.e., 60 dB) when making a decision about the need for contralateral masking during speech audiometry.

Unmasked speech recognition thresholds of 55 dB HL and 10 dB HL were measured for the right and left ears respectively.

Contralateral ear masking is not required when obtaining the SRT in either ear:

$$\text{Presentation level}_T - \text{IA} \geq \text{Best BC}_{NT}$$

Right Ear	55 dB HL − 60 dB ≥ 5 dB HL?	
	−5 dB HL ≥ 5 dB HL?	*No*
Left Ear	10 dB HL − 60 dB ≥ 45 dB HL?	
	−50 dB HL ≥ 45 dB HL?	*No*

FIGURE 8–6 Audiogram presenting normal hearing in the left ear and a moderate, sensorineural hearing loss of flat configuration in the right ear. Contralateral masking is not required when obtaining the SRT in either ear: The obtained SRT does not equal or exceed the best bone-conduction threshold in the nontest ear by the amount of interaural attenuation (i.e., 60 dB). Contralateral masking will be required, however, when measuring suprathreshold speech recognition ability at 40 dB SL in the right ear: The presentation level (i.e., 95 dB HL) exceeds the best bone-conduction threshold in the nontest ear (i.e., 5 dB HL) by the amount of interaural attenuation (i.e., 60 dB).

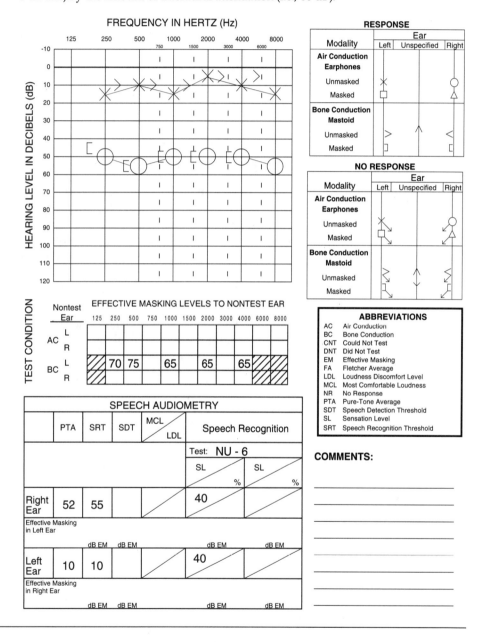

Contralateral masking will be required, however, when measuring suprathreshold speech recognition ability using NU-6. A sensation level of 40 dB will be used in both ears.

$$\text{Presentation level}_T - IA \geq \text{Best BC}_{NT}$$

Right Ear	95 dB HL − 60 dB ≥ 5 dB HL?	
	35 dB HL ≥ 5 dB HL?	*Yes*
Left Ear	50 dB HL − 60 dB ≥ 45 dB HL?	
	−10 dB HL ≥ 45 dB HL?	*No*

Because of the high presentation level (i.e., 95 dB HL) and the good bone-conduction sensitivity in the nontest ear (i.e., best bone-conduction threshold = 5 dB HL), contralateral masking is required when measuring speech recognition ability in the right ear.

Selection of Appropriate Masking Levels

Recall from our discussion in Chapter 6 the formulas for determining minimum (M_{min}) and maximum (M_{max}) masking levels during speech audiometry:

$$M_{min} = \text{Presentation level}_T - IA + \text{Max AB Gap}_{NT}$$
$$M_{max} = \text{Best BC}_T + IA - 5 \text{ dB}$$

The selection of appropriate masking levels involves the same set of formulas regardless of the type of air-conduction transducer used (i.e., supra-aural versus insert). The only modification needed is the use of a greater value of interaural attenuation when calculating minimum and maximum masking levels.

Refer again to the audiogram presented in Figure 8-6. We already have decided that contralateral masking is not needed when measuring speech recognition thresholds in either ear. However, masking is required when assessing suprathreshold speech recognition ability in the right ear. Remember that for this example we are using a single interaural attenuation value of 60 dB. M_{min} and M_{max} are calculated as follows:

$$M_{min} = \text{Presentation level}_T - IA + \text{Max AB Gap}_{NT}$$
$$= 95 \text{ dB HL} - 60 \text{ dB} + 5 \text{ dB (at 250, 1000, 4000 Hz)}$$
$$= 40 \text{ dB EM}$$
$$M_{max} = \text{Best BC}_T + IA - 5 \text{ dB}$$
$$= 45 \text{ dB (at 250 Hz)} + 60 \text{ dB} - 5 \text{ dB}$$
$$= 100 \text{ dB EM}$$

Recall that an optimal masking level during speech audiometry is one that falls above M_{min} yet below M_{max}. Specifically, we want to select a masker level that occurs at the middle of the range (i.e., midplateau). The mid-masking level is calculated as follows:

$$M_{mid} = (M_{max} + M_{min}) / 2$$
$$= (100 + 40) / 2$$
$$= 70 \text{ dB EM}$$

It is important to note that the selected masking level is not required to be *exactly* at midplateau. In this particular example, the width of the masking plateau is very wide because of increased interaural attenuation. Thus, we have some flexibility when selecting the masking level. Ideally, there are two goals when selecting masking levels during speech audiometry. First, the masking level should be at least 10 dB above M_{min} to account for intersubject variability of masker effectiveness. Second, the masking level should fall in the "vicinity" of midplateau. In the above example, we could use a masker level as low as 55 to 60 dB EM and still meet our two goals of masker selection.

Recall from Chapter 6 that a short-cut approach for selecting an appropriate level of masking during suprathreshold speech audiometry can be used *provided that the following two conditions are met*: (1) There are no *significant* air-bone gaps in either ear; (2) suprathreshold speech recognition is evaluated at a *moderate* sensation level (i.e., approximately 40 dB SL). Given these two prerequisites, the selected masking level typically will occur approximately at midplateau. Stated simply, effective masking level is equal to the presentation level of the speech signal at the test ear (PL_T) minus 20 dB:

$$dB\ EM = PL_T - 20\ dB$$

This short-cut procedure can also be applied equally effectively when using insert earphones, assuming that the same two underlying conditions are met. Remember that a major advantage of any procedure based on the principles of the midplateau is that interaural attenuation is eliminated as a source of error when selecting an appropriate masking level. Interaural attenuation for speech differs for supra-aural and insert earphones (e.g., values of approximately 40 dB and 60 dB, respectively). Yet, a midplateau-based procedure (including the "short-cut" approach) will always result in the selection of an appropriate masking level, regardless of the value of interaural attenuation used. Although interaural attenuation affects the width of the masking plateau, the mid-masking level remains unaffected.

It is important to remember that the use of the short-cut approach is not recommended when assessing suprathreshold speech recognition at higher sensation levels (i.e., greater than approximately 50 dB SL). First, the disparity between mid-masking level and the value calculated using the short-cut procedure progressively increases with increasing sensation level (above approximately 40 dB SL). Second, the probability of overmasking increases at high sensation levels. The mid-masking level procedure is preferred in such cases.

Insert Earphones: A Solution to the Masking Dilemma?

The masking dilemma was discussed at length in Chapter 5. Recall that the classic example of the masking dilemma is demonstrated when assessing air- and bone-conduction thresholds in individuals with bilateral conductive hearing loss that exceeds approximately 40 dB. Specifically, a situation can result in which the initial minimum masking level equals or exceeds the maximum masking level. When overmasking occurs, the consequence is *measured* thresholds that are poorer than the *true* thresholds. The use of 3A insert earphones can solve many masking dilemmas.

Consider the examples presented in Figure 8-7. This is a patient with a mild-to-moderate, conductive hearing loss bilaterally. The unmasked pure-tone

FIGURE 8–7   Audiogram presenting a mild-to-moderate, conductive hearing loss bilaterally. The unmasked pure-tone audiogram, obtained with 3A insert earphones, is presented in Figure 8-7A; the masked audiogram is presented in Figure 8-7B. The use of insert earphones has eliminated the need for contralateral masking during air-conduction threshold audiometry.

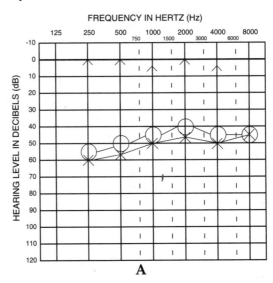

A

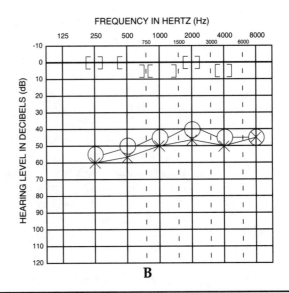

B

audiogram, obtained with 3A insert receivers, is presented in Figure 8-7A . The "true" or correct audiogram is presented in Figure 8-7B. The use of insert earphones has eliminated the need for contralateral masking during air-conduction audiometry in both ears: Unmasked air-conduction thresholds do not equal or exceed the unmasked bone-conduction thresholds at any frequency by the amount of interaural attenuation (i.e., 75 dB at frequencies ≤ 1000, 50 dB at frequencies > 1000 Hz). If traditional supra-aural earphones had been used to measure air-conduction thresholds, contralateral masking would have been required *at all frequencies in both ears*: Unmasked air-conduction thresholds would equal or exceed the unmasked bone-conduction thresholds by the amount of interaural attenuation (i.e., 40 dB). There would be a high probability of overmasking because of the severity of the air-conduction thresholds and the normal bone-conduction thresholds: Initial masking levels would be increased while maximum masking levels would be decreased. We have avoided a masking dilemma during air-conduction audiometry in this example by using 3A insert earphones. Specifically, we have eliminated the need for masking in a situation in which the risk of overmasking is high.

Figure 8-8 illustrates an example in which a masking dilemma is avoided

FIGURE 8–8   Audiogram presenting a mild, conductive hearing loss bilaterally. The unmasked pure-tone audiogram is presented in Figure 8-8*A*; the masked audiogram is presented in Figure 8-8*B*. Although masked bone-conduction thresholds are needed at all frequencies in both ears, the risk of overmasking will be significantly reduced or eliminated with the use of insert earphones for presentation of contralateral masking.

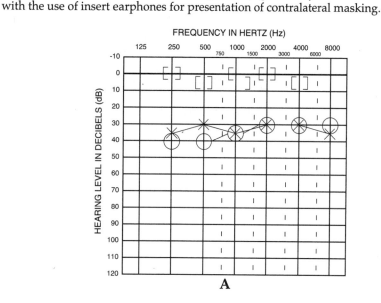

A

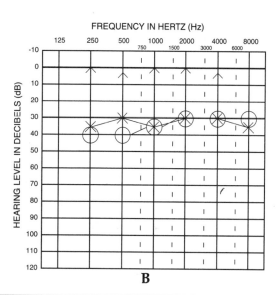

B

during bone-conduction audiometry. This patient exhibits a mild, conductive hearing loss bilaterally. The unmasked pure-tone audiogram, obtained with 3A insert receivers, is presented in Figure 8-8*A*. The "true" or correct audiogram is presented in Figure 8-8*B*. As in our previous example, contralateral masking is not indicated when measuring air-conduction thresholds in either ear: Unmasked air-conduction thresholds do not equal or exceed the unmasked bone-conduction thresholds at any frequency by the amount of interaural attenuation. However, masked bone-conduction thresholds are needed at all frequencies in both ears: Comparison of unmasked bone-conduction thresholds with air-conduction thresholds suggests the presence of significant air-bone gaps (i.e., ≥ 15 dB). The risk of overmasking will be significantly reduced or eliminated, however, with the use of insert earphones for presentation of contralateral masking. Although initial masking level (i.e., $AC_{NT} + OE + 10$ dB) is the same for either type of air-conduction transducer in this example, the maximum masking level will be greatly increased for the 3A insert earphone because of increased interaural attenuation, particularly in the lower frequencies.

Consider the required masking levels when measuring a masked bone-conduction threshold at 250 Hz in the right ear: Contralateral masking will be presented to the left ear through either a supra-aural or insert earphone. Because of the significant air-bone gap of 35 dB in the nontest ear (i.e., masked ear), we do not need to correct for the occlusion effect (OE) when determining initial minimum masking level:

$$M_{min} = AC_{NT} + OE + 10 \text{ dB}$$
$$= 35 \text{ dB HL} + 10 \text{ dB}$$
$$= 45 \text{ dB EM}$$

Although M_{min} is the same when using either air-conduction transducer for the delivery of contralateral masking, significant differences will be observed in the estimates of M_{max}:

$$M_{max} = BC_T + IA - 5 \text{ dB}$$

Supra-aural Earphone	0 dB HL + 40 dB – 5 dB = 35 dB EM
Insert Earphone	0 dB HL + 75 dB – 5 dB = 70 dB EM

It should be apparent that overmasking is a possibility when using the supra-aural earphone: M_{min} (i.e., 45 dB EM) exceeds M_{max} (i.e., 35 dB EM). However, the risk of overmasking is greatly reduced when using the insert earphone because of increased interaural attenuation: M_{max} now *exceeds* M_{min} by 25 dB. Consequently, there is greater probability that a masking plateau can be measured and that the correct bone-conduction threshold will be obtained.

Unfortunately, there is only slightly greater interaural attenuation (i.e., 10 dB) for insert earphones when compared to supra-aural earphones in the higher frequencies (i.e., 2000 and 4000 Hz). Consequently, there is increased probability of overmasking in the higher frequencies when using insert earphones. Refer again to the audiograms presented in Figure 8-8. Consider the required masking levels when measuring a masked bone-conduction threshold at 2000 Hz in the right ear: Contralateral masking will be presented to the left ear through either a supra-aural or insert earphone. Because there is no occlusion effect at 2000 Hz, we can eliminate this component when calculating M_{min}:

$$M_{Min} = AC_{NT} + OE + 10 \text{ dB}$$
$$= 30 \text{ dB HL} + 10 \text{ dB}$$
$$= 40 \text{ dB EM}$$

Because interaural attenuation is very similar for insert and supra-aural earphones in the high frequencies, our estimates of M_{max} will be very similar:

$$M_{max} = BC_T + IA - 5 \text{ dB}$$

Supra-aural Earphone	0 dB HL + 40 dB – 5 dB = 35 dB EM
Insert Earphone	0 dB HL + 50 dB – 5 dB = 45 dB EM

It should be noted that there is only a slight advantage to the use of insert earphones when measuring masked bone-conduction thresholds in the high frequencies. Depending on individual interaural attenuation (which can be considerably greater than the conservative estimates used clinically), overmasking can result when using either type of air-conduction transducer.

It is important to remember that although the use of insert earphones can reduce or eliminate the risk of overmasking, they will not solve *all* masking dilemmas (Hosford-Dunn et al., 1986). There is a higher probability of overmasking whenever there is maximum conductive hearing impairment (i.e., 60 dB), even when using insert earphones: The greater degree of air-conduction hearing loss will require higher levels of masking.

In summary, the use of 3A insert earphones can solve *many* audiometric masking dilemmas. First, the increased interaural attenuation often eliminates the need for contralateral masking during air-conduction audiometry in individuals with bilateral conductive hearing impairment. Second, the increased interaural attenuation (particularly in the lower frequencies) increases the maximum masking level, thereby reducing the risk of overmasking.

Calibration of Effective Masking Level

Recall from Chapter 2 that narrow-band noise and speech spectrum noise are the maskers of choice during pure-tone and speech audiometry, respectively. The calibration of effective masking level is very straightforward whether the 3A insert earphone is used as the primary transducer or as a plug-in substitute for the standard supra-aural earphone.

Insert Earphone as Primary Transducer

When the 3A insert earphone is used as the primary transducer, calibration is performed according to guidelines outlined in the current American National Standard specification for audiometers (ANSI S3.6-1989). If the spectral density of the narrow-band noise meets the specified band limits, *and* the sound pressure level in each one-third octave band centered at each frequency is calibrated to a level 3 dB above the reference equivalent threshold level at the test frequency, then masking level for pure tones is calibrated in dB EM. For example, the interim standard reference equivalent threshold sound pressure level at 250 Hz for the 3A insert earphone (calibrated using a standard 2-cc HA-1 coupler) is 15.5 dB. Consequently, if the narrow-band noise is calibrated to 18.5 dB

SPL (i.e., reference level of 15.5 dB SPL plus 3 dB), then the masker level is specified in dB EM (i.e., 0 dB EM).

Similarly, if the speech spectrum noise has spectral density characteristics as specified by ANSI S3.6-1989 *and* if the sound pressure level is calibrated to the standard reference sound pressure level for speech (i.e., 12.5 dB above the 1000 Hz standard reference sound pressure level threshold), then the masker level for speech will be calibrated in dB EM (Wilber, personal communication, 1992). For example, the interim standard reference equivalent threshold sound pressure level at 1000 Hz for the 3A insert earphone is 3.5 dB (calibrated using the HA-1 coupler). Therefore, the standard reference sound pressure level for speech is specified as 16 dB SPL (i.e., reference level of 3.5 dB SPL at 1000 Hz plus 12.5 dB). If the speech spectrum noise of ANSI-specified spectral density characteristics is calibrated to 16 dB SPL, then the masker level for the 3A insert earphone is specified in dB EM (i.e., 0 dB EM).

Insert Earphone as Plug-in Substitute

When the 3A insert is used as a plug-in substitute for the standard supra-aural earphone, only minor corrections will be required. In fact, we can use the same plug-in correction factors recommended by the manufacturer when correcting for *nominal* versus *actual* dB HL. Table 8-1 presented the plug-in correction factors (in dB) that should be added to the audiometer dial setting (i.e., *nominal dB HL*) to determine the correct or *actual dB HL* presented to the patient. During clinical masking procedures, however, a reverse correction process will be required. Specifically, we initially determine the *desired* (or actual) *dB EM*; a correction factor subsequently is applied to the desired dB EM to determine the *nominal* dB EM (i.e., the dial setting) required. Consequently, the same numerical plug-in correction factors can be used to determine the required dB EM dial setting. However, the correction factors are applied in the opposite direction. The following two hypothetical examples will help illustrate the use of plug-in correction factors during clinical masking procedures.

Example 1: It has been decided that contralateral masking will be required when assessing hearing sensitivity at 1000 Hz; the initial masking level is determined to be 30 dB EM. Because there is a 0 dB correction at 1000 Hz for dB HL (see Table 8-1), no correction factor needs to be applied when determining the nominal dB EM dial setting. Consequently, a dial setting of 30 dB EM will result in the desired effective masking level of 30 dB EM.

Example 2: It has been decided that contralateral masking will be required when assessing hearing sensitivity at 6000 Hz; initial masking level is determined to be 50 dB EM. Because there is a 10-dB correction factor at 6000 Hz for dB HL (see Table 8-1), a correction factor also needs to be applied when determining the nominal dB EM dial setting. Recall that during clinical masking procedures, we will need to apply a reverse correction process. While 10 dB is subtracted from the nominal dB HL dial setting to achieve the actual dB HL, it will be necessary to add a correction factor of 10 dB to the desired dB EM to determine the required dB EM dial setting on the audiometer. Consequently, if the desired effective masking is 50 dB EM, then 10 dB must be added to the dB EM dial setting. A dial setting of 60 dB EM will result in the desired effective masking of 50 dB EM (i.e., the desired effective masking of 50 dB EM + 10 dB correction factor = nominal dial setting of 60 dB EM).

It may be confusing in a clinical setting to apply the same plug-in correction factors differently for dB HL and dB EM dial settings: The use of separate correction tables may prove more efficient. Table 8-4 lists plug-in correction factors for dB EM dial settings. It should be noted that this table is identical to the correction factors for dB HL listed in Table 8-1, with the exception that the correction factors are applied in opposite directions.

Although correction factors are needed during masked pure-tone audiometry, a correction factor applied to effective masking levels should not be required during speech audiometry. Remember that the effective masking level for speech is specified relative to the standard reference sound pressure level of a 1000-Hz pure tone signal. Because there is no standard plug-in correction factor for dB HL at 1000 Hz (see Table 8-1), there should be no need to apply a correction factor for effective masking when using the 3A insert earphone as a plug-in substitute during speech audiometry. If the effective masking level for speech was calibrated using the standard supra-aural earphone, then the 3A insert earphone can be used as a plug-in substitute without the application of a correction factor.

As discussed earlier in this chapter, *verification of the appropriateness of the standard correction factors is recommended each time that the audiometer is calibrated* if the audiologist is using the Tubephone insert earphone as a plug-in substitute for the supra-aural earphone. The same calibration procedure recommended by the manufacturer of the E-A-RTONE 3A insert earphone (Cabot Safety Corporation, Auditory Systems Divisions, 1990) for determining *individual correction factors* can be used for either dB HL and dB EM. Specifically, the difference between the actual (i.e., measured) and the target sound pressure levels for effective masking at each frequency determines the appropriate correction factors for your 3A insert earphone.

Although a correction factor should not be required during speech audiometry, the cautious audiologist can easily verify the speech spectrum noise calibration of the insert earphone using the real ear method (see Chapter 2). When the audiometer is newly calibrated with the standard supra-aural earphones, measure the masked SRT at a fixed masker level for both the supra-aural and insert (i.e., plug-in substitute) earphones using ten to twelve normal-hearing subjects. For example, if the speech spectrum noise is fixed at a dial setting of 50 dB EM, the median masked SRT for both the supra-aural and insert earphones

TABLE 8–4   Plug-in correction factors for effective masking level (dB EM) when using the Etymotic Research ER-3A and E-A-RTONE™ 3A insert earphones as a complement to the Telephonics TDH-39, 49, or 50 earphones or the Telex 1470A earphone.

Transducer	Frequency (in Hz)										
	125	250	500	750	1000	1500	2000	3000	4000	6000	8000
TDH-39, 49, 50	–15	–5	0	5	0	0	0	0	0	10	10
1470A	–15	–5	0	5	0	0	0	5	0	10	15

Decibel (dB) value to be added to the desired dB EM to determine the dB EM dial setting.

Adapted from *Instructions for Use of E-A-RTONE™ 3A Insert Earphones* by Cabot Safety Corporation, Auditory Systems Division, 1990, Indianapolis, Indiana and *ER-3A Tubephone™ Insert Earphone*, Etymotic Research, 1991, Elk Grove Village, Illinois.

should be 50 dB HL. If there is a difference between the two masked speech thresholds, a correction factor will be required to calibrate the effective masking level for speech when using the insert earphone.

Summary

Insert earphones are sometimes substituted for the standard supra-aural configuration during audiometric testing. The Tubephone (ER-3A or E-A-RTONE 3A) currently is the most commonly used clinical audiometric insert earphone (Killion & Villchur, 1989) and has been researched extensively since its development by Etymotic Research in the 1980s. There is considerable empirical evidence suggesting that Tubephone insert earphones offer a valid alternative in many audiometric applications because they solve several of the problems associated with conventional supra-aural earphones. A major advantage of the 3A insert earphone when compared to the conventional supra-aural earphone is *increased interaural attenuation* for air-conducted sound, particularly in the lower frequencies.

The use of an earphone that yields increased interaural attenuation for air-conducted sound provides two major advantages. First, the need for contralateral masking is significantly reduced during air-conduction audiometry. Second, the range between the minimum and maximum masking levels is increased, thereby increasing the width of the masking plateau and the range of permissible masking levels during both air- and bone-conduction audiometry.

Three factors must be considered when making a decision about the need for masking during pure-tone air-conduction testing:

1. Unmasked air-conduction threshold in the test ear (AC_T)
2. Interaural attenuation (IA)
3. Bone-conduction hearing sensitivity in the nontest ear (BC_{NT})

The same rules can be employed when using the 3A insert earphones; the only modification required is the use of a larger value of interaural attenuation than 40 dB, which was appropriate when using the standard supra-aural earphone. Based on currently available data, conservative estimates of interaural attenuation for the 3A insert earphone are 75 dB at 1000 Hz and below and 50 dB at frequencies above 1000 Hz. The rules for when to mask during pure-tone air-conduction audiometry using 3A insert earphones can be restated as follows:

$$AC_T - BC_{NT} \text{ or } AC_{NT} \geq IA$$

or

$$AC_T - IA \geq BC_{NT} \text{ or } AC_{NT}$$

where interaural attenuation is equal to

75 dB at frequencies ≤ 1000 Hz

50 dB at frequencies > 1000 Hz

The recommended interaural attenuation values are appropriate when *deeply inserted* (or at least *intermediately inserted*) foam eartips are used. A decision about when to mask during bone-conduction audiometry is not affected by the transducer type used to deliver contralateral masking.

Regardless of the transducer type used to deliver the contralateral masking, the initial minimum masking level (M_{min}) during air-conduction audiometry is equal to the air-conduction threshold of the nontest ear. No modification is required when using an insert earphone:

$$M_{min} = AC_{NT} + 10 \text{ dB safety factor}$$

Recall that calculation of M_{min} during bone-conduction audiometry includes a correction factor for the occlusion effect (OE) in the low frequencies:

$$M_{min} = AC_{NT} + OE + 10 \text{ dB safety factor}$$

There is evidence, however, suggesting that the occlusion effect is negligible when using intermediately or deeply inserted insert earphones. The clinician can use either *average* or *individual* values when correcting for the occlusion effect. Based on the average occlusion effects reported in the research literature, the following values are recommended for clinical use: 10 dB at 250 Hz and 0 dB at frequencies of 500 Hz and higher.

Although M_{max} is calculated in the same way during masked air- and bone-conduction audiometry when using an 3A insert earphone, the estimated value will be greater because of increased interaural attenuation:

$$M_{max} = B_T + IA - 5 \text{ dB}$$

where interaural attenuation is equal to

75 dB at frequencies ≤ 1000 Hz

50 dB at frequencies > 1000 Hz

Contralateral masking is required during speech audiometry whenever the presentation level of the signal at the test ear (Presentation level $_T$) equals or exceeds the best pure-tone bone-conduction threshold (from 250 to 4000 Hz) in the nontest ear (Best BC_{NT}) by the amount of interaural attenuation (IA):

$$\text{Presentation level}_T - IA \geq \text{Best } BC_{NT}$$

When using 3A insert earphones, we can use a greater value of interaural attenuation for speech. It is necessary to add a correction factor of 20 dB to the interaural attenuation values used with supra-aural earphones. The audiologist can use either a single value of interaural attenuation (i.e., IA = 60 dB) for all speech audiometric measurements or different values for each component of the test battery (i.e., IA = 65 dB for SRT, IA = 55 dB for SDT and suprathreshold speech recognition). The rules for when to mask during speech audiometry using 3A insert earphones can be summarized as follows:

$$\text{Presentation level}_T - IA \geq \text{Best } BC_{NT}$$
or
$$\text{Presentation level}_T - \text{Best } BC_{NT} \geq IA$$

where interaural attenuation values for speech are equal to

65 dB	Speech recognition threshold
55 dB	Speech detection threshold
55 dB	Suprathreshold speech recognition

or

| 60 dB | All speech audiometric measurements |

The formulas for determining minimum (M_{min}) and maximum (M_{max}) masking levels during speech audiometry remain the same when using 3A insert earphones:

$$M_{min} = \text{Presentation level}_T - IA + \text{Max AB gap}_{NT}$$
$$M_{max} = \text{Best BC}_T + IA - 5 \text{ dB}$$

The only modification needed is a greater value of interaural attenuation than that used with supra-aural earphones. The width of the masking plateau will be increased because of increased interaural attenuation.

A masking dilemma can result when assessing air- and bone-conduction thresholds in individuals with bilateral conductive hearing loss that exceeds approximately 40 dB. Although the use of 3A insert earphones can reduce or eliminate the risk of overmasking, they will not solve all masking dilemmas.

When the 3A insert earphone is used as the primary transducer, calibration of the effective masking level is performed according to guidelines outlined in the current standard specification for audiometers. When the 3A insert is used as a plug-in substitute for the standard supra-aural earphone, correction factors should be applied when determining the effective masking levels during pure-tone audiometry. Although correction factors are needed during masked pure-tone audiometry, a correction factor applied to the effective masking levels typically is not required during speech audiometry.

Study Questions

1. There are several limitations of traditional supra-aural earphones. Briefly discuss.

2. Explain why insert earphones result in increased interaural attenuation when compared to conventional supra-aural earphones.

3. The use of a transducer that yields increased interaural attenuation for air-conducted sound is advantageous. Briefly discuss.

4. What are conservative estimates of interaural attenuation for pure-tone stimuli when using 3A insert earphones? State the rule for when to mask during pure-tone air-conduction audiometry using 3A insert earphones with foam plugs.

5. The minimum masking level (M_{min}) during pure-tone air-conduction audiometry is always equal to air-conduction threshold of the nontest ear, regardless of the transducer used to deliver contralateral masking. The maximum masking level (M_{max}) is significantly increased, however, when using 3A insert earphones. Why?

6. There is evidence that the occlusion effect is significantly reduced when using deeply inserted insert earphones. What theories have been proposed to explain the reduced occlusion effect when using insert earphones?

7. Calculation of the minimum masking level during bone-conduction audiometry requires a correction factor for the occlusion effect. Based on currently available data, what values are recommended for clinical use when correcting for the occlusion effect?

8. What interaural attenuation values are recommended during speech audiometry using 3A insert earphones?

9. Although the use of insert earphones can reduce or eliminate the risk of overmasking, they will not solve all masking dilemmas. Briefly discuss.

10. Describe the procedure for calculating the correction factors for the effective masking level when using 3A insert earphones as a plug-in substitute.

Endnotes

1. The MX-41/AR supra-aural earphone cushion has been the standard for audiological testing for several years (ANSI S3.6-1969). The two-piece cushion is composed of a rubber base and a sponge neoprene cap. However, considerable acoustic performance differences have been observed across different MX-41/AR cushions. These differences are attributable to aging characteristics, material compounds, and the effectiveness of the cementing process required for the two-piece construction (Michael & Bienvenue, 1980).

   Approximately fifteen years ago, Telephonics Corporation developed a new supra-aural cushion, Model 51, in an effort to minimize the problems associated with the MX-41/AR. Michael and Bienvenue (1980) reported that the acoustic performance of the Telephonics Model 51 cushion does not differ significantly from the MX-41/AR. In addition, the noise attenuation characteristics provided by the Model 51 and MX-41/AR cushions are generally equivalent (Franks et al., 1992; Michael & Bienvenue, 1981). There also is indication that the one-piece cushion will result in more reliable performance between units and greater long-term stability. The MX-41/AR supra-aural cushion is no longer being manufactured; the Model 51 is now considered the standard supra-aural earphone cushion (Franks et al., 1992). The standard physical dimensions of the MX-41/AR and Model 51 cushion are specified in ANSI S3.6-1989.

2. The Etymotic Research ER-3A insert earphone can be coupled to the ear by two methods. The use of the disposable foam eartip is recommended by the manufacturer. An impedance tip adapter is also provided and can be used with most rubber impedance (or immittance) probe tips (Etymotic Research, 1991). However, the maximum external noise exclusion and interaural attenuation should be achieved with the foam eartip (Hosford-Dunn et al., 1986; Killion, personal communication, 1993).

9
Case Studies

The final chapter of this book presents eight case studies that will facilitate an understanding of clinical masking procedures. Each case study will include a series of audiograms that will take you step by step from the initial audiological results (i.e., *unmasked* air- and bone-conduction audiometry) through the completed audiological evaluation using appropriate contralateral masking (i.e., the final audiogram including interpretation of results from both pure-tone and speech audiometry). In addition, each presentation will provide commentary that emphasizes important concepts in clinical masking.

Although each component of an individual case study can be reviewed sequentially from the initial through the final audiograms, you also can focus on a particular aspect of clinical masking. The following classification system will be used to identify each aspect of the clinical masking process:

A. When to Mask: Pure-Tone Air-Conduction Audiometry

B. How Much Masking: Pure-Tone Air-Conduction Audiometry

C. When to Mask: Pure-Tone Bone-Conduction Audiometry

D. How Much Masking: Pure-Tone Bone-Conduction Audiometry

E. When To Mask: Threshold Speech Audiometry

F. How Much Masking: Threshold Speech Audiometry

G. When to Mask: Suprathreshold Speech Audiometry

H. How Much Masking: Suprathreshold Speech Audiometry

I. Use of Insert Earphones

J. Audiogram Interpretation

For example, if you wish to focus on when to mask during pure-tone bone-conduction audiometry, audiograms for each case study labeled with the alphabetical letter *C* should be reviewed. If you need more experience in deciding how much masking to use during suprathreshold speech audiometry, study the audiograms for each case presentation labeled with the letter *H*, and so on. For your convenience, a directory of case studies has been provided as an appendix at the end of this chapter.

In a survey of current audiologic practices in the United States conducted by Martin and Morris (1989), audiologists were asked to rank audiological tests in the order in which they are typically performed. Although the order of tests is often modified for a particular patient, the order typically followed was:

1. Pure-tone air-conduction audiometry

2. Speech threshold (SRT or SDT)

3. Suprathreshold speech recognition (i.e., speech discrimination)
4. Pure-tone bone-conduction audiometry

This particular order of audiological tests is undoubtedly popular because of its time efficiency. Pure-tone air-conduction audiometry, traditionally conducted first, is followed by speech audiometric tests because all involve the use of the same air-conduction transducer (i.e., earphones). The evaluation is completed by substituting the air-conduction transducer with a bone vibrator and measuring bone-conduction thresholds. A major disadvantage of this typically followed order is that the audiologist has no information about bone-conduction sensitivity. Bone-conduction thresholds can influence not only a correct decision about the need for masking during air-conduction audiometry, but also can contribute to the calculation of appropriate masking levels.

Appropriate decisions about the need for contralateral masking during air-conduction audiometry frequently can be made without information about bone-conduction sensitivity. However, there are some clinical situations in which unmasked bone-conduction thresholds are essential and can alter a preliminary decision about the need for masking based only on air-conduction responses (e.g., the presence of an air-bone gap in the nontest ear). In addition, calculation of appropriate masking levels often requires estimates of bone-conduction sensitivity in both the test and nontest ears, particularly during speech audiometry. Consequently, it is recommended that unmasked bone-conduction thresholds be obtained relatively early in the audiological evaluation.

The following sequence of audiological procedures is recommended for routine clinical use because it results in the greatest clinical efficiency:

1. Unmasked pure-tone bone-conduction thresholds
2. Unmasked pure-tone air-conduction thresholds
3. Masked pure-tone air-conduction thresholds, if required
4. Masked pure-tone bone conduction thresholds, if required
5. Speech recognition thresholds (SRT) using contralateral masking, where required
6. Suprathreshold speech recognition (i.e., "discrimination") using contralateral masking, where required.

Unmasked pure-tone bone conduction audiometry is generally recommended as the first audiometric test. In many situations, it will not be necessary to obtain masked bone-conduction thresholds (Step 4). Consequently, the audiologist can proceed directly from pure-tone air conduction audiometry (Steps 2, 3) to speech audiometry (Steps 5, 6) without the need for changing transducers. Ideally, unmasked air- and bone-conduction threshold audiometry should be the first audiometric tests. It is important to keep in mind, however, that it may be appropriate to modify the recommended order of audiometric tests for a particular case.

Before performing any audiometric testing, a case history and acoustic immittance measurements should be conducted. The case studies that follow include case history information as well as the results of acoustic immittance measurements.[1] These initial tests in the audiological evaluation provide invaluable information on the probable audiologic diagnosis (e.g., conductive versus sensorineural hearing impairment). In fact, preliminary information about gross site of lesion, particularly when conductive involvement is suspected, can help the audiologist develop testing strategies during clinical masking procedures.

Although the case studies that follow will facilitate an understanding of the decision-making processes required for clinical masking, ultimately hands on experience will be required to become proficient with clinical masking procedures. Practice with pure-tone audiometric simulators has proven invaluable when learning the masking plateau procedure. The ultimate test, however, is the ability to apply the concepts of masking in the clinical setting *and* to modify clinical masking procedures where appropriate.

Case 1

History

Your patient is a 21-year-old female college student who was referred to your hearing clinic for routine audiological evaluation. She reports no hearing difficulty and no history of middle ear disorders. Other medical history is negative.

Acoustic Immittance Measurements

	Right Ear	Left Ear
Tympanometry		
Static acoustic immittance (mmho)	1.1	1.2
Tympanometric peak pressure (daPa)	0	−10
Equivalent ear canal volume (mmho)	0.8	0.9
Contralateral Acoustic Reflexes (dB HL)		
500 Hz	85	90
1000 Hz	90	90
2000 Hz	85	85

Tympanometry revealed normal admittance (Van Camp, Margolis, Wilson, Creten, & Shanks, 1986), peak pressure (Silman & Silverman, 1991), and equivalent ear canal volume (Margolis & Heller, 1987) in both ears. Contralateral acoustic reflexes were elicited at hearing levels consistent with normal hearing (Gelfand, Schwander, & Silman, 1990). In summary, the preliminary results of acoustic immittance measurements support the patient's report of normal hearing and negative history of middle ear disorders. *Results do not suggest the presence of significant conductive pathology in either ear.*

Case 1-A

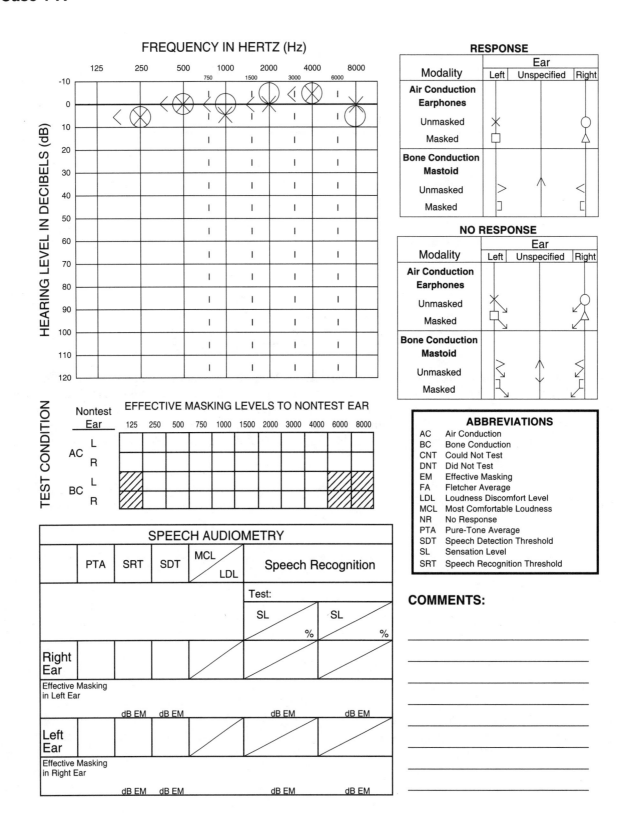

FREQUENCY IN HERTZ (Hz)

HEARING LEVEL IN DECIBELS (dB)

TEST CONDITION

EFFECTIVE MASKING LEVELS TO NONTEST EAR

Nontest Ear

	125	250	500	750	1000	1500	2000	3000	4000	6000	8000
AC L											
AC R											
BC L											
BC R											

SPEECH AUDIOMETRY

	PTA	SRT	SDT	MCL / LDL	Speech Recognition	
					Test:	
					SL %	SL %
Right Ear						
Effective Masking in Left Ear		dB EM	dB EM		dB EM	dB EM
Left Ear						
Effective Masking in Right Ear		dB EM	dB EM		dB EM	dB EM

RESPONSE

Modality	Ear		
	Left	Unspecified	Right
Air Conduction Earphones			
Unmasked	✕		◯
Masked	☐		△
Bone Conduction Mastoid			
Unmasked	>	∧	<
Masked	⊐		⊏

NO RESPONSE

Modality	Ear		
	Left	Unspecified	Right
Air Conduction Earphones			
Unmasked	✕		◯
Masked	☐		△
Bone Conduction Mastoid			
Unmasked	>	∧	<
Masked	⊐	∨	⊏

ABBREVIATIONS

AC	Air Conduction
BC	Bone Conduction
CNT	Could Not Test
DNT	Did Not Test
EM	Effective Masking
FA	Fletcher Average
LDL	Loudness Discomfort Level
MCL	Most Comfortable Loudness
NR	No Response
PTA	Pure-Tone Average
SDT	Speech Detection Threshold
SL	Sensation Level
SRT	Speech Recognition Threshold

COMMENTS:

_____
_____
_____
_____
_____
_____
_____
_____

A. When to Mask: Pure-Tone Air-Conduction Audiometry

Is contralateral masking required when measuring air-conduction thresholds in either ear?

No, contralateral masking is not required when measuring air-conduction thresholds in either ear. Recall our rules for when to mask during pure-tone air-conduction audiometry:

$$AC_T - BC_{NT} \geq IA \quad or \quad AC_T - IA \geq BC_{NT}$$

Measured air-conduction threshold does not exceed or equal bone-conduction threshold in the nontest ear (i.e., unmasked bone-conduction threshold) by the amount of interaural attenuation (IA) (i.e., our conservative estimate of 40 dB). We will use the following equation when making a decision about the need for masking:

$$AC_T - 40\ dB \geq BC_{NT} \qquad\qquad AC_T - 40\ dB \geq BC_{NT}$$

Right Ear (Test Ear)		Masking Needed?	Left Ear (Test Ear)		Masking Needed?
250 Hz	$5 - 40 \geq 5$?	No	250 Hz	$5 - 40 \geq 5$?	No
500 Hz	$0 - 40 \geq 0$?	No	500 Hz	$0 - 40 \geq 0$?	No
1000 Hz	$0 - 40 \geq 0$?	No	1000 Hz	$5 - 40 \geq 0$?	No
2000 Hz	$-5 - 40 \geq 0$?	No	2000 Hz	$0 - 40 \geq -5$?	No
4000 Hz	$-5 - 40 \geq -5$?	No	4000 Hz	$-5 - 40 \geq -5$?	No
8000 Hz	$5 - 40 \geq 5^*$?	No	8000 Hz	$0 - 40 \geq 0^*$?	No

*Estimated bone-conduction threshold

Commentary

1. *This case study illustrates that contralateral masking will never be required during pure-tone air-conduction threshold audiometry whenever there is normal hearing sensitivity bilaterally.* If we assume that interaural attenuation can be as small as 40 dB, then the nontest ear would require bone-conduction hearing sensitivity that is 40 dB better than the air-conduction threshold of the test ear. Consequently, if pure-tone air conduction thresholds are approximately 0 dB HL, then bone-conduction thresholds in the nontest ear would have to be approximately –40 dB HL in order for cross hearing to occur!

2. When testing the left ear at 2000 Hz during assessment of the need for contralateral masking, it should be noted that we used a value of –5 dB HL as our estimate of bone-conduction threshold in the nontest ear (i.e., right ear). The unmasked bone-conduction threshold theoretically can reflect hearing in either ear. However, the unmasked bone-conduction threshold of 0 dB HL is 5 dB *poorer* than the air-conduction threshold of –5 dB HL in the right (i.e., nontest) ear. Although a measured bone-conduction threshold that is poorer than air-conduction threshold is observed clinically, theoretically this should not occur (Studebaker, 1967b). Consequently, a more accurate estimate of bone-conduction threshold of the right ear is the measured air-conduction threshold. *When you are estimating the bone-conduction threshold of the nontest ear, use either the unmasked bone-conduction threshold or the air-conduction threshold of the nontest ear, whichever is better.*

3. When determining the need for contralateral masking at 8000 Hz, we do not have an unmasked bone-conduction threshold to consider. Consequently, it will be necessary to predict a probable bone-conduction threshold for the nontest ear. Unmasked bone-conduction thresholds at other frequencies do not suggest the presence of significant air-bone gaps. Therefore, we can also assume that a significant air-bone gap probably does not exist at 8000 Hz. We can use the air-conduction thresholds in each ear as our estimates of bone-conduction threshold. For example, the air-conduction thresholds of 5 dB HL and 0 dB HL for the right and left ears, respectively, were used as estimates of bone-conduction thresholds at 8000 Hz.

Case 1-C

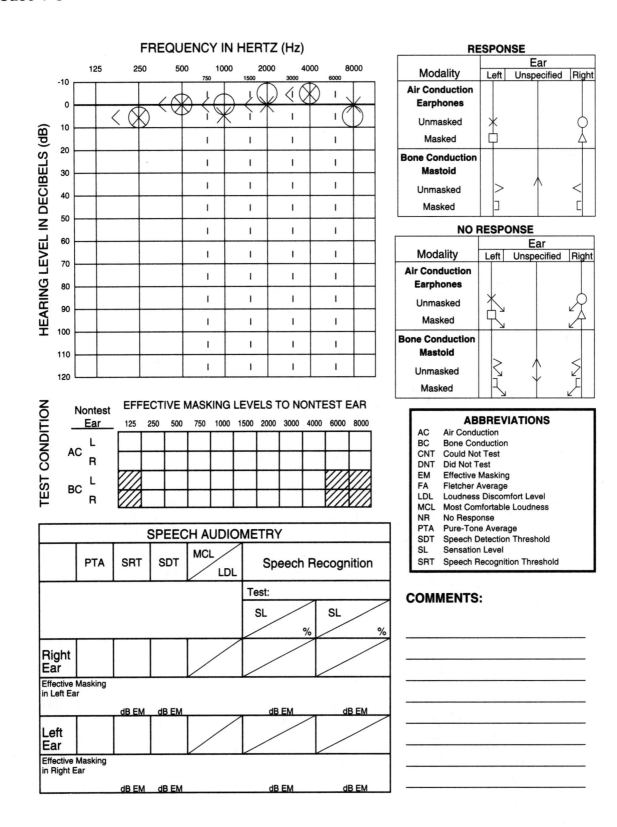

C. When to Mask: Pure-Tone Bone-Conduction Audiometry

Is contralateral masking required when measuring bone-conduction thresholds in either ear?

No, contralateral masking is not required when measuring bone-conduction thresholds in either ear. Recall our rule for when to mask during pure-tone bone conduction audiometry:

$$\text{AB Gap}_T \geq 15 \text{ dB}$$

Contralateral masking is required during bone-conduction audiometry whenever comparison of the unmasked bone-conduction threshold (Unmasked BC) and the air-conduction threshold in the test ear (AC_T) at that frequency reveals a potential air-bone gap (AB Gap_T) of 15 dB or greater.

$$\text{AB Gap}_T \geq 15 \text{ dB?}$$
$$\text{AC}_T - \text{Unmasked BC} \geq 15 \text{ dB?}$$

Right Ear	AB Gap$_T$	AB Gap$_T$ ≥15 dB?
250 Hz	5 – 5 = 0	No
500 Hz	0 – 0 = 0	No
1000 Hz	0 – 0 = 0	No
2000 Hz	–5 – 0 = –5	No
4000 Hz	–5 – 5 = 0	No
Left Ear	**AB Gap$_T$**	**AB Gap$_T$ ≥15 dB?**
250 Hz	5 – 5 = 0	No
500 Hz	0 – 0 = 0	No
1000 Hz	5 – 0 = 5	No
2000 Hz	0 – 0 = 0	No
4000 Hz	–5 – (–5) = 0	No

Case 1-E

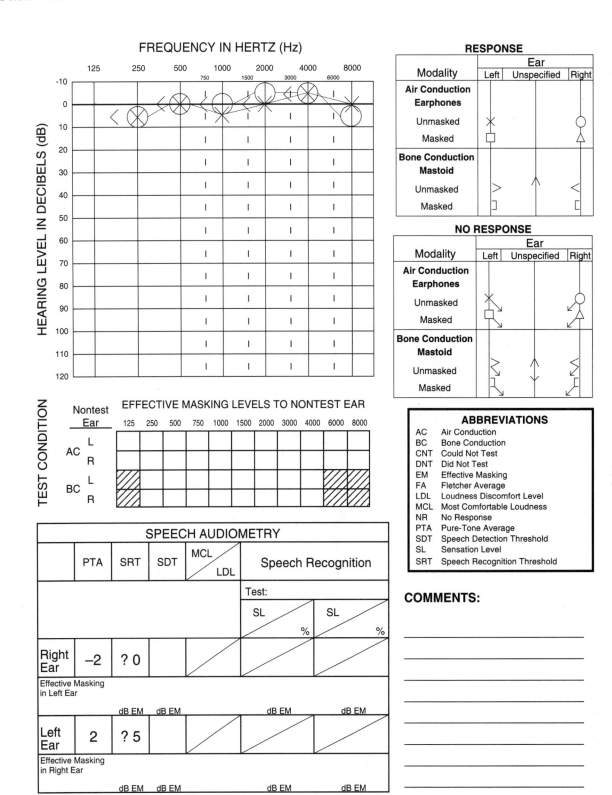

FREQUENCY IN HERTZ (Hz)

HEARING LEVEL IN DECIBELS (dB)

TEST CONDITION

EFFECTIVE MASKING LEVELS TO NONTEST EAR

Nontest Ear		125	250	500	750	1000	1500	2000	3000	4000	6000	8000
AC	L											
	R											
BC	L											
	R											

SPEECH AUDIOMETRY

	PTA	SRT	SDT	MCL / LDL	Speech Recognition			
					Test:			
					SL	%	SL	%
Right Ear	–2	? 0						
Effective Masking in Left Ear		dB EM	dB EM			dB EM		dB EM
Left Ear	2	? 5						
Effective Masking in Right Ear		dB EM	dB EM			dB EM		dB EM

RESPONSE

Modality	Ear		
	Left	Unspecified	Right
Air Conduction Earphones			
Unmasked	✕		◯
Masked	▢		△
Bone Conduction Mastoid			
Unmasked	>	∧	<
Masked	⊐		⊏

NO RESPONSE

Modality	Ear		
	Left	Unspecified	Right
Air Conduction Earphones			
Unmasked	✕↘		◯↙
Masked	▢↘		△↙
Bone Conduction Mastoid			
Unmasked	>↘	∧↕	<↙
Masked	⊐↘		⊏↙

ABBREVIATIONS

AC	Air Conduction
BC	Bone Conduction
CNT	Could Not Test
DNT	Did Not Test
EM	Effective Masking
FA	Fletcher Average
LDL	Loudness Discomfort Level
MCL	Most Comfortable Loudness
NR	No Response
PTA	Pure-Tone Average
SDT	Speech Detection Threshold
SL	Sensation Level
SRT	Speech Recognition Threshold

COMMENTS:

_____

_____

_____

_____

_____

_____

_____

_____

_____

E. When to Mask: Threshold Speech Audiometry

We have already decided that contralateral masking is not required during pure-tone audiometry.

Is contralateral masking required when measuring speech recognition threshold (SRT)?

SRTs are measured at 0 dB HL and 5 dB HL for the right and left ears respectively, findings that confirm the pure-tone results. Contralateral masking is not needed because the presentation level of speech in the test ear does not equal or exceed the bone-conduction thresholds at frequencies between 250 through 4000 Hz in the nontest ear by the amount of interaural attenuation (IA):

$$\text{Presentation level}_T - \text{IA} \geq \text{Best BC}_{NT}$$

Recall from Chapter 4 that there are two approaches to selecting interaural attenuation values during speech audiometry. In the first approach, we can use 45 dB as the estimate of interaural attenuation for spondaic words (i.e., SRT) and the more conservative value of 35 dB for suprathreshold speech measures. In the second approach, we can use a single interaural attenuation value of 40 dB for all threshold and suprathreshold speech measures. *For this particular case study, we will use 45 dB as the estimated value of interaural attenuation for spondaic words.*

Right Ear	0 dB HL – 45 dB	$\geq$ –5 dB HL?	
	– 45 dB HL	$\geq$ –5 dB HL?	*No*
Left Ear	5 dB HL – 45 dB	$\geq$ –5 dB HL?	
	– 40 dB HL	$\geq$ –5 dB HL?	*No*

When assessing the right ear, the predicted cross-hearing level of the speech signal reaching the nontest (i.e., left) ear is *–45 dB HL*! It should be clear that there is no need for contralateral masking because the predicted level of the cross-hearing signal (i.e., –45 dB HL) is considerably lower than the best bone-conduction threshold in the left (i.e., nontest) ear (i.e., –5 dB HL at 4000 Hz). Consequently, if the SRT is approximately 0 dB HL, then bone-conduction thresholds in the nontest ear would have to be approximately *–45 dB HL* in order for cross hearing to occur! A similar situation results when measuring the SRT in the left ear.

Commentary

1. *This case study illustrates that contralateral masking is not required when measuring speech recognition thresholds in individuals with normal hearing sensitivity in both ears.*

Case 1-GH

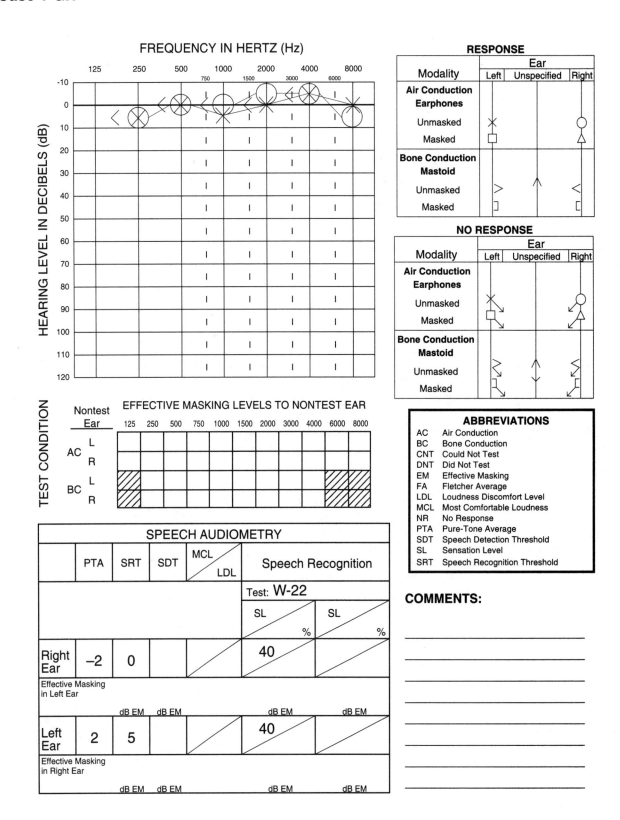

FREQUENCY IN HERTZ (Hz)

RESPONSE

Modality	Ear		
	Left	Unspecified	Right
Air Conduction Earphones			
Unmasked	✕		◯
Masked	▢		△
Bone Conduction Mastoid			
Unmasked	>	∧	<
Masked	⊏		⊐

NO RESPONSE

Modality	Ear		
	Left	Unspecified	Right
Air Conduction Earphones			
Unmasked	✕↙		◯↘
Masked	▢↙		△↘
Bone Conduction Mastoid			
Unmasked	>↙	↕	<↘
Masked	⊏↙		⊐↘

ABBREVIATIONS
AC   Air Conduction
BC   Bone Conduction
CNT   Could Not Test
DNT   Did Not Test
EM   Effective Masking
FA   Fletcher Average
LDL   Loudness Discomfort Level
MCL   Most Comfortable Loudness
NR   No Response
PTA   Pure-Tone Average
SDT   Speech Detection Threshold
SL   Sensation Level
SRT   Speech Recognition Threshold

EFFECTIVE MASKING LEVELS TO NONTEST EAR

Nontest Ear		125	250	500	750	1000	1500	2000	3000	4000	6000	8000
AC	L											
	R											
BC	L											
	R											

SPEECH AUDIOMETRY

	PTA	SRT	SDT	MCL / LDL	Speech Recognition	
					Test: W-22	
					SL / %	SL / %
Right Ear	−2	0			40	
Effective Masking in Left Ear		dB EM	dB EM		dB EM	dB EM
Left Ear	2	5			40	
Effective Masking in Right Ear		dB EM	dB EM		dB EM	dB EM

COMMENTS:

_____
_____
_____
_____
_____
_____
_____
_____
_____

G. When to Mask: Suprathreshold Speech Audiometry

Suprathreshold speech recognition will be assessed using a traditional, open-set monosyllabic word test: CID W-22 (monitored live-voice presentation). The majority of audiologists present monosyllabic words at a fixed sensation level (SL) referenced to the SRT, typically at 40 dB SL (Martin, Armstrong et al., 1994). In this particular case, we will present the test words at 40 dB SL re: SRT. The patient reported that speech (at 40 dB SL) was presented at a comfortable loudness.

Is contralateral masking required when assessing suprathreshold speech recognition ability at 40 dB SL?
Recall our rule for when to mask during speech audiometry:

$$\text{Presentation level}_T - IA \geq \text{Best BC}_{NT}$$

Presentation level during suprathreshold speech audiometry is determined by simply adding the selected sensation level (e.g., 40 dB SL) to the SRT in the test ear.

Right Ear	Presentation level = 0 dB HL + 40 dB SL = 40 dB HL
Left Ear	Presentation level = 5 dB HL + 40 dB SL = 45 dB HL

In this example, we will use the more conservative value of 35 dB as our estimate of interaural attenuation for suprathreshold speech (i.e., IA of 45 dB for spondaic words minus a correction factor of 10 dB for suprathreshold measures). Is contralateral masking required in either ear?

Right Ear	40 dB HL – 35 dB ≥ –5 dB HL?	
	5 dB HL ≥ –5 dB HL?	*Yes*
Left Ear	45 dB HL – 35 dB ≥ –5 dB HL?	
	10 dB HL ≥ –5 dB HL?	*Yes*

Contralateral masking will be required when assessing suprathreshold speech recognition ability in both ears. When speech is presented at 40 dB HL in the right ear and if we assume that interaural attenuation can be as small as 35 dB, then theoretically a cross-hearing signal of 5 dB HL can be reaching the opposite ear. Because there is an apparent bone-conduction threshold of –5 dB HL at 4000 Hz, theoretically the estimated cross-hearing signal of 5 dB HL could be perceived in the nontest ear. A similar situation also occurs when assessing suprathreshold speech recognition ability in the left ear.

Commentary

1. There is a common misconception that contralateral masking is not required when assessing suprathreshold speech recognition ability using traditional monosyllabic test materials *in individuals with normal hearing sensitivity*. This case study illustrates that contralateral masking is often required during suprathreshold speech audiometry, particularly when presenting speech at moderate to high intensity levels. The need for contralateral masking can be sometimes be eliminated, however, by using a lower sensation level (e.g., 30 dB SL).

H. How Much Masking: Suprathreshold Speech Audiometry

There are two goals to consider when selecting an appropriate masking level during speech audiometry. First, the masking level should be placed at approximately the middle of the range of correct values (i.e., the middle of the masking plateau). Second, the masking level *ideally* should be placed at least 10 dB above the minimum masking level (i.e., a 10-dB safety factor) to account for intersubject variability in the calibration of the effective masking level. If the calculated masking plateau is very narrow, however, this second goal may be difficult to achieve.

Recall that mid-masking level (M_{mid}) is the midpoint between the minimum (M_{min}) and maximum (M_{max}) masking levels. Mid-masking level can be calculated as follows:

$$M_{mid} = (M_{max} + M_{min}) / 2$$

where

$$M_{min} = \text{Presentation level}_T - IA + \text{Max AB Gap}_{NT}$$
$$M_{max} = \text{Best BC}_T + IA - 5 \text{ dB}$$

Remember that bone-conduction sensitivity is always considered at frequencies from 250 through 4000 Hz.

How much contralateral masking should be used when assessing suprathreshold speech recognition ability in both ears?

Right Ear	$M_{min} = 40 \text{ dB HL} - 35 \text{ dB} + 5 \text{ dB}$ (at 1000 Hz)
	$= 10 \text{ dB EM}$
	$M_{max} = -5 \text{ dB HL}$ (at 4000 Hz) $+ 35 \text{ dB} - 5 \text{ dB}$
	$= 25 \text{ dB EM}$
	$M_{mid} = (25 \text{ dB} + 10 \text{ dB}) / 2$
	$= 17.5 \text{ dB EM}$
Left Ear	$M_{min} = 45 \text{ dB HL} - 35 \text{ dB} + 0 \text{ dB}$
	$= 10 \text{ dB EM}$
	$M_{max} = -5 \text{ dB HL}$ (at 4000 Hz) $+ 35 \text{ dB} - 5 \text{ dB}$
	$= 25 \text{ dB EM}$
	$M_{mid} = (25 \text{ dB} + 10 \text{ dB}) / 2$
	$= 17.5 \text{ dB EM}$

The mid-masking level is calculated as 17.5 dB EM for both ears. Consequently, we will select a masking level of *20 dB EM* when assessing suprathreshold speech recognition ability in each ear. In addition to falling at mid-plateau, a value of 20 dB EM is at least 10 dB above the minimum masking level required.

Commentary

1. Recall from Chapter 6 that a short-cut approach for selecting an appropriate level of masking during suprathreshold speech audiometry can be used *provided that the following two conditions are met*: (a) There are no *significant* air-bone gaps in either ear and (b) suprathreshold speech recognition is evaluated at a *moderate* sensation level (i.e., approximately 40 dB SL). Given these two prerequisites, the selected masking level usually will occur approximately at midplateau. These two requirements are met in the current case study. Thus, we should be able to use the short-cut approach when selecting an appropriate level of masking.

The effective masking level is equal to the presentation level of the speech signal at the test ear (PL_T) minus 20 dB:

$$\text{dB EM} = PL_T - 20 \text{ dB}$$

This equation is basically a modification of Studebaker's original equation for calculating the effective masking level.

Let us calculate effective masking levels during suprathreshold speech audiometry using this short-cut approach.

Right Ear   40 dB HL – 20 dB = 20 dB EM
Left Ear   45 dB HL – 20 dB = 25 dB EM

It should be noted that the effective masking levels calculated using the short-cut approach are essentially the same (within 5 dB) as those values calculated using the midplateau procedure. Appropriate levels of masking have been selected when using the short-cut approach in this particular example.

Case 1-J

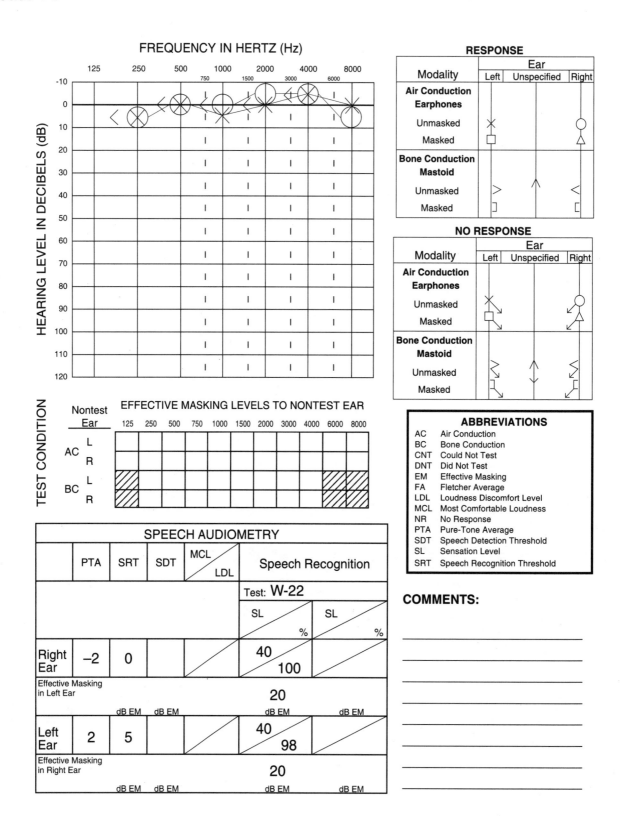

FREQUENCY IN HERTZ (Hz)

RESPONSE

Modality	Ear		
	Left	Unspecified	Right
Air Conduction Earphones			
Unmasked	✕		◯
Masked	☐		△
Bone Conduction Mastoid			
Unmasked	>	∧	<
Masked	⊏		⊐

NO RESPONSE

Modality	Ear		
	Left	Unspecified	Right
Air Conduction Earphones			
Unmasked	✕		◯
Masked	☐		△
Bone Conduction Mastoid			
Unmasked	⟩	∧	⟨
Masked			

ABBREVIATIONS

AC	Air Conduction
BC	Bone Conduction
CNT	Could Not Test
DNT	Did Not Test
EM	Effective Masking
FA	Fletcher Average
LDL	Loudness Discomfort Level
MCL	Most Comfortable Loudness
NR	No Response
PTA	Pure-Tone Average
SDT	Speech Detection Threshold
SL	Sensation Level
SRT	Speech Recognition Threshold

EFFECTIVE MASKING LEVELS TO NONTEST EAR

Nontest Ear	125	250	500	750	1000	1500	2000	3000	4000	6000	8000
AC L											
AC R											
BC L											
BC R											

SPEECH AUDIOMETRY

	PTA	SRT	SDT	MCL / LDL	Speech Recognition	
					Test: W-22	
					SL	SL
					%	%
Right Ear	−2	0			40 / 100	
Effective Masking in Left Ear					20	
		dB EM	dB EM		dB EM	dB EM
Left Ear	2	5			40 / 98	
Effective Masking in Right Ear					20	
		dB EM	dB EM		dB EM	dB EM

COMMENTS:

_____
_____
_____
_____
_____
_____
_____
_____

J. Audiogram Interpretation

Pure-tone testing revealed normal hearing sensitivity bilaterally. Speech recognition thresholds confirmed the pure-tone findings. Suprathreshold word recognition ability assessed using traditional monosyllabic words was excellent bilaterally.

Tympanometry revealed normal admittance and peak pressure bilaterally. Contralateral acoustic reflex thresholds were elicited bilaterally at hearing levels consistent with the presence of normal hearing.

Case 2

History

Your patient is a 42-year-old man who reports a unilateral "nerve" hearing loss in his right ear of unknown etiology since childhood. He has noted increasing hearing difficulty over the past two years, however, and is concerned that the hearing in his better (i.e., left) ear has deteriorated. There is no history of middle ear disorders; other medical history is negative.

Acoustic Immittance Measurements

	Right Ear	Left Ear
Tympanometry		
Static acoustic immittance (mmho)	0.9	1.4
Tympanometric peak pressure (daPa)	−25	−20
Equivalent ear canal volume (mmho)	1.4	1.3
Contralateral Acoustic Reflexes (dB HL)		
500 Hz	100	90
1000 Hz	115	85
2000 Hz	NR	85

NR = no response

Tympanometry revealed normal admittance (Van Camp et al., 1986), peak pressure (Silman & Silverman, 1991), and equivalent ear canal volume (Margolis & Heller, 1987) bilaterally. Contralateral acoustic reflexes were elicited at normal hearing levels (Gelfand et al., 1990) in the left ear. Acoustic reflexes were present at elevated hearing levels at 500 and 1000 Hz in the right ear; no response was measured at 2000 Hz. In summary, the preliminary results of acoustic immittance measurements *do not suggest the presence of significant conductive pathology in either ear.*

Case 2-AB

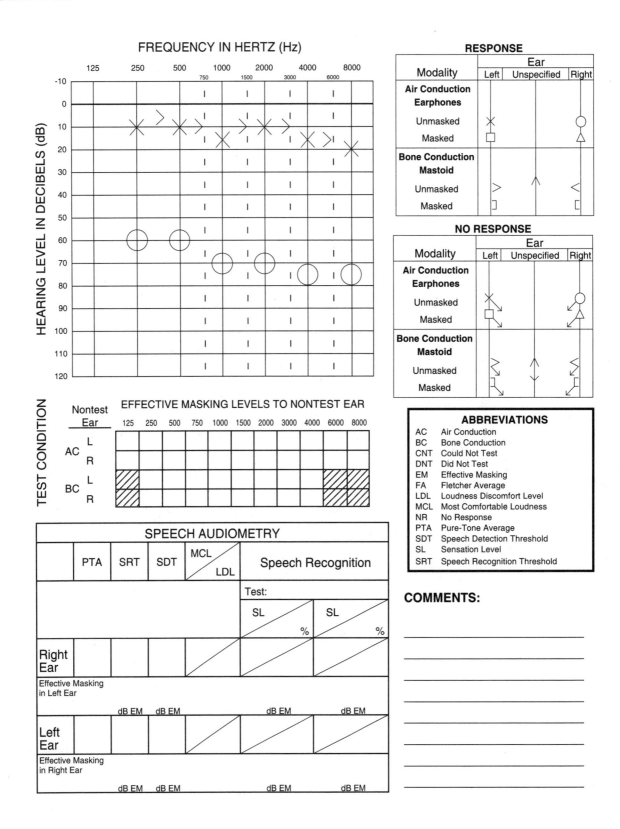

A. When to Mask: Pure-Tone Air-Conduction Audiometry

Is contralateral masking required when measuring air-conduction thresholds in either ear?

Contralateral masking is not required when measuring air-conduction thresholds in the left ear: Measured air-conduction threshold does not exceed or equal bone-conduction threshold in the nontest ear (i.e., unmasked bone-conduction threshold) by the amount of interaural attenuation (i.e., 40 dB). However, contralateral masking will be required when measuring air-conduction thresholds *at all frequencies* in the right ear. We will use the following equation when making a decision about the need for masking:

$$AC_T - BC_{NT} \geq 40 \text{ dB}$$

Right Ear (Test Ear)		Masking Needed?
250 Hz	$60 - 5 \geq 40$?	Yes
500 Hz	$60 - 10 \geq 40$?	Yes
1000 Hz	$70 - 10 \geq 40$?	Yes
2000 Hz	$70 - 10 \geq 40$?	Yes
4000 Hz	$75 - 15 \geq 40$?	Yes
8000 Hz	$75 - 20^* \geq 40$?	Yes

Left Ear (Test Ear)		Masking Needed?
250 Hz	$10 - 5 \geq 40$?	No
500 Hz	$10 - 10 \geq 40$?	No
1000 Hz	$15 - 10 \geq 40$?	No
2000 Hz	$10 - 10 \geq 40$?	No
4000 Hz	$15 - 15 \geq 40$?	No
8000 Hz	$20 - 20^* \geq 40$?	No

*Estimated bone-conduction threshold

Commentary

1. Because bone-conduction thresholds cannot be measured at 8000 Hz, we again will make some assumptions about bone-conduction sensitivity. There is normal hearing in the better (i.e., left) ear, and unmasked bone-conduction thresholds do not suggest the presence of a significant air-bone gap in that ear. Thus, it is reasonable to assume that bone-conduction sensitivity at 8000 Hz is approximately equal to the air-conduction threshold of the better ear (i.e., 20 dB HL).

2. Theoretically, although information about bone-conduction sensitivity is required, we often can make a correct decision about the need to mask during pure-tone air-conduction audiometry by considering only the *air-conduction thresholds* in the two ears:

$$AC_T - AC_{NT} \geq IA$$

Specifically, contralateral masking is required when measuring air-conduction threshold in the poorer ear if the difference between the *unmasked* air-conduction thresholds in the two ears equals or exceeds interaural attenuation (i.e., 40 dB). In this particular case, there exists a difference of 40 dB or greater between the unmasked air-conduction thresholds at all frequencies. Consequently, contralateral masking will be required when measuring air-conduction thresholds in the poorer (i.e., right) ear. Whenever there exists a 40 dB or greater difference between the two air-conduction thresholds, there already is evidence that contralateral masking will be required when testing the *poorer* ear.

B. How Much Masking: Pure-Tone Air-Conduction Audiometry

We have decided that contralateral masking will be required when measuring air-conduction thresholds at all frequencies in the right ear. We will use the plateau procedure for establishing masked pure-tone thresholds. We will calculate the initial minimum masking levels using Martin's (1967, 1974) recommendation. Recall that initial minimum masking level (M_{min}) is simply equal to the air-conduction threshold of the nontest ear (AC_{NT}) plus a safety factor of 10 dB to account for intersubject variability with respect to effectiveness of masking levels:

$$M_{min} = AC_{NT} + 10 \text{ dB}$$

Right Ear (Test Ear)		How Much Masking (Nontest Ear)?
250 Hz	10 dB HL + 10 dB	20 dB EM
500 Hz	10 dB HL + 10 dB	20 dB EM
1000 Hz	15 dB HL + 10 dB	25 dB EM
2000 Hz	10 dB HL + 10 dB	20 dB EM
4000 Hz	15 dB HL + 10 dB	25 dB EM
8000 Hz	20 dB HL + 10 dB	30 dB EM

We will introduce masking during the plateau procedure using the levels calculated above.

Case 2-CD

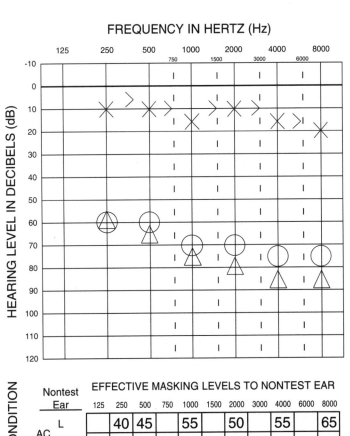

FREQUENCY IN HERTZ (Hz)

RESPONSE

Modality	Ear		
	Left	Unspecified	Right
Air Conduction Earphones			
Unmasked	X		◯
Masked	▢		△
Bone Conduction Mastoid			
Unmasked	>	∧	<
Masked	⊐		⊏

NO RESPONSE

Modality	Ear		
	Left	Unspecified	Right
Air Conduction Earphones			
Unmasked	X↙		◯↙
Masked	▢↙		△↙
Bone Conduction Mastoid			
Unmasked	>↙	∧↕	<↙
Masked	⊐↙	∨	⊏↙

EFFECTIVE MASKING LEVELS TO NONTEST EAR

Nontest Ear		125	250	500	750	1000	1500	2000	3000	4000	6000	8000
AC	L		40	45		55		50		55		65
	R											
BC	L											
	R											

ABBREVIATIONS

AC	Air Conduction
BC	Bone Conduction
CNT	Could Not Test
DNT	Did Not Test
EM	Effective Masking
FA	Fletcher Average
LDL	Loudness Discomfort Level
MCL	Most Comfortable Loudness
NR	No Response
PTA	Pure-Tone Average
SDT	Speech Detection Threshold
SL	Sensation Level
SRT	Speech Recognition Threshold

SPEECH AUDIOMETRY

	PTA	SRT	SDT	MCL / LDL	Speech Recognition	
					Test:	
					SL / %	SL / %
Right Ear						
Effective Masking in Left Ear		dB EM	dB EM		dB EM	dB EM
Left Ear						
Effective Masking in Right Ear		dB EM	dB EM		dB EM	dB EM

COMMENTS:

_____

_____

_____

_____

_____

_____

_____

_____

C. When to Mask: Pure-Tone Bone-Conduction Audiometry

Masked air-conduction thresholds have been obtained in the right ear using the plateau procedure and are presented on the adjacent audiogram. The final masking level used to obtain masked threshold at each frequency is also reported for the nontest (i.e., left) ear.

Is contralateral masking required when measuring bone-conduction thresholds in either ear?

When comparing unmasked bone-conduction thresholds to the air-conduction thresholds, it is important to remember that *masked* air-conduction thresholds are always considered because they represent the true thresholds for that ear. For example, contralateral masking was required at all frequencies when measuring air-conduction thresholds in the right ear. Thus, we must considered the *masked* air-conduction thresholds in the right ear when making a decision about the need for contralateral masking during bone-conduction audiometry in that ear. Remember that contralateral masking is required during bone-conduction audiometry whenever comparison of the unmasked bone-conduction threshold (Unmasked BC) and the air-conduction threshold in the test ear (AC_T) at that frequency suggests a potential air-bone gap (AB Gap_T) of 15 dB or greater:

$$AB\ Gap_T \geq 15\ dB?$$
$$AC_T - Unmasked\ BC \geq 15\ dB?$$

Right Ear	AB Gap_T	AB $Gap_T \geq$15 dB?
250 Hz	60 – 5 = 55	Yes
500 Hz	65 – 10 = 55	Yes
1000 Hz	75 – 10 = 65	Yes
2000 Hz	80 – 10 = 70	Yes
4000 Hz	85 – 15 = 70	Yes
Left Ear	**AB Gap_T**	**AB $Gap_T \geq$15 dB?**
250 Hz	10 – 5 = 5	No
500 Hz	10 – 10 = 0	No
1000 Hz	15 – 10 = 5	No
2000 Hz	10 – 10 = 0	No
4000 Hz	15 – 15 = 0	No

Commentary

1. It should be noted that the maximum conductive hearing loss will result in an air-bone gap of approximately 60 dB. Calculation of potential air-bone gaps in the right ear reveal air-bone gaps at 1000, 2000, and 4000 Hz that are greater than the theoretical maximum. This example simply demonstrates that there are potentially very large air-bone gaps in the right ear at all frequencies.

D. How Much Masking: Pure-Tone Bone-Conduction Audiometry

We have decided that contralateral masking will be required at all frequencies when measuring bone-conduction thresholds in the right ear. We again will use the plateau procedure for establishing masked pure-tone thresholds. The initial minimum masking levels will be calculated using Martin's (1967, 1974) recommendation. Recall that the initial minimum masking level (M_{min}) during bone-conduction audiometry is simply equal to air-conduction threshold of the nontest ear (AC_{NT}) plus compensation for the occlusion effect (OE) plus a safety factor of 10 dB:

$$M_{min} = AC_{NT} + OE + 10 \text{ dB}$$

Recall that patients with either normal hearing or a sensorineural hearing loss will exhibit an occlusion effect. The left ear will be covered (i.e., occluded) when contralateral masking is introduced during measurement of masked bone-conduction thresholds in the right ear. Because this patient exhibits normal hearing (and no evidence of significant air-bone gaps) in the masked (i.e., occluded) ear, he theoretically will exhibit an occlusion effect. In this particular example, we will use *average* values when compensating for the occlusion effect: 30 dB at 250 Hz, 20 dB at 500 Hz, 10 dB at 1000 Hz, and 0 dB at frequencies above 1000 Hz.

$$M_{min} = AC_{NT} + OE + 10 \text{ dB}$$

Right Ear (Test Ear)		How Much Masking (Nontest Ear)?
250 Hz	10 dB HL + 30 dB + 10 dB	50 dB EM
500 Hz	10 dB HL + 20 dB + 10 dB	40 dB EM
1000 Hz	15 dB HL + 10 dB + 10 dB	35 dB EM
2000 Hz	10 dB HL + 0 dB + 10 dB	20 dB EM
4000 Hz	15 dB HL + 0 dB + 10 dB	25 dB EM

We will introduce masking during the plateau procedure using the levels calculated above.

Case 2-EF

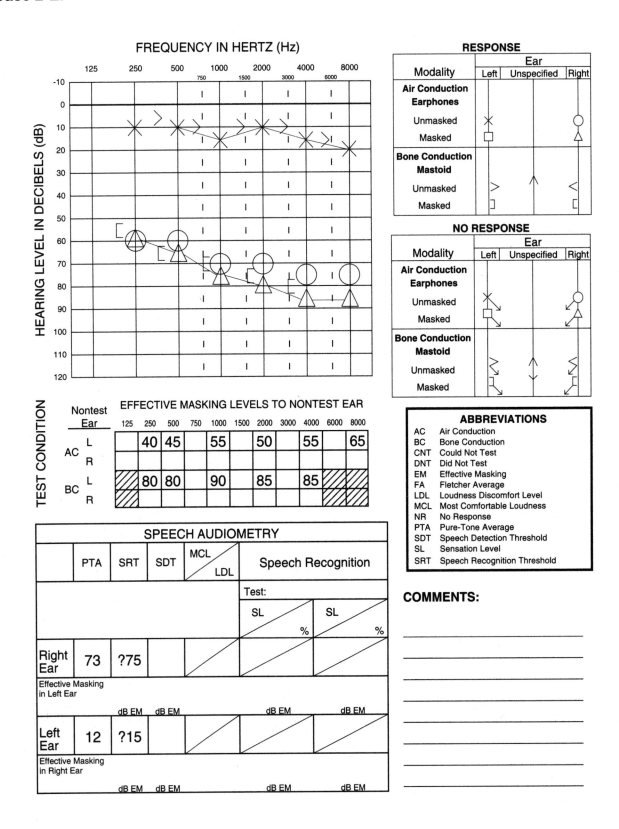

FREQUENCY IN HERTZ (Hz)

EFFECTIVE MASKING LEVELS TO NONTEST EAR

TEST CONDITION

Nontest Ear		125	250	500	750	1000	1500	2000	3000	4000	6000	8000
AC	L		40	45		55		50		55		65
	R											
BC	L		80	80		90		85		85		
	R											

RESPONSE

Modality	Ear		
	Left	Unspecified	Right
Air Conduction Earphones			
Unmasked	✕		○
Masked	☐		△
Bone Conduction Mastoid			
Unmasked	>	∧	<
Masked	⊐		⊏

NO RESPONSE

Modality	Ear		
	Left	Unspecified	Right
Air Conduction Earphones			
Unmasked	✕		○
Masked	☐		△
Bone Conduction Mastoid			
Unmasked	>	∧	<
Masked	⊐		⊏

ABBREVIATIONS

AC	Air Conduction
BC	Bone Conduction
CNT	Could Not Test
DNT	Did Not Test
EM	Effective Masking
FA	Fletcher Average
LDL	Loudness Discomfort Level
MCL	Most Comfortable Loudness
NR	No Response
PTA	Pure-Tone Average
SDT	Speech Detection Threshold
SL	Sensation Level
SRT	Speech Recognition Threshold

SPEECH AUDIOMETRY

	PTA	SRT	SDT	MCL / LDL	Speech Recognition
					Test:
					SL / %	SL / %
Right Ear	73	?75			
Effective Masking in Left Ear			dB EM	dB EM	dB EM	dB EM
Left Ear	12	?15			
Effective Masking in Right Ear			dB EM	dB EM	dB EM	dB EM

COMMENTS:

_____
_____
_____
_____
_____
_____
_____
_____
_____

E. When to Mask: Threshold Speech Audiometry

Masked bone-conduction thresholds have been obtained in the right ear using the plateau procedure and are presented on the adjacent audiogram. The final masking level used to obtain masked threshold at each frequency is also reported for the nontest (i.e., left) ear.

Is contralateral masking required when obtaining speech recognition threshold in either ear?

Based upon the pure-tone averages, it is predicted that SRTs will be measured at approximately 75 dB HL and 15 dB HL for the right and left ears, respectively. Prior to measurement of speech recognition thresholds, we can determine whether contralateral masking will likely be required:

$$\text{Presentation level}_T - \text{IA} \geq \text{Best BC}_{NT}$$

We will use a value of 45 dB as our estimate of interaural attenuation for spondaic words (and the more conservative value of 35 dB when subsequently measuring suprathreshold speech recognition).

Right Ear	75 dB HL – 45 dB ≥ 5 dB HL?	
	30 dB HL ≥ 5 dB HL?	*Yes*
Left Ear	15 dB HL – 45 dB ≥ 55 dB HL?	
	–30 dB HL ≥ 55 dB HL?	*No*

When measuring SRT in the right ear, the predicted cross-hearing level of the speech signal reaching the nontest (i.e., left) ear is 30 dB HL. Because the best bone-conduction threshold in the nontest ear is 5 dB HL, cross hearing theoretically will occur. Consequently, it will be necessary to use contralateral masking when measuring the SRT in the right ear.

There will be no need for contralateral masking, however, when measuring SRT in the left ear. The predicted level of the cross-hearing signal (i.e., –30 dB HL) is considerably lower than the best bone-conduction threshold in the nontest ear (i.e., 55 dB HL at 250 Hz). Because of the predicted SRT at a very low intensity level in the left ear and the poor bone-conduction sensitivity in the nontest ear, contralateral masking will not be required.

Commentary

1. In some instances, a correct decision about the need for contralateral masking can be made without consideration of bone-conduction thresholds. Recall from Chapter 4 that masking is required when testing the poorer ear whenever the speech recognition thresholds in the two ears differ by at least the amount of interaural attenuation.

$$\text{SRT}_T - \text{SRT}_{NT} \geq \text{IA}$$
or
$$\text{SRT}_T - \text{IA} \geq \text{SRT}_{NT}$$

Even without information about bone-conduction hearing sensitivity, there is sufficient indication that contralateral masking will be required when measuring the SRT in the poorer (i.e., right) ear. The predicted SRT of 75 dB HL in the right ear could reflect a cross-hearing response from the left ear; there is a difference of 60 dB between the predicted speech thresholds, a value that equals or exceeds interaural attenuation (i.e., 45 dB).

$$\text{SRT}_T - \text{SRT}_{NT} \geq \text{IA}$$
$$75 \text{ dB HL} - 15 \text{ dB HL} \geq 45 \text{ dB?}$$
$$60 \text{ dB} \geq 45 \text{ dB?}$$

F. How Much Masking: Threshold Speech Audiometry

We have decided that contralateral masking will be required when measuring speech recognition threshold in the right ear. Recall from Chapter 6 that we can use either a psychoacoustic or acoustic approach when determining masking requirements during assessment of SRT. In this example, we will use an acoustic approach. That is, the required masking level is derived by calculating the estimated levels of the test and maker signals in the test and nontest ears. Specifically, we will calculate mid-masking level:

$$M_{mid} = (M_{max} + M_{min}) / 2$$

where

$$M_{min} = \text{Presentation level}_T - IA + \text{Max AB gap}_{NT}$$
$$M_{max} = \text{Best BC}_T + IA - 5\ dB$$

How much contralateral masking should be used when measuring speech recognition threshold in the right ear?

$$M_{min} = 75\ dB\ HL - 45\ dB + 5\ dB\ (\text{at } 250\ Hz)$$
$$= 35\ dB\ EM$$
$$M_{max} = 55\ dB\ HL\ (\text{at } 250\ Hz) + 45\ dB - 5\ dB$$
$$= 95\ dB\ EM$$
$$M_{mid} = (95\ dB + 35\ dB) / 2$$
$$= 65\ dB\ EM$$

Commentary

1. The mid-masking level was calculated as 65 dB EM. In addition to falling at mid-plateau, a value of 65 dB EM is 30 dB above the minimum masking level required. Consequently, there is "reserve" masking available should speech be presented at levels higher than the predicted SRT of 75 dB HL. In fact, depending on the particular SRT procedure, it is likely that spondees will be presented at levels that are higher than the estimated SRT. It is important to consider your SRT procedure when evaluating the appropriateness of the selected masking level.

2. Although it is not necessary, some audiologists initially will obtain an unmasked SRT in the poorer ear even though it is expected that contralateral masking will be required. An unmasked SRT can be useful in two ways. First, an unmasked SRT is recommended if functional hearing impairment is suspected. In this particular example, if we assume that interaural attenuation for spondaic words can be as small as 45 dB, then an unmasked SRT could be measured at a level 45 dB above the best bone-conduction threshold in the nontest ear (i.e., 5 dB). Consequently, we expect to measure an unmasked SRT at an intensity level of 50 dB HL or greater. If an unmasked SRT were measured at 30 dB HL in the right ear, for example, we would have strong evidence that the pure-tone thresholds in that ear are invalid.

Second, an unmasked SRT can provide a more accurate estimate of interaural attenuation for speech. This information can be useful, particularly when the width of the masking plateau is very narrow. Consider the following hypothetical example for this case study. Assume that unmasked SRTs are measured at 65 dB HL and 15 dB HL for the right and left ears, respectively. Because the unmasked SRT in the right ear is equal to 65 dB HL and the best bone-conduction threshold in the nontest ear is equal to 5 dB HL, a more accurate estimate of interaural attenuation for this patient may be 60 dB (i.e., estimated IA = Unmasked SRT$_T$ – Best BC$_{NT}$). It is sometimes difficult to know, however, what aspect of hearing sensitivity in the nontest ear should be considered when estimating interaural attenuation (e.g., best bone-conduction threshold, average bone-conduction threshold, SRT, etc.). At the very least, interaural attenuation cannot be smaller than the difference between the two SRTs. Recall that the value of interaural attenuation used when determining the minimum and maximum masking levels does not affect the calculated mid-masking level: Interaural attenuation has equal yet opposite effects on the minimum and maximum masking levels. Although the use of a larger value of interaural attenuation will not change the calculated mid-masking level, it will result in an estimated masking plateau that is wider. This information can be useful when determining the appropriateness of a selected masking level, particularly when the masking plateau is narrow.

Case 2-GH

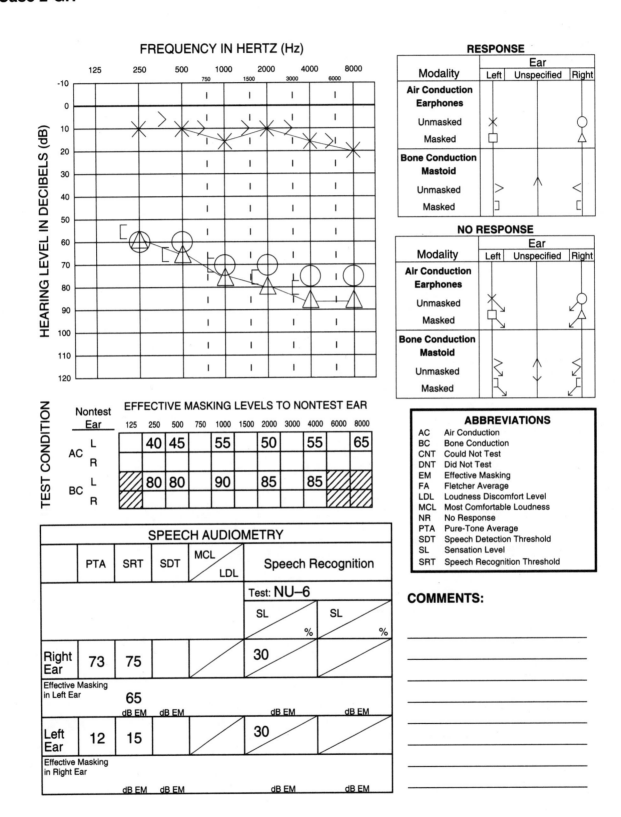

FREQUENCY IN HERTZ (Hz)

RESPONSE

Modality	Ear		
	Left	Unspecified	Right
Air Conduction Earphones			
Unmasked	X		O
Masked	□		△
Bone Conduction Mastoid			
Unmasked	>	∧	<
Masked	⊏		⊐

NO RESPONSE

Modality	Ear		
	Left	Unspecified	Right
Air Conduction Earphones			
Unmasked	X		O
Masked	□		△
Bone Conduction Mastoid			
Unmasked	>	∧	<
Masked	⊏		⊐

EFFECTIVE MASKING LEVELS TO NONTEST EAR

Nontest Ear		125	250	500	750	1000	1500	2000	3000	4000	6000	8000
AC	L		40	45		55		50		55		65
	R											
BC	L		80	80		90		85		85		
	R											

ABBREVIATIONS

AC	Air Conduction
BC	Bone Conduction
CNT	Could Not Test
DNT	Did Not Test
EM	Effective Masking
FA	Fletcher Average
LDL	Loudness Discomfort Level
MCL	Most Comfortable Loudness
NR	No Response
PTA	Pure-Tone Average
SDT	Speech Detection Threshold
SL	Sensation Level
SRT	Speech Recognition Threshold

SPEECH AUDIOMETRY

	PTA	SRT	SDT	MCL / LDL	Speech Recognition
					Test: NU–6
					SL ___ % ___ | SL ___ % ___
Right Ear	73	75			30
Effective Masking in Left Ear		65 dB EM	dB EM		dB EM | dB EM
Left Ear	12	15			30
Effective Masking in Right Ear		dB EM	dB EM		dB EM | dB EM

COMMENTS:

_____
_____
_____
_____
_____
_____
_____
_____

G. When to Mask: Suprathreshold Speech Audiometry

Suprathreshold speech recognition will be assessed using a traditional, open-set monosyllabic word test: Northwestern University Auditory Test #6 (NU-6). A monitored-live voice presentation will be used. In this particular case, we will present the test words at 30 dB SL re: SRT. The patient reported that speech was presented at a comfortable loudness at 30 dB SL in both ears.

Is contralateral masking required when assessing suprathreshold speech recognition ability at 30 dB SL?
Recall our rule for when to mask during speech audiometry:

$$\text{Presentation level}_T - IA \geq \text{Best BC}_{NT}$$

Presentation level during suprathreshold speech audiometry is determined by simply adding the selected sensation level (e.g., 30 dB SL) to the SRT in the test ear.

Right Ear	Presentation level = 75 dB HL + 30 dB SL = 105 dB HL
Left Ear	Presentation level = 15 dB HL + 30 dB SL = 45 dB HL

Remember that in this example we will be using the more conservative value of 35 dB as our estimate of interaural attenuation for suprathreshold speech. Is contralateral masking required in either ear?

Right Ear	105 dB HL − 35 dB ≥ 5 dB HL?	
	70 dB HL ≥ 5 dB HL?	*Yes*
Left Ear	45 dB HL − 35 dB ≥ 55 dB HL?	
	10 dB HL ≥ 55 dB HL?	*No*

Contralateral masking will be required when assessing suprathreshold speech recognition ability in the right ear. This is not unexpected because contralateral masking was required during *threshold* testing in the right ear.

H. How Much Masking: Suprathreshold Speech Audiometry

Ideally, the selected masking level should be placed at approximately the middle of the masking plateau (i.e., midplateau). Recall that the mid-masking level (M_{mid}) is the midpoint between the minimum (M_{min}) and maximum (M_{max}) masking levels. The mid-masking level can be calculated as follows:

$$M_{mid} = (M_{max} + M_{min}) / 2$$
$$\text{where}$$
$$M_{min} = \text{Presentation level}_T - IA + \text{Max AB Gap}_{NT}$$
$$M_{max} = \text{Best BC}_T + IA - 5 \text{ dB}$$

Remember that bone-conduction sensitivity is always considered at frequencies from 250 through 4000 Hz.

How much contralateral masking should be used when assessing suprathreshold speech recognition ability in the right ear?

Right Ear	M_{min} = 105 dB HL − 35 dB + 5 dB (at 250 Hz)
	= 75 dB EM
	M_{max} = 55 dB HL (at 250 Hz) + 35 dB − 5 dB
	= 85 dB EM
	M_{mid} = (85 dB + 75 dB) / 2
	= 80 dB EM

The mid-masking level is calculated as 80 dB EM. Ideally, the selected masking level should be at least 10 dB above the minimum required (i.e., 10-dB safety factor). It should be noted that the estimated width of the masking plateau is very narrow (i.e., only 10 dB). Consequently, there is not much flexibility in selecting an appropriate masking level. In this particular case, a masking level of 85 dB EM is recommended when assessing suprathreshold speech recognition ability in the right ear. In addition to falling approximately at midplateau, a value of 85 dB EM is at least 10 dB above the minimum masking level required and it does not exceed the estimated maximum.

Commentary

1. If the patient's actual interaural attenuation for speech is greater than the conservative estimate of 35 dB, then a wider masking plateau will exist. Given this assumption, a selected masking level of 80 dB EM (the "precise" mid-masking level) can be justified: A value of 80 dB EM would likely be at least 10 dB greater than the minimum. It is important to remember, however, that the mid-masking level is not a precise value, but only an *estimate*. Thus, the mid-masking level should not be considered a single value, but rather a range of values. The selected masking level will be influenced by a combination of variables that often are unique for a particular case. For example, if the patient reports that the selected masking level is uncomfortably loud, it will be necessary to reduce the intensity level of the masker.

2. Recall from Chapter 6 that a short-cut approach for selecting an appropriate level of masking during suprathreshold speech audiometry can be used *provided that the following two conditions are met*: (1) There are no *significant* air-bone gaps in either ear (2) suprathreshold speech recognition is evaluated at a *moderate* sensation level (i.e., approximately 40 dB SL). Given these two prerequisites, the selected masking level typically will occur at midplateau. These two requirements are met in the current example. Thus, the short-cut approach should prove effective when selecting an appropriate masking level.

Recall that the effective masking level using the short-cut approach is equal to the presentation level of the speech signal at the test ear (PL_T) minus 20 dB:

$$dB\ EM = PL_T - 20\ dB$$

Let us calculate the effective masking level using this short-cut approach when evaluating suprathreshold speech recognition in the right ear:

$$\text{Right Ear} \quad 105\ dB\ HL - 20\ dB = 85\ dB\ EM$$

It should be noted that the effective masking level calculated using the short-cut approach is essentially the same (within 5 dB) as that value calculated using the midplateau procedure. Recall our earlier calculations using the midplateau procedure:

$$M_{min} = 75\ dB\ EM$$
$$M_{max} = 85\ dB\ EM$$
$$M_{mid} = 80\ dB\ EM$$

The masking level of 85 dB EM calculated using the short-cut approach is clearly appropriate given the underlying assumptions of the midplateau procedure.

Case 2-J

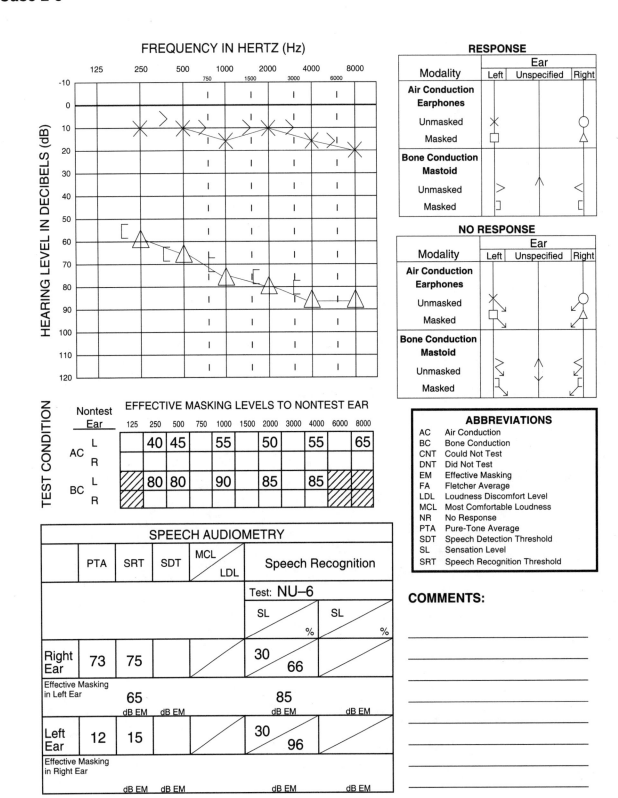

FREQUENCY IN HERTZ (Hz)

RESPONSE

Modality	Ear		
	Left	Unspecified	Right
Air Conduction Earphones			
Unmasked	X		O
Masked	□		△
Bone Conduction Mastoid			
Unmasked	>	∧	<
Masked	⊏		⊐

NO RESPONSE

Modality	Ear		
	Left	Unspecified	Right
Air Conduction Earphones			
Unmasked	X↘		O↘
Masked	□↘		△↘
Bone Conduction Mastoid			
Unmasked	>↘	∨	<↘
Masked	⊏↘		⊐↘

EFFECTIVE MASKING LEVELS TO NONTEST EAR

Nontest Ear		125	250	500	750	1000	1500	2000	3000	4000	6000	8000
AC	L		40	45		55		50		55		65
	R											
BC	L		80	80		90		85		85		
	R											

ABBREVIATIONS

AC	Air Conduction
BC	Bone Conduction
CNT	Could Not Test
DNT	Did Not Test
EM	Effective Masking
FA	Fletcher Average
LDL	Loudness Discomfort Level
MCL	Most Comfortable Loudness
NR	No Response
PTA	Pure-Tone Average
SDT	Speech Detection Threshold
SL	Sensation Level
SRT	Speech Recognition Threshold

SPEECH AUDIOMETRY

	PTA	SRT	SDT	MCL / LDL	Speech Recognition
					Test: NU–6
					SL / % — SL / %
Right Ear	73	75			30 / 66
Effective Masking in Left Ear	65 dB EM	dB EM			85 dB EM — dB EM
Left Ear	12	15			30 / 96
Effective Masking in Right Ear	dB EM	dB EM			dB EM — dB EM

COMMENTS:

_____

_____

_____

_____

_____

_____

_____

_____

J. Audiogram Interpretation

Pure-tone testing revealed normal hearing sensitivity in the left ear. There is a severe, sensorineural hearing loss of gradually sloping configuration in the right ear. Speech recognition thresholds confirmed the pure-tone findings. Suprathreshold word recognition ability assessed using traditional monosyllabic words was excellent in the left ear and fair in the right ear.

Tympanometry revealed normal admittance and peak pressure bilaterally. Contralateral acoustic reflex thresholds were elicited at hearing levels consistent with the presence of normal hearing in the left ear and a severe, cochlear hearing impairment in the right ear (Gelfand et al., 1990).

Case 3

History

Your patient is a 67-year-old woman who reports bilateral hearing impairment of gradual onset and progression over the past four years. Her primary communicative complaint is difficulty understanding speech, particularly in noisy situations. She also reports the relatively sudden onset of "muffled" hearing in her left ear following a recent upper respiratory infection and believes that her hearing has deteriorated in that ear. The results of a current otologic examination suggested the presence of otitis media with effusion in the left ear. There is no prior history of middle ear disorders; other medical history is negative.

Acoustic Immittance Measurements

	Right Ear	Left Ear
Tympanometry		
Static acoustic admittance (mmho)	1.2	0.1
Tympanometric peak pressure (daPa)	–5	—
Equivalent ear canal volume (mmho)	1.0	1.1
Contralateral Acoustic Reflexes (dB HL)		
500 Hz	NR	NR
1000 Hz	NR	NR
2000 Hz	NR	NR
Ipsilateral Acoustic Reflexes (dB HL)		
500 Hz	80	NR
1000 Hz	85	NR
2000 Hz	80	NR

NR = no response

Tympanometry revealed normal admittance (Van Camp et al., 1986) and peak pressure (Silman & Silverman, 1991) in the right ear. The tympanogram in the left ear was flat (i.e., Type B). Measures of ear-canal acoustic admittance were within the normal range bilaterally (Margolis & Heller, 1987). Contralateral acoustic reflexes were absent bilaterally. Ipsilateral acoustic reflexes were elicited at normal hearing levels in the right ear (Wiley, Oviatt, & Block, 1987) and were absent in the left ear. In summary, the preliminary results of acoustic immittance measurements *suggest the presence of conductive pathology in the left ear.*

Case 3-AB

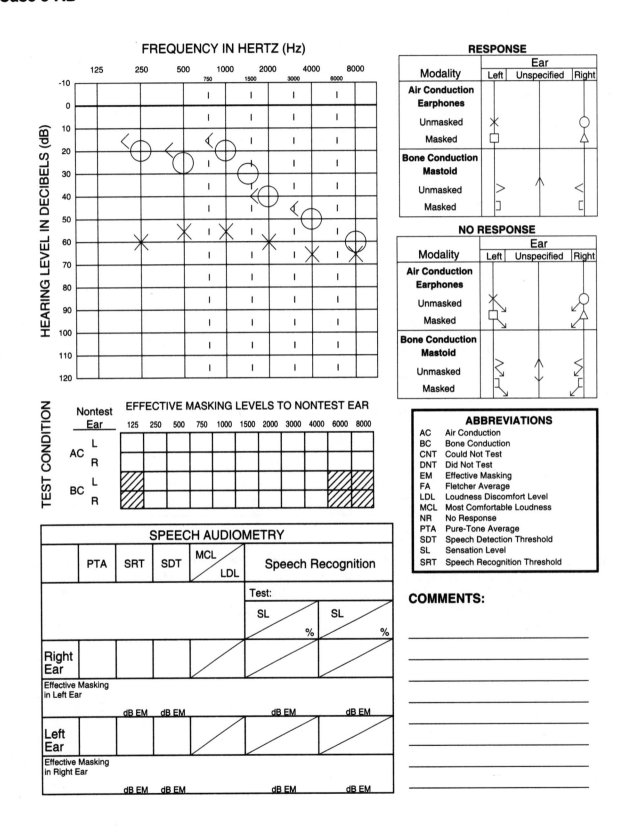

FREQUENCY IN HERTZ (Hz)

HEARING LEVEL IN DECIBELS (dB)

EFFECTIVE MASKING LEVELS TO NONTEST EAR

TEST CONDITION

Nontest Ear	125	250	500	750	1000	1500	2000	3000	4000	6000	8000
AC L											
AC R											
BC L											
BC R											

RESPONSE

Modality	Ear		
	Left	Unspecified	Right
Air Conduction Earphones			
Unmasked	✕		◯
Masked	☐		△
Bone Conduction Mastoid			
Unmasked	>	∧	<
Masked	⊐		⊏

NO RESPONSE

Modality	Ear		
	Left	Unspecified	Right
Air Conduction Earphones			
Unmasked	✕↘		◯↙
Masked	☐↘		△↙
Bone Conduction Mastoid			
Unmasked	>↘	⇕	<↙
Masked	⊐↘		⊏↙

ABBREVIATIONS

AC	Air Conduction
BC	Bone Conduction
CNT	Could Not Test
DNT	Did Not Test
EM	Effective Masking
FA	Fletcher Average
LDL	Loudness Discomfort Level
MCL	Most Comfortable Loudness
NR	No Response
PTA	Pure-Tone Average
SDT	Speech Detection Threshold
SL	Sensation Level
SRT	Speech Recognition Threshold

SPEECH AUDIOMETRY

	PTA	SRT	SDT	MCL / LDL	Speech Recognition			
					Test:			
					SL	%	SL	%
Right Ear								
Effective Masking in Left Ear		dB EM	dB EM		dB EM		dB EM	
Left Ear								
Effective Masking in Right Ear		dB EM	dB EM		dB EM		dB EM	

COMMENTS:

_____

_____

_____

_____

_____

_____

_____

_____

_____

A. When to Mask: Pure-Tone Air-Conduction Audiometry

Is contralateral masking required when measuring air-conduction thresholds in either ear?

Contralateral masking is not required when measuring air-conduction thresholds in the right ear: Measured air-conduction thresholds do not equal or exceed bone-conduction thresholds in the nontest ear (i.e., unmasked bone-conduction threshold) by the amount of interaural attenuation (i.e., 40 dB). However, contralateral masking will be required when measuring air-conduction thresholds at 250 and 1000 Hz in the left ear. We will use the following equation when making a decision about the need for masking:

$$AC_T - 40 \text{ dB} \geq BC_{NT}$$

Right Ear (Test Ear)		Masking Needed?
250 Hz	$20 - 40 \geq 15$?	No
500 Hz	$25 - 40 \geq 20$?	No
1000 Hz	$20 - 40 \geq 15$?	No
2000 Hz	$40 - 40 \geq 40$?	No
4000 Hz	$50 - 40 \geq 45$?	No
8000 Hz	$60 - 40 \geq 60$?*	No
Left Ear (Test Ear)		**Masking Needed?**
250 Hz	$55 - 40 \geq 15$?	Yes
500 Hz	$55 - 40 \geq 20$?	No
1000 Hz	$60 - 40 \geq 15$?	Yes
2000 Hz	$60 - 40 \geq 40$?	No
4000 Hz	$65 - 40 \geq 45$?	No
8000 Hz	$65 - 40 \geq 60$?*	No

*Estimated bone-conduction threshold

Commentary

1. Because an unmasked bone-conduction threshold is unavailable at 8000 Hz, it will be necessary to estimate a probable threshold at that frequency. It should be noted that unmasked bone-conduction thresholds at 250 through 4000 Hz interweave with air-conduction thresholds in the right ear (i.e., there is no evidence of significant air-bone gaps in the right ear). Consequently, it is reasonable to conclude that an unmasked bone-conduction threshold at 8000 Hz would probably occur at an intensity level equal to the air-conduction threshold in the right ear (i.e., about 60 dB HL).

B. How Much Masking: Pure-Tone Air-Conduction Audiometry

We have decided that contralateral masking will be required when measuring air-conduction thresholds at 250 and 1000 Hz in the left ear. We will use the plateau procedure for establishing masked pure-tone thresholds. We will calculate initial minimum masking levels using Martin's (1967, 1974) recommendation. Recall that initial minimum masking level (M_{min}) is simply equal to the air-conduction threshold of the nontest ear (AC_{NT}) plus a safety factor of 10 dB to account for intersubject variability in the effectiveness of masking levels:

$$M_{min} = AC_{NT} + 10 \text{ dB}$$

Right Ear (Test Ear)		How Much Masking (Nontest Ear)?
250 Hz	20 dB HL + 10 dB	30 dB EM
1000 Hz	20 dB HL + 10 dB	30 dB EM

We will introduce masking during the plateau procedure using the levels calculated above.

Case 3-CD

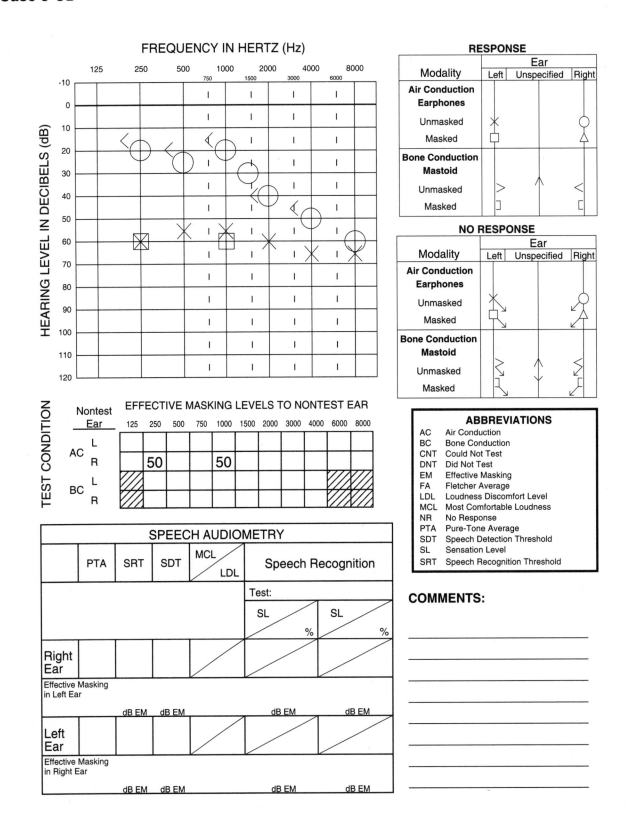

FREQUENCY IN HERTZ (Hz)

HEARING LEVEL IN DECIBELS (dB)

EFFECTIVE MASKING LEVELS TO NONTEST EAR

TEST CONDITION

Nontest Ear		125	250	500	750	1000	1500	2000	3000	4000	6000	8000
AC	L											
	R		50			50						
BC	L											
	R											

RESPONSE

Modality	Ear		
	Left	Unspecified	Right
Air Conduction Earphones			
Unmasked	X		◯
Masked	□		△
Bone Conduction Mastoid			
Unmasked	>	∧	<
Masked	⊏		⊐

NO RESPONSE

Modality	Ear		
	Left	Unspecified	Right
Air Conduction Earphones			
Unmasked	X		◯
Masked	□		△
Bone Conduction Mastoid			
Unmasked	>	∨	<
Masked	⊏		⊐

ABBREVIATIONS

AC	Air Conduction
BC	Bone Conduction
CNT	Could Not Test
DNT	Did Not Test
EM	Effective Masking
FA	Fletcher Average
LDL	Loudness Discomfort Level
MCL	Most Comfortable Loudness
NR	No Response
PTA	Pure-Tone Average
SDT	Speech Detection Threshold
SL	Sensation Level
SRT	Speech Recognition Threshold

SPEECH AUDIOMETRY

	PTA	SRT	SDT	MCL / LDL	Speech Recognition	
					Test:	
					SL _____ %	SL _____ %
Right Ear						
Effective Masking in Left Ear		dB EM	dB EM		dB EM	dB EM
Left Ear						
Effective Masking in Right Ear		dB EM	dB EM		dB EM	dB EM

COMMENTS:

_____

_____

_____

_____

_____

_____

_____

_____

C. When to Mask: Pure-Tone Bone-Conduction Audiometry

Masked air-conduction thresholds have been obtained at 250 and 1000 Hz in the left ear using the plateau procedure and are presented on the adjacent audiogram. The final masking level used to obtain masked threshold at each frequency is also reported for the nontest (i.e., right) ear.

Is contralateral masking required when measuring bone-conduction thresholds in either ear?

When comparing unmasked bone-conduction thresholds to air-conduction thresholds, it is important to remember that *masked* air-conduction thresholds are always considered because they represent the true thresholds for that ear. Remember that contralateral masking is required during bone-conduction audiometry whenever comparison of the unmasked bone-conduction threshold (Unmasked BC) and the air-conduction threshold in the test ear (AC_T) at that frequency reveals a potential air-bone gap (AB Gap_T) of 15 dB or greater:

$$AB\ Gap_T \geq 15\ dB?$$
$$AC_T - Unmasked\ BC \geq 15\ dB?$$

Right Ear	AB Gap_T	AB $Gap_T \geq$15 dB?
250 Hz	20 – 15 = 5	No
500 Hz	25 – 20 = 5	No
1000 Hz	20 – 15 = 5	No
2000 Hz	40 – 40 = 0	No
4000 Hz	50 – 45 = 5	No
Left Ear	**AB Gap_T**	**AB $Gap_T \geq$15 dB?**
250 Hz	60 – 15 = 45	Yes
500 Hz	55 – 20 = 35	Yes
1000 Hz	60 – 15 = 45	Yes
2000 Hz	60 – 40 = 20	Yes
4000 Hz	65 – 45 = 20	Yes

Commentary

1. It should be noted that when contralateral masking was applied to the nontest (i.e., right ear) during air-conduction audiometry at 250 and 1000 Hz, masked thresholds were obtained at levels essentially equivalent to the unmasked responses (i.e., within 5 dB). Contralateral masking has confirmed that the unmasked thresholds at 250 and 1000 Hz represented true hearing responses in the left ear. Remember that the introduction of contralateral masking can produce a small threshold shift in the test ear even when masking intensity is insufficient to produce overmasking. The threshold shift that may be produced by "central masking" is generally considered to be about 5 dB. The threshold shift of 5 dB that resulted at 1000 Hz when using contralateral masking may reflect the effect of central masking and probably does not represent a significant shift in hearing. The majority of audiologists do not subtract 5 dB from the obtained threshold in order to compensate for a central masking effect during threshold pure-tone audiometry (Martin et al., 1994). Consequently, we have reported the masked threshold of 60 dB HL at 1000 Hz as the "true" threshold.

D. How Much Masking: Pure-Tone Bone-Conduction Audiometry

We have decided that contralateral masking will be required at all frequencies when measuring bone-conduction thresholds in the left ear. We again will use the plateau procedure for establishing masked pure-tone thresholds. Initial minimum masking levels will be calculated using Martin's (1967, 1974) recommendation:

$$M_{min} = AC_{NT} + OE + 10 \text{ dB}$$

Recall that patients with either normal hearing or a sensorineural hearing loss will exhibit an occlusion effect. The right ear will be covered (i.e., occluded) when contralateral masking is introduced during measurement of masked bone-conduction thresholds in the left ear. Because this patient exhibits a sensorineural (i.e., no evidence of significant air-bone gaps) in the masked (i.e., occluded) ear, she theoretically will exhibit an occlusion effect. In this particular example, we will use *average* values when compensating for the occlusion effect: 30 dB at 250 Hz, 20 dB at 500 Hz, 10 dB at 1000 Hz, and 0 dB at frequencies above 1000 Hz.

$$M_{min} = AC_{NT} + OE + 10 \text{ dB}$$

Left Ear (Test Ear)		How Much Masking (Nontest Ear)?
250 Hz	20 dB HL + 30 dB + 10 dB	60 dB EM
500 Hz	25 dB HL + 20 dB + 10 dB	55 dB EM
1000 Hz	20 dB HL + 10 dB + 10 dB	40 dB EM
2000 Hz	40 dB HL + 0 dB + 10 dB	50 dB EM
4000 Hz	50 dB HL + 0 dB + 10 dB	60 dB EM

We will introduce masking during the plateau procedure using the levels calculated above. Masked bone-conduction responses for the left ear are presented in the next section.

Case 3-DI

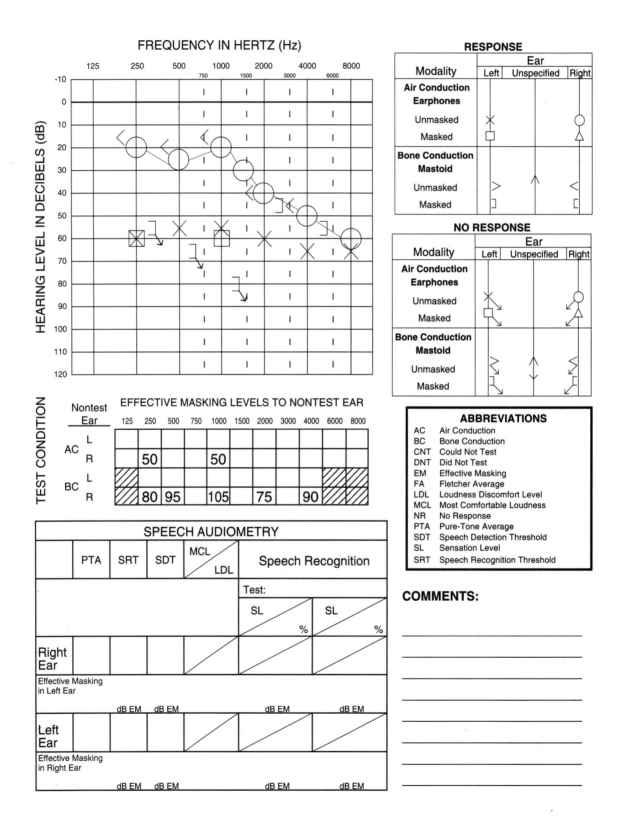

D. How Much Masking: Pure-Tone Bone-Conduction Audiometry (continued)

I. Use of Insert Earphones

A masking plateau was obtained at 2000 and 4000 Hz when measuring bone-conduction thresholds in the left ear. However, a masking plateau could not be obtained at 250, 500, and 1000 Hz. Masked bone-conduction thresholds shifted progressively with each increment in masking level until equipment limits of the pure-tone signal were reached. A masking plateau was not obtained and "no responses" were recorded at equipment limits. The results of masked bone-conduction audiometry in the left ear strongly suggest the possibility of over-masking in the lower frequencies. First, the results of masked bone-conduction audiometry are not consistent with acoustic immittance measurements that suggest the presence of significant conductive pathology in the left ear. Second, "no responses" to bone-conducted sound were obtained at hearing levels significantly greater than the air-conduction thresholds at 500 and 1000 Hz. Although there is variability associated with measurement of bone-conduction thresholds and the air-bone gap (Studebaker, 1967b), theoretically bone-conduction thresholds cannot be poorer than those measured by air conduction. In fact, the progressive shift of a masked bone-conduction threshold to hearing levels greater than the measured air-conduction threshold is a red flag for over-masking. This is particularly evident at 1000 Hz.

The solution to this masking dilemma during bone-conduction audiometry is the use of insert earphones to deliver contralateral masking; we will remeasure bone-conduction thresholds at 250, 500, and 1000 Hz in the left ear. The 3A insert earphone will be used to deliver contralateral masking because of its increased interaural attenuation for air-conducted sound in the low frequencies. Recall from Chapter 8 that interaural attenuation is increased by approximately 35 dB at frequencies of 1000 Hz and below when compared to the traditional supra-aural earphone.

We again will use the plateau procedure for establishing masked pure-tone thresholds. Initial minimum masking levels will be calculated using Martin's (1967, 1974) recommendation:

$$M_{min} = AC_{NT} + OE + 10\ dB$$

Remember that the occlusion effect is minimal when using 3A insert earphones with either deep or intermediate insertion. In this particular example, we again will use *standard* values when compensating for the occlusion effect: 10 dB at 250 Hz and 0 dB at frequencies of 500 Hz and above.

$$M_{min} = AC_{NT} + OE + 10\ dB$$

Left Ear (Test Ear)		How Much Masking (Nontest Ear)?
250 Hz	20 dB HL + 10 dB + 10 dB	40 dB EM
500 Hz	25 dB HL + 0 dB + 10 dB	35 dB EM
1000 Hz	20 dB HL + 0 dB + 10 dB	30 dB EM

The risk of overmasking will be greatly reduced for two reasons. First, smaller correction factors for the occlusion effect will result in lower levels of M_{min}. Second, increased interaural attenuation for the air-conducted masking stimulus will greatly increase M_{max}.

Commentary

1. We will use the 3A insert earphones as plug-in substitutes for the traditional supra-aural earphones. Consequently, it will be necessary to use appropriate correction factors for both dB HL and dB EM (refer to Tables 8-1 and 8-4 in Chapter 8).

Case 3-EI

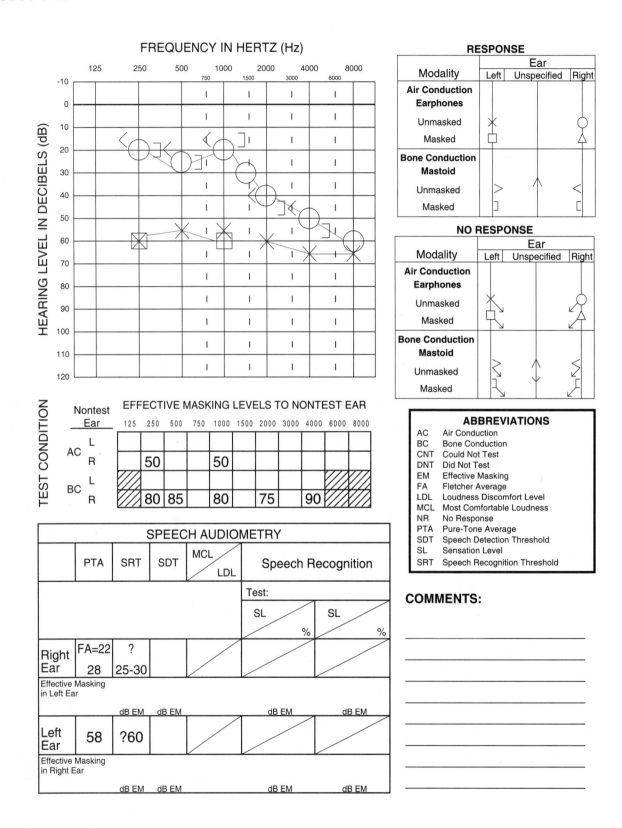

FREQUENCY IN HERTZ (Hz)

HEARING LEVEL IN DECIBELS (dB)

RESPONSE

Modality	Ear		
	Left	Unspecified	Right
Air Conduction Earphones			
Unmasked	X		O
Masked	□		△
Bone Conduction Mastoid			
Unmasked	>	∧	<
Masked	□		□

NO RESPONSE

Modality	Ear		
	Left	Unspecified	Right
Air Conduction Earphones			
Unmasked	X		O
Masked	□		△
Bone Conduction Mastoid			
Unmasked	>	∧	<
Masked	□		□

TEST CONDITION

EFFECTIVE MASKING LEVELS TO NONTEST EAR

Nontest Ear	125	250	500	750	1000	1500	2000	3000	4000	6000	8000
AC L											
AC R		50			50						
BC L											
BC R		80	85		80		75		90		

ABBREVIATIONS

AC Air Conduction
BC Bone Conduction
CNT Could Not Test
DNT Did Not Test
EM Effective Masking
FA Fletcher Average
LDL Loudness Discomfort Level
MCL Most Comfortable Loudness
NR No Response
PTA Pure-Tone Average
SDT Speech Detection Threshold
SL Sensation Level
SRT Speech Recognition Threshold

SPEECH AUDIOMETRY

	PTA	SRT	SDT	MCL / LDL	Speech Recognition		
					Test:		
					SL		SL
						%		%
Right Ear	FA=22 / 28	? / 25-30					
Effective Masking in Left Ear			dB EM	dB EM		dB EM	dB EM
Left Ear	58	?60					
Effective Masking in Right Ear			dB EM	dB EM		dB EM	dB EM

COMMENTS:

_____
_____
_____
_____
_____
_____
_____
_____
_____

E. When to Mask: Threshold Speech Audiometry

I. Use of Insert Earphones

Masked bone-conduction thresholds have been obtained in the left ear using the plateau procedure and are presented on the adjacent audiogram (see Commentary 1 below). The final masking levels used to obtain masked thresholds at each frequency are also reported for the nontest (i.e., right) ear. Recall that masked bone-conduction thresholds were remeasured at 250, 500, and 1000 Hz using the 3A insert earphone for delivering contralateral masking; masked bone-conduction thresholds at 2000 and 4000 Hz were obtained using the standard supra-aural earphone for presentation of contralateral masking. When using the 3A insert earphone for contralateral masking, it was possible to establish a masking plateau when measuring bone-conduction thresholds because of the elimination of overmasking. *Masked bone-conduction thresholds now indicate the presence of air-bone gaps ranging from 30 to 45 dB in the low frequencies, a finding consistent with the patient's case history and the results of acoustic immittance.*

It should be noted that pure-tone audiometry reveals a moderate-to-severe hearing loss in the left ear with relatively good bone-conduction hearing sensitivity in the lower frequencies. To avoid the need for contralateral masking and to reduce the potential for overmasking when contralateral masking is required during speech audiometry, we will continue to use the 3A insert earphones for the remainder of the audiological evaluation.

Is contralateral masking required when obtaining speech recognition threshold in either ear?

Based on the pure-tone averages, it is predicted that SRTs will be measured at approximately 25 to 30 dB HL and 60 dB HL for the right and left ears respectively. Prior to measurement of SRTs, we can predict whether contralateral masking will be required:

$$\text{Presentation level}_T - \text{IA} \geq \text{Best BC}_{NT}$$

Because we are using 3A insert earphones, there will be increased interaural attenuation for speech. Recall from Chapter 8 that 65 dB is a conservative estimate of interaural attenuation for spondaic words. We have increased interaural attenuation by 20 dB by using insert earphones rather than the conventional supra-aural configuration. *We will use 65 dB as our estimate of interaural attenuation for spondaic words (and the more conservative value of 55 dB when subsequently measuring suprathreshold speech recognition).*

Right Ear	30 dB HL – 65 dB ≥ 15 dB HL (1000 Hz)?	
	–35 dB HL ≥ 15 dB HL?	*No*
Left Ear	60 dB HL– 65 dB ≥ 15 dB HL (250, 1000 Hz)?	
	–5 dB HL ≥ 15 dB HL?	*No*

There will be no need for contralateral masking when measuring the SRT in either ear. The predicted level of the cross-hearing signal is lower than the best bone-conduction threshold in the nontest ear.

Commentary

1. The need for contralateral masking was eliminated during measurement of speech recognition thresholds because of the use of 3A insert earphones. A different situation would have resulted if traditional supra-aural earphones were used. We will use a value of 45 dB as our estimate of interaural attenuation when making a decision about the need for contralateral masking when measuring the SRT:

Right Ear	30 dB HL – 45 dB ≥ 15 dB HL (1000 Hz)?	
	–15 dB HL ≥ 15 dB HL?	*No*
Left Ear	60 dB HL – 45 dB ≥ 15 dB HL (250, 1000 Hz)?	
	15 dB HL ≥ 15 dB HL?	*Yes*

If supra-aural earphones had been used, contralateral masking would have been required when measuring the SRT in the left ear. Because of increased interaural attenuation of 3A insert earphones, however, the need for contralateral masking was eliminated.

Case 3-GHI

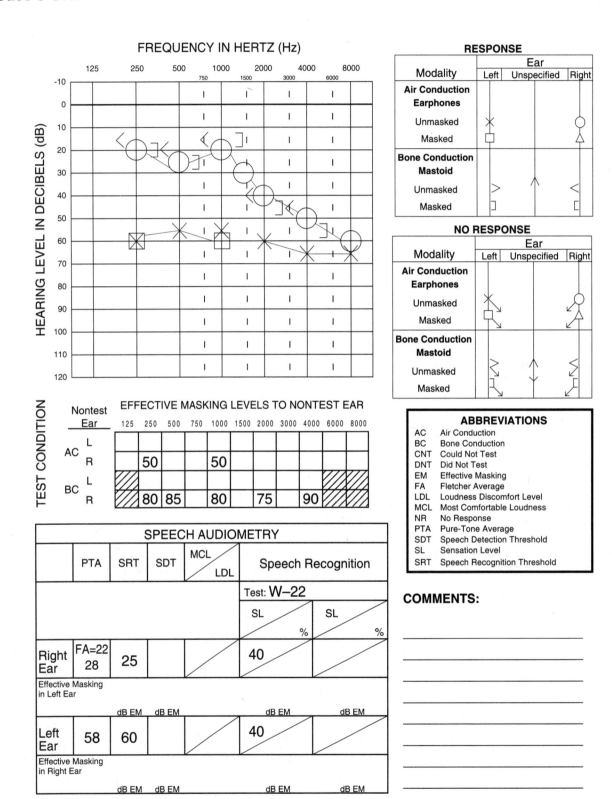

FREQUENCY IN HERTZ (Hz)

	RESPONSE		
		Ear	
Modality	Left	Unspecified	Right
Air Conduction Earphones			
Unmasked	╳		◯
Masked	▢		△
Bone Conduction Mastoid			
Unmasked	>	∧	<
Masked	⊐		⊏

	NO RESPONSE		
		Ear	
Modality	Left	Unspecified	Right
Air Conduction Earphones			
Unmasked	╳		◯
Masked	▢		△
Bone Conduction Mastoid			
Unmasked	>	∧	<
Masked	⊐		⊏

EFFECTIVE MASKING LEVELS TO NONTEST EAR

Nontest Ear	125	250	500	750	1000	1500	2000	3000	4000	6000	8000
AC L											
AC R		50			50						
BC L											
BC R		80	85		80		75		90		

ABBREVIATIONS

AC	Air Conduction
BC	Bone Conduction
CNT	Could Not Test
DNT	Did Not Test
EM	Effective Masking
FA	Fletcher Average
LDL	Loudness Discomfort Level
MCL	Most Comfortable Loudness
NR	No Response
PTA	Pure-Tone Average
SDT	Speech Detection Threshold
SL	Sensation Level
SRT	Speech Recognition Threshold

SPEECH AUDIOMETRY

	PTA	SRT	SDT	MCL / LDL	Speech Recognition	
					Test: W–22	
					SL / %	SL / %
Right Ear	FA=22 28	25			40	
Effective Masking in Left Ear						
		dB EM	dB EM		dB EM	dB EM
Left Ear	58	60			40	
Effective Masking in Right Ear						
		dB EM	dB EM		dB EM	dB EM

COMMENTS:

_____
_____
_____
_____
_____
_____
_____
_____
_____

G. When to Mask: Suprathreshold Speech Audiometry

I. Use of Insert Earphones

Speech recognition thresholds were obtained at 25 dB HL and 60 dB HL in the right and left ears respectively. Suprathreshold speech recognition will be assessed using a traditional, open-set monosyllabic word test: CID W-22. A monitored-live voice presentation will be used. In this particular case, we will present the test words at 40 dB SL re: SRT. The patient reported that speech was presented at a comfortable loudness at 40 dB SL.

Is contralateral masking required when assessing suprathreshold speech recognition ability at 40 dB SL? Recall our rule for when to mask during suprathreshold speech audiometry:

$$\text{Presentation level}_T - IA \geq \text{Best BC}_{NT}$$

Presentation level during suprathreshold speech audiometry is determined by simply adding the selected sensation level (e.g., 40 dB SL) to the measured SRT in the test ear:

Right Ear	Presentation level = 25 dB HL + 40 dB SL = 65 dB HL
Left Ear	Presentation level = 60 dB HL + 40 dB SL = 100 dB HL

In this example, we will use the very conservative value of 55 dB as our estimate of interaural attenuation for suprathreshold speech. Recall from Chapters 4 and 8 that there is some evidence that a more conservative estimate of interaural attenuation should be used when measuring suprathreshold speech recognition. More specifically, we will use a 10-dB more conservative value of interaural attenuation than that used for the SRT (i.e., IA of 65 dB – 10 dB = 55 dB). Is contralateral masking required in either ear?

Right Ear	65 dB HL – 55 dB ≥ 15 dB HL?	
	10 dB HL ≥ 15 dB HL?	*No*
Left Ear	100 dB HL – 55 dB ≥ 15 dB HL?	
	45 dB HL ≥ 15 dB HL?	*Yes*

Contralateral masking will be required when assessing suprathreshold speech recognition ability in the left ear. This is not unexpected given the high presentation level in the left ear (i.e., 100 dB HL) and the relative good bone-conduction sensitivity in the low frequencies in the nontest (i.e., right) ear.

Commentary

1. It should be noted that contralateral masking would also have been required when assessing suprathreshold speech recognition ability in the right ear *if traditional supra-aural earphones had been used*. Remember that when assessing the need for masking using supra-aural earphones, we would use a value of *35 dB* (i.e., interaural attenuation for spondaic words of 45 dB – 10 dB).

	$\text{Presentation level}_T - IA \geq \text{Best BC}_{NT}$	
Right Ear	65 dB HL – 35 dB ≥ 15 dB HL?	
	30 dB HL ≥ 15 dB HL?	*Yes*

The need for contralateral masking when testing the right ear was eliminated because of our use of insert earphones.

H. How Much Masking: Suprathreshold Speech Audiometry

I. Use of Insert Earphones

How much contralateral masking should be used when assessing suprathreshold speech recognition ability in the left ear?

Ideally, the selected masking level should be placed at approximately the middle of the masking plateau (i.e., midplateau). Recall that mid-masking level (M_{mid}) is the midpoint between the minimum (M_{min}) and maximum (M_{max}) masking levels. Mid-masking level can be calculated as follows:

$$M_{mid} = (M_{max} + M_{min}) / 2$$

$$\text{where}$$

$$M_{min} = \text{Presentation level}_T - IA + \text{Max AB Gap}_{NT}$$

$$M_{max} = \text{Best BC}_T + IA - 5 \text{ dB}$$

Bone-conduction sensitivity is always considered at frequencies from 250 through 4000 Hz.

$$\text{Left Ear} \quad M_{min} = 100 \text{ dB HL} - 55 \text{ dB} + 5 \text{ dB}$$
$$= 50 \text{ dB EM}$$
$$M_{max} = 15 \text{ dB HL (at 1000 Hz)} + 55 \text{ dB} - 5 \text{ dB}$$
$$= 65 \text{ dB EM}$$
$$M_{mid} = (65 \text{ dB} + 50 \text{ dB}) / 2$$
$$= 57.5 \text{ dB EM}$$

The mid-masking level is calculated as 57.5 dB EM. Ideally, the selected masking level should be at least 10 dB above the minimum required (i.e., 10 dB safety factor). It should be noted that the estimated width of the masking plateau is very narrow (i.e., only 15 dB). Consequently, there is not much flexibility in selecting an appropriate masking level. In this particular case, a masking level of 60 dB EM is recommended when assessing suprathreshold speech recognition ability in the left ear. In addition to falling approximately at midplateau, a value of 60 dB EM is at least 10 dB above the minimum masking level required and it does not exceed the estimated maximum.

Commentary

1. It was previously stated that contralateral masking would have been required when assessing suprathreshold speech recognition ability in both ears *if supra-aural earphones had been used*. The use of traditional earphones, however, would have resulted in a masking dilemma in both ears. Let us calculate how much contralateral masking would have been required when using supra-aural earphones. Again we will use the mid-masking method. A value of 35 dB will be used as a conservative estimate of interaural attenuation during suprathreshold speech recognition testing when using traditional supra-aural earphones.

$$\text{Right Ear} \quad M_{min} = 65 \text{ dB HL} - 35 \text{ dB} + 45 \text{ dB (at 1000 Hz)}$$
$$= 75 \text{ dB EM}$$
$$M_{max} = 15 \text{ dB HL (at 250, 1000 Hz)} + 35 \text{ dB} - 5 \text{ dB}$$
$$= 45 \text{ dB EM}$$
$$\text{Left Ear} \quad M_{min} = 100 \text{ dB HL} - 35 \text{ dB} + 5 \text{ dB}$$
$$= 70 \text{ dB EM}$$
$$M_{max} = 15 \text{ dB HL (at 1000 Hz)} + 35 \text{ dB} - 5 \text{ dB}$$
$$= 45 \text{ dB EM}$$

In both cases, M_{min} greatly exceeds the estimated M_{max}. Consequently, the minimum required masking level theoretically would result in overmasking. When testing the right ear, a high M_{min} is required because of the large air-bone gap (45 dB at 1000 Hz) that must be compensated for in the nontest (i.e., left) ear. In the left ear, a high M_{min} is required because of the high presentation level (i.e., 100 dB HL). When testing either ear, M_{max} is reduced because of good bone-conduction hearing sensitivity in the low frequencies. The use of 3A insert earphones has avoided a masking dilemma in both ears.

2. Recall that the short-cut approach for selecting an appropriate level of masking during suprathreshold speech audiometry can be used *provided that the following two conditions are met*: (1) There are no *significant* air-bone gaps in either ear; (2) suprathreshold speech recognition is evaluated at a *moderate* sensation level (i.e., approximately 40 dB SL). The short-cut approach for selecting masking level during suprathreshold speech audiometry is not appropriate in this particular example because the first prerequisite has not been met. It is apparent from the pure-tone audiogram that there are significant air-bone gaps in the left ear. The use of the short-cut approach would have resulted in the selection of an inappropriate masking level.

Recall the equation for calculating effective masking level using the short-cut approach:

$$dB\ EM = PL_T - 20\ dB$$

In this case study, contralateral masking is required when assessing suprathreshold speech recognition in the left ear. The effective masking level in the nontest (i.e., right) ear would be calculated as follows using the short-cut approach:

$$100\ dB\ HL - 20\ dB = 80\ dB\ EM$$

Recall our earlier calculations using the midplateau procedure:

$$M_{min} = 50\ dB\ EM$$
$$M_{max} = 65\ dB\ EM$$
$$M_{mid} = 57.5\ dB\ EM$$

It should be apparent that the selected masking level of 80 dB EM calculated using the short-cut approach theoretically could result in overmasking. Although the short-cut approach can simplify the calculations required for determination of the mid-masking level, it should only be used when appropriate (i.e., prerequisite conditions have been met).

Case 3-J

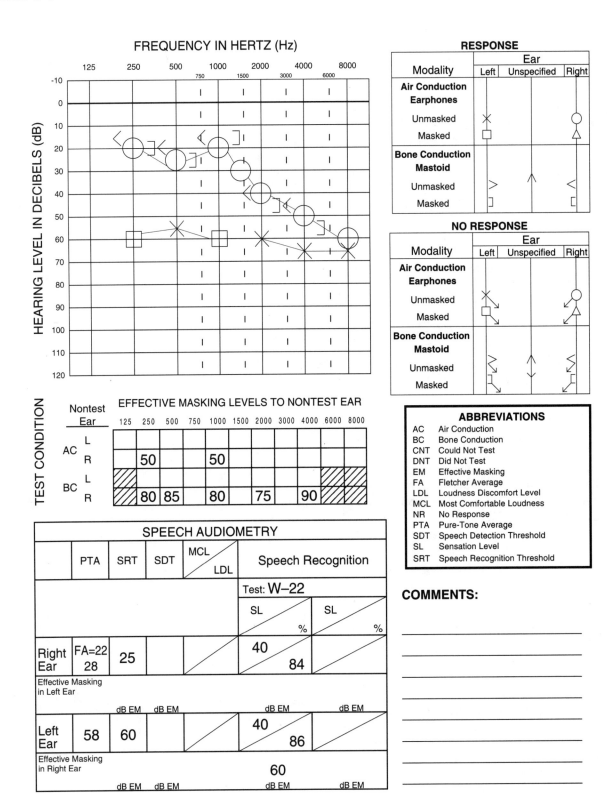

RESPONSE

Modality	Ear		
	Left	Unspecified	Right
Air Conduction Earphones			
Unmasked	X		O
Masked	☐		△
Bone Conduction Mastoid			
Unmasked	>	∧	<
Masked	⸤		⸣

NO RESPONSE

Modality	Ear		
	Left	Unspecified	Right
Air Conduction Earphones			
Unmasked	X		O
Masked	☐		△
Bone Conduction Mastoid			
Unmasked	>	∧	<
Masked	⸤		⸣

ABBREVIATIONS

AC	Air Conduction
BC	Bone Conduction
CNT	Could Not Test
DNT	Did Not Test
EM	Effective Masking
FA	Fletcher Average
LDL	Loudness Discomfort Level
MCL	Most Comfortable Loudness
NR	No Response
PTA	Pure-Tone Average
SDT	Speech Detection Threshold
SL	Sensation Level
SRT	Speech Recognition Threshold

COMMENTS:

_____
_____
_____
_____
_____
_____
_____
_____

J. Audiogram Interpretation

Pure-tone testing revealed borderline normal hearing through 1000 Hz in the right ear, sloping to a mild-to-moderate, sensorineural hearing loss in the high frequencies. There is a moderate-to-severe, mixed hearing loss of flat configuration in the left ear; air-bone gaps of 30 to 45 dB in the low frequencies suggest substantial conductive involvement. Speech recognition thresholds confirmed the pure-tone findings. Suprathreshold word recognition ability assessed using traditional monosyllabic words was good bilaterally.

Tympanometry revealed normal admittance and peak pressure in the right ear. The flat tympanogram with normal equivalent ear canal volume in the left ear is consistent with the medical diagnosis of middle ear effusion. Ipsilateral acoustic reflexes were elicited at normal hearing levels in the right ear, a finding consistent with the presence of cochlear hearing impairment. Absent ipsilateral acoustic reflex thresholds in the left ear and absent contralateral reflexes bilaterally are consistent with conductive pathology in the left ear.

Commentary

1. It should be noted that the bone-conduction thresholds in the left ear are similar to the air-conduction thresholds in the right ear. Therefore, sensorineural acuity is similar in both ears. *Without the addition of the conductive component in the left ear*, it would appear that the hearing loss is symmetrical.

Case 4

History

Your patient is a 73-year-old man who reports a bilateral hearing impairment of gradual onset. He has noted increasing hearing difficulty over the past five years. The patient states that "speech does not sound clear." Although he reports that he can hear people talking, he experiences considerable difficulty understanding speech, particularly in noisy backgrounds. The patient has inquired about the possible benefits of amplification. There is no history of middle ear disorders; other medical history is negative. The results of a recent otologic examination were within normal limits.

Acoustic Immittance Measurements

	Right Ear	Left Ear
Tympanometry		
Static acoustic immittance (mmho)	1.1	1.3
Tympanometric peak pressure (daPa)	–5	–25
Equivalent ear canal volume (mmho)	1.6	1.7
Contralateral Acoustic Reflexes (dB HL)		
500 Hz	95	90
1000 Hz	90	90
2000 Hz	105	110

Tympanometry revealed normal admittance (Van Camp et al., 1986), peak pressure (Silman & Silverman, 1991), and equivalent ear canal volume (Margolis & Heller, 1987) in both ears. The preliminary results of acoustic immittance measurements *do not suggest the presence of significant conductive involvement in either ear*.

Case 4-A

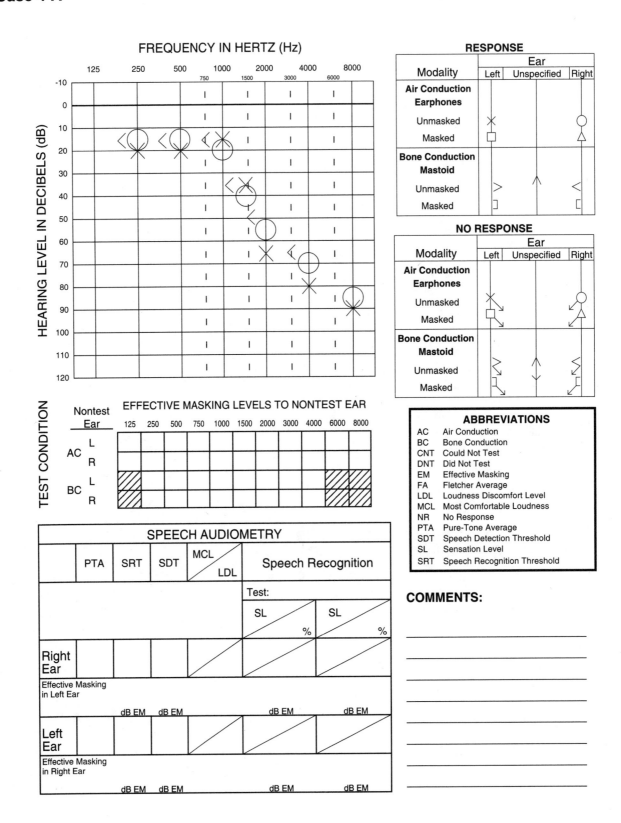

A. When to Mask: Pure-Tone Air-Conduction Audiometry

Is contralateral masking required when measuring air-conduction thresholds in either ear?

Contralateral masking is not required when measuring air-conduction thresholds in either ear: Measured air-conduction thresholds do not equal or exceed bone-conduction threshold in the nontest ear (i.e., unmasked bone-conduction threshold) by the amount of interaural attenuation (i.e., 40 dB). We will use the following equation when making a decision about the need for masking:

$$AC_T - BC_{NT} \geq 40 \text{ dB}$$

Right Ear (Test Ear)		Masking Needed?
250 Hz	$10 - 15 \geq 40$?	No
500 Hz	$15 - 15 \geq 40$?	No
1000 Hz	$20 - 15 \geq 40$?	No
1500 Hz	$40 - 35 \geq 40$?	No
2000 Hz	$55 - 50 \geq 40$?	No
4000 Hz	$70 - 65 \geq 40$?	No
8000 Hz	$85 - 80^* \geq 40$?	No
Left Ear (Test Ear)		**Masking Needed?**
250 Hz	$20 - 15 \geq 40$?	No
500 Hz	$20 - 15 \geq 40$?	No
1000 Hz	$15 - 15 \geq 40$?	No
1500 Hz	$35 - 35 \geq 40$?	No
2000 Hz	$65 - 50 \geq 40$?	No
4000 Hz	$80 - 65 \geq 40$?	No
8000 Hz	$90 - 80^* \geq 40$?	No

*Estimated bone-conduction threshold

Commentary

1. Because bone-conduction thresholds cannot be measured at 8000 Hz, we will need to make some assumptions about bone-conduction sensitivity. It should be noted that the unmasked bone-conduction thresholds interweave with air-conduction thresholds in each ear at frequencies from 250 through 4000 Hz. The difference between the unmasked bone-conduction thresholds and air-conduction thresholds in either ear is small, not exceeding 15 dB. In fact, the largest difference between the unmasked bone-conduction threshold and the air-conduction threshold of the better ear equals 5 dB. Thus, it is reasonable to assume that a similar relationship would also exist at 8000 Hz. Given this assumption, we will use a value of 80 dB HL as our estimate of unmasked bone-conduction threshold.

Case 4-CD

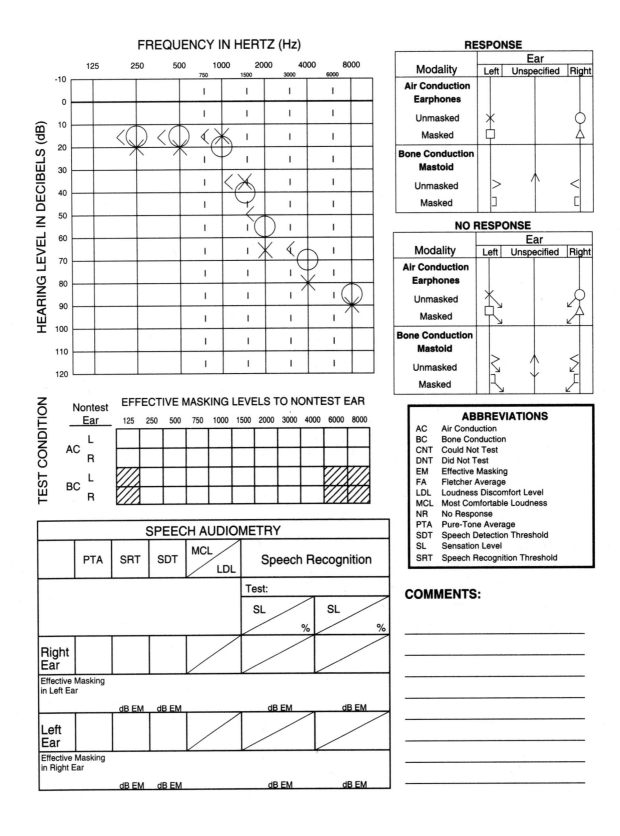

C. When to Mask: Pure-Tone Bone-Conduction Audiometry

It has been decided that masked air-conduction thresholds are not required in either ear.

Is contralateral masking required when measuring bone-conduction thresholds in either ear?

Remember that contralateral masking is required during bone-conduction audiometry whenever comparison of the unmasked bone-conduction threshold (Unmasked BC) and the air-conduction threshold in the test ear (AC_T) at that frequency reveals a potential air-bone gap (AB Gap_T) of 15 dB or greater:

$$AB\ Gap_T \geq 15\ dB?$$

$$AC_T - Unmasked\ BC \geq 15\ dB?$$

Right Ear	AB Gap$_T$	AB Gap$_T$ ≥15 dB?
250 Hz	15 – 15 = 0	No
500 Hz	15 – 15 = 0	No
1000 Hz	20 – 15 = 5	No
1500 Hz	40 – 35 = 5	No
2000 Hz	55 – 50 = 5	No
4000 Hz	70 – 65 = 5	No
Left Ear	**AB Gap$_T$**	**AB Gap$_T$ ≥15 dB?**
250 Hz	20 – 15 = 5	No
500 Hz	20 – 15 = 5	No
1000 Hz	15 – 15 = 0	No
1500 Hz	35 – 35 = 0	No
2000 Hz	65 – 50 = 15	Yes
4000 Hz	80 – 65 = 15	Yes

Masked bone-conduction thresholds will not be required in the right ear; potential air-bone gaps do not equal or exceed 15 dB. However, it will be necessary to use contralateral masking when measuring bone-conduction thresholds at 2000 and 4000 Hz in the left ear.

D. How Much Masking: Pure-Tone Bone-Conduction Audiometry

We have decided that contralateral masking will be required when measuring bone-conduction thresholds at 2000 and 4000 Hz in the left ear. We again will use the plateau procedure for establishing masked pure-tone thresholds. Recall that initial minimum masking level (M_{min}) during bone-conduction audiometry is simply equal to air-conduction threshold of the nontest ear (AC_{NT}) plus compensation for the occlusion effect (OE) plus a safety factor of 10 dB:

$$M_{min} = AC_{NT} + OE + 10\ dB$$

Recall that patients with either normal hearing or a sensorineural hearing loss will exhibit an occlusion effect at frequencies of 1000 Hz and below. Therefore, we do not need to compensate for the occlusion effect in the non-test ear when measuring masked bone-conduction thresholds at 2000 and 4000 Hz.

$$M_{min} = AC_{NT} + OE + 10 \text{ dB}$$

Left Ear (Test Ear)		How Much Masking (Nontest Ear)?
2000 Hz	55 dB HL + 10 dB	65 dB EM
4000 Hz	70 dB HL + 10 dB	80 dB EM

We will introduce masking during the plateau procedure using the levels calculated above.

Case 4-E

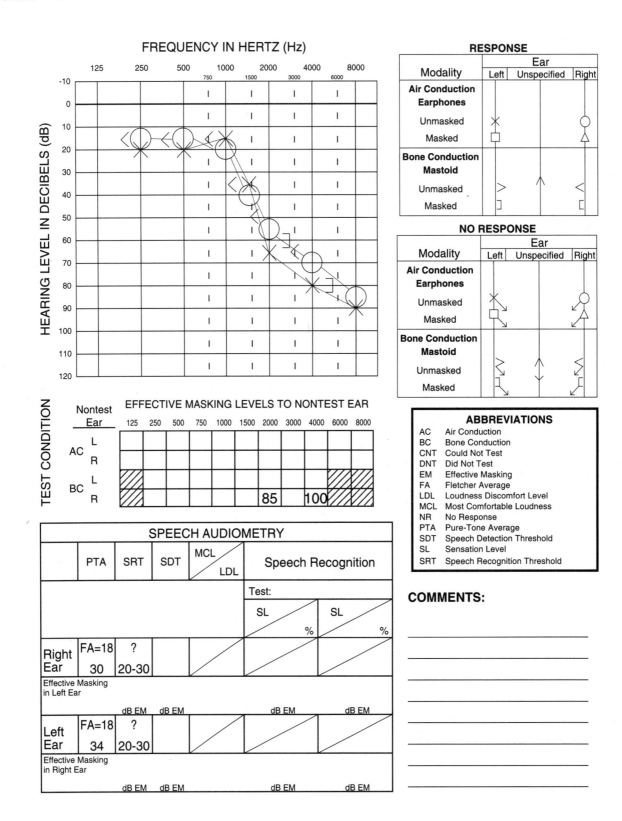

E. When to Mask: Threshold Speech Audiometry

Masked bone-conduction thresholds have been obtained in the left ear at 2000 and 4000 Hz using the plateau procedure and are presented on the adjacent audiogram. The final masking level used to obtain masked threshold at each frequency is also reported for the nontest (i.e., right) ear.

Is contralateral masking required when obtaining speech recognition threshold in either ear?

Based on the pure-tone averages, it is predicted that SRTs will be measured at approximately 20 to 30 dB HL in both ears. Prior to measurement of speech recognition thresholds, we can determine whether contralateral masking is likely to be required:

$$\text{Presentation level}_T - \text{IA} \geq \text{Best BC}_{NT}$$

Recall from Chapter 4 that there are two approaches to selecting interaural attenuation values during speech audiometry. In the first approach, we can use 45 dB as the estimate of interaural attenuation for spondaic words (i.e., SRT) and the more conservative value of 35 dB for suprathreshold speech measures. In the second approach, we can use a single interaural attenuation value of 40 dB for *all* threshold and suprathreshold speech measures. *For this particular case study, we will use a single value of 40 dB as our estimate of interaural attenuation for all speech audiometric measures.*

Right Ear   30 dB HL – 40 dB ≥ 15 dB HL?

–10 dB HL ≥ 15 dB HL?   *No*

Left Ear   30 dB HL – 40 dB ≥ 15 dB HL?

–10 dB HL ≥ 15 dB HL?   *No*

When measuring SRT in either ear, the predicted cross-hearing level of the speech signal reaching the nontest (i.e., left) ear is approximately –10 dB HL. Because the best bone-conduction threshold in the nontest ear is 15 dB HL (unmasked bone-conduction thresholds at 250, 500, and 1000 Hz), theoretically cross hearing cannot occur. Thus, it will not be necessary to use contralateral masking when measuring the SRT in either ear.

Case 4-GH (Part 1)

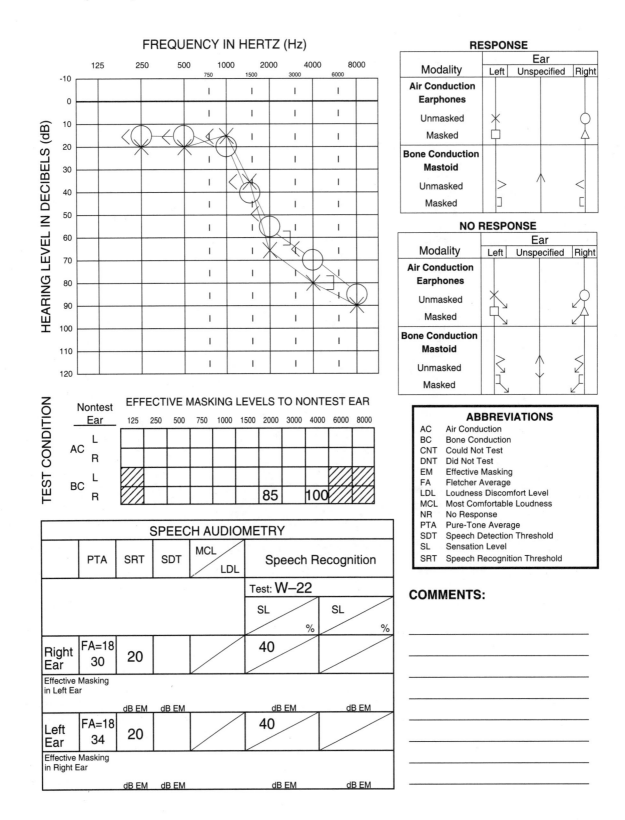

FREQUENCY IN HERTZ (Hz)

HEARING LEVEL IN DECIBELS (dB)

TEST CONDITION

EFFECTIVE MASKING LEVELS TO NONTEST EAR

Nontest Ear		125	250	500	750	1000	1500	2000	3000	4000	6000	8000
AC	L											
	R											
BC	L											
	R							85		100		

RESPONSE

Modality	Ear		
	Left	Unspecified	Right
Air Conduction Earphones			
Unmasked	×		○
Masked	☐		△
Bone Conduction Mastoid			
Unmasked	>	∧	<
Masked	⊐		⊏

NO RESPONSE

Modality	Ear		
	Left	Unspecified	Right
Air Conduction Earphones			
Unmasked	×↙		○↘
Masked	☐↙		△↘
Bone Conduction Mastoid			
Unmasked	>↙	∧↕	<↘
Masked	⊐↙		⊏↘

ABBREVIATIONS

AC	Air Conduction
BC	Bone Conduction
CNT	Could Not Test
DNT	Did Not Test
EM	Effective Masking
FA	Fletcher Average
LDL	Loudness Discomfort Level
MCL	Most Comfortable Loudness
NR	No Response
PTA	Pure-Tone Average
SDT	Speech Detection Threshold
SL	Sensation Level
SRT	Speech Recognition Threshold

SPEECH AUDIOMETRY

	PTA	SRT	SDT	MCL / LDL	Speech Recognition	
					Test: W–22	
					SL / %	SL / %
Right Ear	FA=18 / 30	20			40	
Effective Masking in Left Ear			dB EM	dB EM	dB EM	dB EM
Left Ear	FA=18 / 34	20			40	
Effective Masking in Right Ear			dB EM	dB EM	dB EM	dB EM

COMMENTS:

_____

_____

_____

_____

_____

_____

_____

_____

G. When to Mask: Suprathreshold Speech Audiometry (Part 1)

Suprathreshold speech recognition will be assessed using a traditional, open-set monosyllabic word test: W-22 (Auditec recording). We will present the test words at 40 dB SL re: SRT.

Is contralateral masking required when assessing suprathreshold speech recognition ability at 40 dB SL? Recall our rule for when to mask during suprathreshold speech audiometry:

$$\text{Presentation level}_T - IA \geq \text{Best BC}_{NT}$$

The presentation level during suprathreshold speech audiometry is determined by simply adding the selected sensation level (i.e., 40 dB SL) to the SRT in the test ear .

> Right Ear Presentation level = 20 dB HL + 40 dB SL = 60 dB HL
>
> Left Ear Presentation level = 20 dB HL + 40 dB SL = 60 dB HL

Remember that we will use the value of 40 dB as our estimate of interaural attenuation for suprathreshold speech. Is contralateral masking required in either ear?

> Right Ear 60 dB HL – 40 dB ≥ 15 dB HL?
>
> 20 dB HL ≥ 15 dB HL? *Yes*
>
> Left Ear 60 dB HL – 40 dB ≥ 15 dB HL?
>
> 20 dB HL ≥ 15 dB HL? *Yes*

Contralateral masking will be required when assessing suprathreshold speech recognition ability in both ears.

Commentary

1. Speech recognition thresholds were measured at 20 dB HL bilaterally. These results are consistent with the best two-frequency averages (i.e., the Fletcher Average, FA) in each ear. When there is a sloping audiometric configuration, the SRT typically will correlate with the two-frequency average (i.e., the average of the best *two* air-conduction thresholds at 500, 1000, and 2000 Hz) rather than the pure-tone average (i.e., the average of the air-conduction thresholds at 500, 1000, and 2000 Hz). Stated differently, the SRT will correspond to the better hearing sensitivity in the lower frequencies.

2. There is a common misconception that contralateral masking is not required during assessment of suprathreshold speech recognition whenever there is a symmetrical sensorineural hearing loss. This clearly is not the case as is demonstrated in this particular clinical example. Contralateral masking may be required even when using typical sensation levels (i.e., 40 dB). *Always evaluate the need for contralateral masking during assessment of suprathreshold speech recognition. Never make assumptions!*

H. How Much Masking: Suprathreshold Speech Audiometry (Part 1)

We will use the mid-masking method for selecting an appropriate masking level during assessment of suprathreshold speech recognition. Recall that the mid-masking level (M_{mid}) is the midpoint between the minimum (M_{min}) and the maximum (M_{max}) masking levels. Mid-masking level can be calculated as follows:

$$M_{mid} = (M_{max} + M_{min}) / 2$$

where

$$M_{min} = \text{Presentation level}_T - IA + \text{Max AB Gap}_{NT}$$

$$M_{max} = \text{Best BC}_T + IA - 5 \text{ dB}$$

Remember that bone-conduction sensitivity is always considered at frequencies from 250 through 4000 Hz.

How much contralateral masking should be used when assessing suprathreshold speech recognition ability?

Right Ear M_{min} = 60 dB HL – 40 dB + 5 dB (at 250, 500 Hz)

= 25 dB EM

M_{max} = 15 dB HL (at 250, 500, 1000 Hz) + 40 dB – 5 dB

= 50 dB EM

M_{mid} = (50 dB + 25 dB) / 2

= 37.5 dB EM

Left Ear M_{min} = 60 dB HL – 40 dB + 5 dB (at 1000 Hz)

= 25 dB EM

M_{max} = 15 dB HL (at 250, 500, 1000 Hz) + 40 dB – 5 dB

= 50 dB EM

M_{mid} = (50 dB + 25 dB) / 2

= 37.5 dB EM

The mid-masking level is calculated as 37.5 dB EM. Ideally, the selected masking level should be at least 10 dB above the minimum required (i.e., 10 dB safety factor). In this particular case, a masking level of either 35 or 40 dB EM is appropriate when assessing suprathreshold speech recognition ability in both ears. In addition to falling approximately at midplateau, a value of either 35 or 40 dB EM is at least 10 dB above the minimum masking level required and it does not exceed the estimated maximum. In this particular case, we arbitrarily will select the lower masking level of 35 dB EM.

Commentary

1. The short-cut approach for selecting an appropriate level of masking during suprathreshold speech audiometry can be used *provided that the following two conditions are met*: (a) There are no *significant* air-bone gaps in either ear; and (b) suprathreshold speech recognition is evaluated at a *moderate* sensation level (i.e., approximately 40 dB SL). Given these two prerequisites, the selected masking level typically will occur at midplateau. These two requirements are met in the current example. Consequently, the short-cut approach should prove effective when selecting appropriate masking levels. Effective masking levels are calculated as follows when using the short-cut procedure:

dB EM = PL_T – 20 dB

Right Ear   = 60 dB HL – 20 dB

= 40 dB

Left Ear   = 60 dB HL – 20 dB

= 40 dB

It should be noted that the effective masking levels calculated using the short-cut approach (i.e., 40 dB EM) are essentially the same (within 5 dB) as those values calculated using the midplateau procedure (i.e., 37.5 dB EM). Appropriate levels of masking would have been selected using the short-cut approach in this particular example.

Case 4-GH (Part 2)

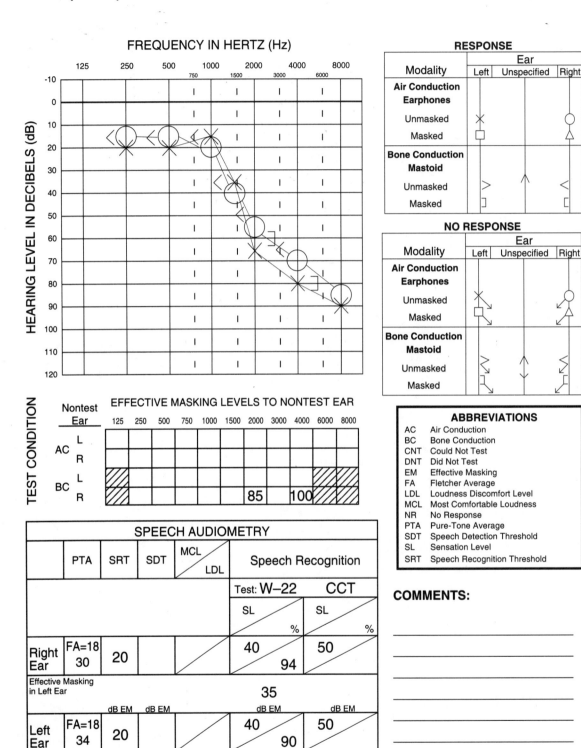

FREQUENCY IN HERTZ (Hz)

HEARING LEVEL IN DECIBELS (dB)

RESPONSE

Modality	Ear		
	Left	Unspecified	Right
Air Conduction Earphones			
Unmasked	✗		◯
Masked	☐		△
Bone Conduction Mastoid			
Unmasked	>	∧	<
Masked	⊐		⊏

NO RESPONSE

Modality	Ear		
	Left	Unspecified	Right
Air Conduction Earphones			
Unmasked	✗↘		◯↙
Masked	☐↘		△↙
Bone Conduction Mastoid			
Unmasked	>↘	∨	<↙
Masked	⊐↘		⊏↙

TEST CONDITION

EFFECTIVE MASKING LEVELS TO NONTEST EAR

Nontest Ear		125	250	500	750	1000	1500	2000	3000	4000	6000	8000
AC	L											
	R											
BC	L	░									░	░
	R	░						85		100	░	░

ABBREVIATIONS

AC	Air Conduction
BC	Bone Conduction
CNT	Could Not Test
DNT	Did Not Test
EM	Effective Masking
FA	Fletcher Average
LDL	Loudness Discomfort Level
MCL	Most Comfortable Loudness
NR	No Response
PTA	Pure-Tone Average
SDT	Speech Detection Threshold
SL	Sensation Level
SRT	Speech Recognition Threshold

SPEECH AUDIOMETRY

	PTA	SRT	SDT	MCL / LDL	Speech Recognition	
					Test: W–22	CCT
					SL / %	SL / %
Right Ear	FA=18 / 30	20			40 / 94	50
Effective Masking in Left Ear					35	
	dB EM	dB EM			dB EM	dB EM
Left Ear	FA=18 / 34	20			40 / 90	50
Effective Masking in Right Ear					35	
	dB EM	dB EM			dB EM	dB EM

COMMENTS:

_____

_____

_____

_____

_____

_____

_____

_____

G. When to Mask: Suprathreshold Speech Audiometry (Part 2)

Suprathreshold speech recognition was excellent bilaterally when measured using traditional, monosyllabic word lists. Yet this patient reports difficulty understanding speech in everyday life. It has been reported that patients with high-frequency, sensorineural hearing impairment often will achieve high scores on traditional (i.e., W-22, NU-6) monosyllabic word tests (Schwartz & Surr, 1979; Sher & Owens, 1974), yet will exhibit reduced word recognition scores on the California Consonant Test (CCT) (Schwartz & Surr, 1979). The CCT is a multiple-choice, consonant identification test that is comprised of one hundred CNC monosyllabic words presented in a closed-set format. It was developed by Owens and Schubert in 1977 for use with hearing-impaired listeners. Historically, the CCT was based on earlier research on consonant identification by hearing-impaired listeners conducted by Owens and associates. The research of Schwartz and Surr (1979) suggests that the CCT is more sensitive to the phoneme recognition difficulties of listeners with high-frequency, sensorineural hearing loss than the traditional monosyllabic word test NU-6. In addition to using the traditional, monosyllabic speech recognition test W-22, we will also evaluate speech recognition ability using the CCT. The results of Schwartz and Surr (1979) indicate that the performance of both normal-hearing listeners and subjects with high-frequency hearing impairment does not reach asymptote until a sensation level of 50 dB SL. Consequently, we will present the test words at 50 dB SL re: SRT in this particular case. The patient reported that speech was comfortably loud when presented at 50 dB SL.

Is contralateral masking required when assessing suprathreshold speech recognition ability at 50 dB SL?

We have already decided that contralateral masking was required when measuring suprathreshold speech recognition in both ears when presenting W-22 word lists at 40 dB SL. Consequently, we know that contralateral masking will also be required when presenting the CCT (Auditec recording) at a 10-dB higher sensation level (i.e., 50 dB SL). Because speech is being presented at a higher sensation level, there is even greater potential for cross hearing to occur. It actually is not necessary to calculate whether contralateral masking will be required. However, the information that follows will provide additional practice in applying the rules for when to mask.

Recall our rule for when to mask during suprathreshold speech audiometry:

$$\text{Presentation level}_T - IA \geq \text{Best BC}_{NT}$$

The presentation level during suprathreshold speech audiometry is determined by adding the selected sensation level (e.g., 50 dB SL) to the SRT in the test ear .

Right Ear	Presentation level = 20 dB HL + 50 dB SL = 70 dB HL
Left Ear	Presentation level = 20 dB HL + 50 dB SL = 70 dB HL

Recall that we are using a value of 40 dB as our estimate of interaural attenuation for suprathreshold speech. Is contralateral masking required in either ear?

Right Ear	70 dB HL – 40 dB ≥ 15 dB HL?	
	30 dB HL ≥ 15 dB HL?	*Yes*
Left Ear	70 dB HL – 40 dB ≥ 15 dB HL?	
	30 dB HL ≥ 15 dB HL?	*Yes*

Contralateral masking will be required when assessing suprathreshold speech recognition ability in both ears.

H. How Much Masking: Suprathreshold Speech Audiometry (Part 2)

Remember that the mid-masking level is calculated as follows:

$$M_{mid} = (M_{max} + M_{min}) / 2$$
where
$$M_{min} = \text{Presentation level}_T - IA + \text{Max AB Gap}_{NT}$$
$$M_{max} = \text{Best BC}_T + IA - 5 \text{ dB}$$

How much contralateral masking should be used when assessing suprathreshold speech recognition ability?

Right Ear M_{min} = 70 dB HL – 40 dB + 5 dB (at 250, 500 Hz)

                     = 35 dB EM

           M_{max} = 15 dB HL (at 250, 500,1000 Hz) + 40 dB – 5 dB

                     = 50 dB EM

           M_{mid} = (50 dB + 35 dB) / 2

                     = 42.5 dB EM

Left Ear M_{min} = 70 dB HL – 40 dB + 5 dB (at 1000 Hz)

                     = 35 dB EM

           M_{max} = 15 dB HL (at 250, 500, 1000 Hz) + 40 dB – 5 dB

                     = 50 dB EM

           M_{mid} = (45 dB + 40 dB) / 2

                     = 42.5 dB EM

The mid-masking level is calculated as 42.5 dB EM. Remember that the selected masking level should be at least 10 dB above the minimum required (i.e., 10-dB safety factor). In this particular case, a masking level of 45 dB EM is recommended when assessing suprathreshold speech recognition ability in both ears. In addition to falling approximately at midplateau, a value of 45 dB EM is at least 10 dB above the minimum masking level required and it does not exceed the estimated maximum.

Commentary

1. Previously we determined that when speech (i.e., W-22) was presented at 40 dB SL, M_{min} and M_{max} were estimated to be 25 dB EM and 50 dB EM, respectively; the mid-masking level was calculated as 37.5 dB EM. We now are presenting the CCT at a 10-dB higher sensation level. It should be noted that while M_{min} increases by 10 dB because of the 10-dB higher presentation level, M_{max} remains unchanged. Thus, the mid-masking level will be increased by only 5 dB (i.e., 42.5 dB EM). *It is important to remember that in cases in which more than one presentation level is used, it is necessary to recalculate only M_{min}; M_{max} remains unaffected by changes in presentation level.*

2. The short-cut approach for selecting masking levels during suprathreshold speech audiometry again can be substituted in this example because both required conditions have been met: (a) There are no *significant* air-bone gaps in either ear; and (b) suprathreshold speech recognition is evaluated at a *moderate* (although slightly higher) sensation level (i.e., 50 dB SL). Effective masking levels are calculated as follows when using the short-cut approach:

                     dB EM = PL_T – 20 dB

Right Ear   = 70 dB HL – 20 dB

                      = 50 dB

Left Ear   = 70 dB HL – 20 dB

                      = 50 dB

It should be noted that the effective masking levels calculated using the short-cut approach (i.e., 50 dB EM) are somewhat higher than those values calculated using the midplateau procedure (i.e., 42.5 dB or 45 dB EM). This has occurred because a somewhat higher sensation level (i.e., 50 dB SL) was used. However, appropriate levels of masking would have been selected using the short-cut approach in this particular example: The selected values are relatively close to the mid-masking level and do not exceed M_{max}. Recall from Chapter 6 that the use of the short-cut procedure is not recommended when assessing suprathreshold speech recognition at higher sensation levels (i.e., greater than approximately 50 dB SL) because of the increased likelihood of overmasking. In fact, the disparity between mid-masking level and the value calculated using the short-cut procedure progressively increases when increasing sensation level (above approximately 40 dB SL).

Case 4-J

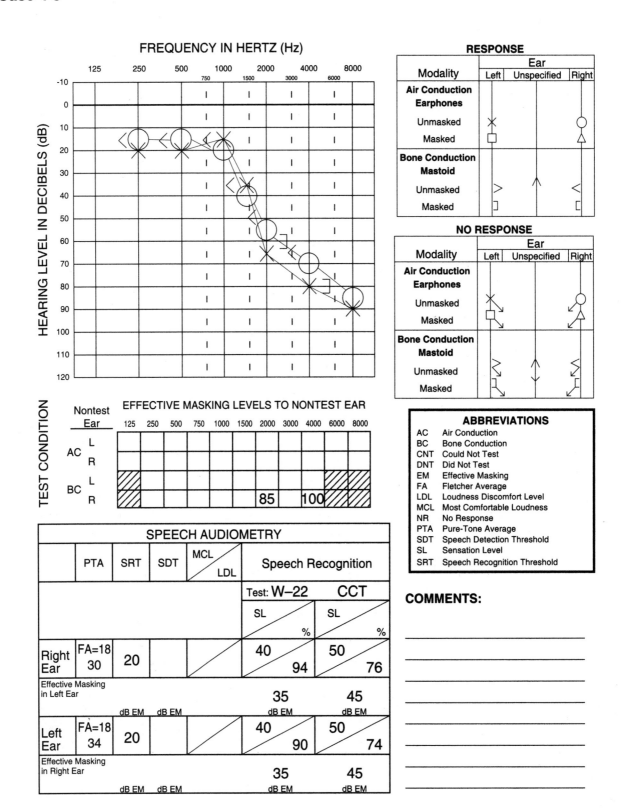

			Ear	
RESPONSE Modality		Left	Unspecified	Right
Air Conduction Earphones				
Unmasked		✕		○
Masked		□		△
Bone Conduction Mastoid				
Unmasked		>	⋀	<
Masked		⊐		⊏

NO RESPONSE

Modality	Left	Unspecified	Right
Air Conduction Earphones			
Unmasked	✕		○
Masked	□		△
Bone Conduction Mastoid			
Unmasked	>	⋀	<
Masked	⊐		⊏

ABBREVIATIONS

AC	Air Conduction
BC	Bone Conduction
CNT	Could Not Test
DNT	Did Not Test
EM	Effective Masking
FA	Fletcher Average
LDL	Loudness Discomfort Level
MCL	Most Comfortable Loudness
NR	No Response
PTA	Pure-Tone Average
SDT	Speech Detection Threshold
SL	Sensation Level
SRT	Speech Recognition Threshold

EFFECTIVE MASKING LEVELS TO NONTEST EAR

Nontest Ear	125	250	500	750	1000	1500	2000	3000	4000	6000	8000
AC L											
AC R											
BC L											
BC R								85	100		

SPEECH AUDIOMETRY

	PTA	SRT	SDT	MCL / LDL	Speech Recognition	
					Test: W–22	CCT
					SL %	SL %
Right Ear	FA=18 30	20			40 / 94	50 / 76
Effective Masking in Left Ear		dB EM	dB EM		35 / dB EM	45 / dB EM
Left Ear	FA=18 34	20			40 / 90	50 / 74
Effective Masking in Right Ear		dB EM	dB EM		35 / dB EM	45 / dB EM

COMMENTS:

_____
_____
_____
_____
_____
_____
_____
_____

J. Audiogram Interpretation

Pure-tone testing revealed borderline normal hearing sensitivity through 1000 Hz, sloping sharply to a severe-to-profound, sensorineural hearing loss in the high frequencies bilaterally. Speech recognition thresholds confirmed the pure-tone findings. Suprathreshold word recognition ability assessed using traditional monosyllabic words (W-22) was excellent bilaterally. Consonant recognition ability was reduced in both ears, however, when measured with the CCT.

Tympanometry revealed normal admittance and peak pressure in both ears. Contralateral acoustic reflex thresholds were elicited at hearing levels consistent with the presence of cochlear hearing impairment bilaterally (Gelfand et al., 1990).

Case 5

History

Your patient is a 28-year-old woman who reports a gradually progressive hearing loss in her left ear for the past three years. No hearing difficulty is reported in the right ear. She also has noted a "ringing" tinnitus in her left ear for the past year. The patient reports that her mother and sister are hearing impaired due to otosclerosis. There is no other history of middle ear disorders; other medical history is negative.

Acoustic Immittance Measurements

	Right Ear	Left Ear
Tympanometry		
Static acoustic immittance (mmho)	0.9	0.4
Tympanometric peak pressure (daPa)	0	−10
Equivalent ear canal volume (mmho)	0.9	0.8
Contralateral Acoustic Reflexes (dB HL)		
500 Hz	NR	NR
1000 Hz	NR	NR
2000 Hz	NR	NR
Ipsilateral Acoustic Reflexes (dB HL)		
500 Hz	85	NR
1000 Hz	85	NR
2000 Hz	90	NR

NR = no response

Tympanometry revealed normal static admittance in the right ear and reduced admittance in the left ear (Van Camp et al., 1986); peak pressure (Silman & Silverman, 1991) and equivalent ear canal volume (Margolis & Heller, 1987) were normal bilaterally. Contralateral acoustic reflexes were absent bilaterally. Ipsilateral acoustic reflexes were present at normal hearing levels in the right ear (Wiley et al., 1987) and were absent in the left ear. In summary, the preliminary results of acoustic immittance measurements *may suggest the presence of conductive pathology in the left ear.*

Case 5-AB

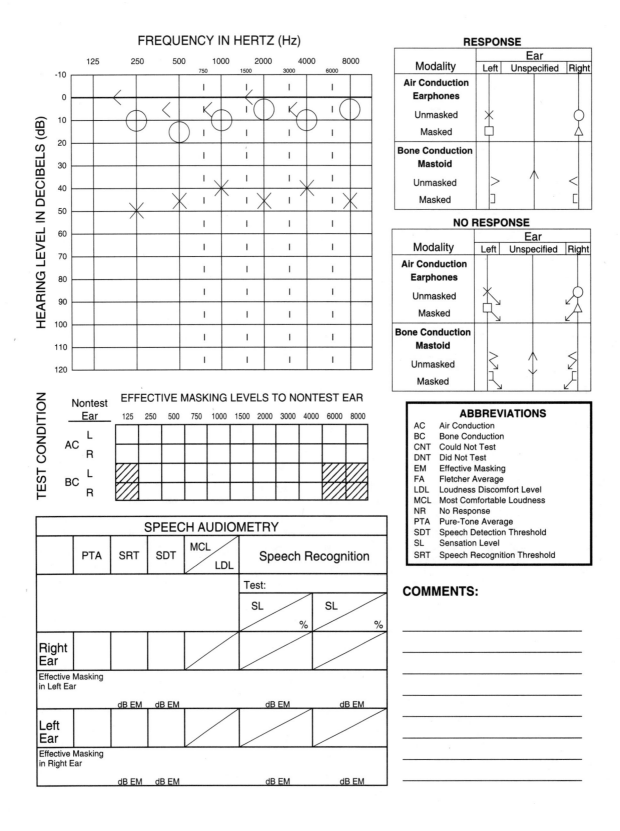

A. When to Mask: Pure-Tone Air-Conduction Audiometry

Is contralateral masking required when measuring air-conduction thresholds in either ear?

Contralateral masking is not required when measuring air-conduction thresholds in the right ear: Measured air-conduction threshold does not equal or exceed bone-conduction threshold in the nontest ear (i.e., unmasked bone-conduction threshold) by the amount of interaural attenuation (i.e., 40 dB). However, contralateral masking will be required when measuring air-conduction thresholds in the right ear. We will use the following equation when making a decision about the need for masking:

$$AC_T - BC_{NT} \geq 40 \text{ dB}$$

Right Ear (Test Ear)		Masking Needed?
250 Hz	$10 - 0 \geq 40?$	No
500 Hz	$15 - 5 \geq 40?$	No
1000 Hz	$10 - 5 \geq 40?$	No
2000 Hz	$5 - 0 \geq 40?$	No
4000 Hz	$10 - 5 \geq 40?$	No
8000 Hz	$5 - 5^* \geq 40?$	No

Left Ear (Test Ear)		Masking Needed?
250 Hz	$50 - 0 \geq 40?$	Yes
500 Hz	$45 - 5 \geq 40?$	Yes
1000 Hz	$40 - 5 \geq 40?$	No
2000 Hz	$45 - 0 \geq 40?$	Yes
4000 Hz	$40 - 5 \geq 40?$	No
8000 Hz	$45 - 5^* \geq 40?$	Yes

*Estimated bone-conduction threshold

Commentary

1. Because bone-conduction thresholds cannot be measured at 8000 Hz, we will make some assumptions about bone-conduction sensitivity. There is normal hearing in the better (i.e., right) ear, and unmasked bone-conduction thresholds do not suggest the presence of significant air-bone gaps in that ear. Thus, it is reasonable to assume that bone-conduction sensitivity at 8000 Hz is approximately equal to the air-conduction threshold of the better ear (i.e., 5 dB HL).

2. Although information about bone-conduction sensitivity ideally is required, we often can make a correct decision about the need to mask during pure-tone air-conduction audiometry by considering only the *air-conduction thresholds* in the two ears:

$$AC_T - AC_{NT} \geq IA$$

Specifically, contralateral masking is required when measuring air-conduction threshold in the poorer ear if the difference between the *unmasked* air-conduction thresholds in the two ears equals or exceeds interaural attenuation (i.e., 40 dB). In this particular case, there exists a difference of 40 dB or greater between the unmasked air-conduction thresholds at frequencies of 250, 2000, and 8000 Hz; consequently, there is indication that contralateral masking will be required when measuring air-conduction threshold in the poorer (i.e., left) ear. However, an unmasked bone-conduction threshold *is* required at 500 Hz in order to make a correct decision about the need for contralateral masking; comparison of only air-conduction thresholds does not suggest the need for masking.

B. How Much Masking: Pure-Tone Air-Conduction Audiometry

We have decided that contralateral masking will be required when measuring air-conduction thresholds at 250, 500, 2000, and 8000 Hz in the left ear. We will use the plateau procedure for establishing masked pure-tone thresholds. We will calculate initial minimum masking levels using Martin's (1967, 1974) recommendation. Recall that the initial minimum masking level (M_{min}) is simply equal to air-conduction threshold of the nontest ear (AC_{NT}) plus a safety factor of 10 dB:

$$M_{min} = AC_{NT} + 10 \text{ dB}$$

Left Ear (Test Ear)		How Much Masking (Nontest Ear)?
250 Hz	10 dB HL + 10 dB	20 dB EM
500 Hz	15 dB HL + 10 dB	25 dB EM
2000 Hz	5 dB HL + 10 dB	15 dB EM
8000 Hz	5 dB HL + 10 dB	15 dB EM

We will introduce masking during the plateau procedure using the levels calculated above.

Case 5-CD

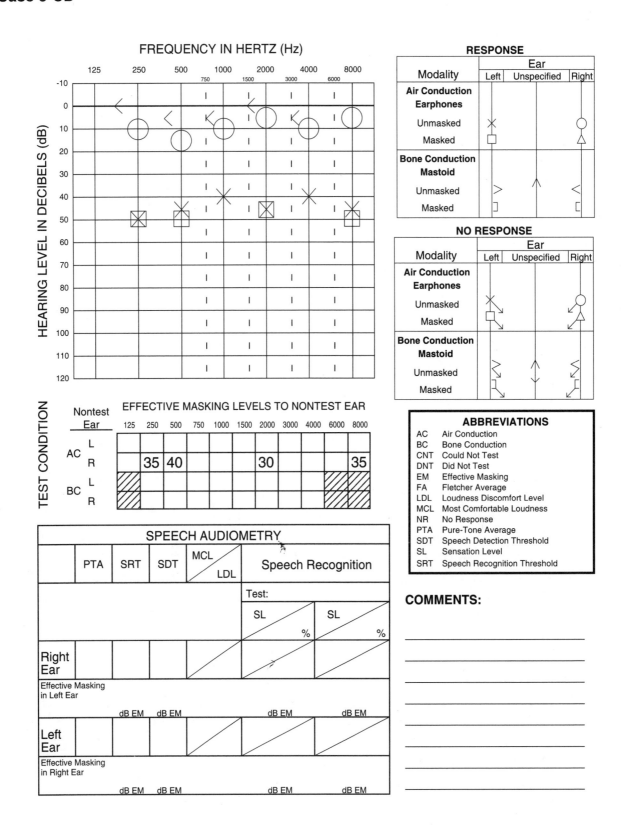

FREQUENCY IN HERTZ (Hz)

RESPONSE

Modality	Ear		
	Left	Unspecified	Right
Air Conduction Earphones			
Unmasked	✕		◯
Masked	☐		△
Bone Conduction Mastoid			
Unmasked	>	∧	<
Masked	☐		☐

NO RESPONSE

Modality	Ear		
	Left	Unspecified	Right
Air Conduction Earphones			
Unmasked	✕		◯
Masked	☐		△
Bone Conduction Mastoid			
Unmasked	⌄	∨	⌄
Masked			

ABBREVIATIONS

AC	Air Conduction
BC	Bone Conduction
CNT	Could Not Test
DNT	Did Not Test
EM	Effective Masking
FA	Fletcher Average
LDL	Loudness Discomfort Level
MCL	Most Comfortable Loudness
NR	No Response
PTA	Pure-Tone Average
SDT	Speech Detection Threshold
SL	Sensation Level
SRT	Speech Recognition Threshold

EFFECTIVE MASKING LEVELS TO NONTEST EAR

Nontest Ear	125	250	500	750	1000	1500	2000	3000	4000	6000	8000
AC L											
AC R		35	40				30				35
BC L											
BC R											

SPEECH AUDIOMETRY

	PTA	SRT	SDT	MCL / LDL	Speech Recognition		
					Test:		
					SL		SL
						%	%
Right Ear							
Effective Masking in Left Ear		dB EM	dB EM		dB EM		dB EM
Left Ear							
Effective Masking in Right Ear		dB EM	dB EM		dB EM		dB EM

COMMENTS:

_____

_____

_____

_____

_____

_____

_____

C. When to Mask: Pure-Tone Bone-Conduction Audiometry

Masked air-conduction thresholds have been obtained in the left ear using the plateau procedure and are presented on the adjacent audiogram. The final masking level used to obtain masked threshold at each frequency is also reported for the nontest (i.e., left) ear.

Is contralateral masking required when measuring bone-conduction thresholds in either ear?

When comparing unmasked bone-conduction thresholds to the air-conduction thresholds, it is important to remember that *masked* air-conduction thresholds are always considered because they represent the true thresholds for that ear. Remember that contralateral masking is required during bone-conduction audiometry whenever comparison of the unmasked bone-conduction threshold (Unmasked BC) and the air-conduction threshold in the test ear (AC_T) at that frequency reveals a potential air-bone gap (AB Gap_T) of 15 dB or greater:

$$AB\ Gap_T \geq 15\ dB?$$
$$AC_T - Unmasked\ BC \geq 15\ dB?$$

Right Ear	AB Gap$_T$	AB Gap$_T$ ≥15 dB?
250 Hz	10 – 0 = 10	No
500 Hz	15 – 5 = 10	No
1000 Hz	10 – 5 = 5	No
2000 Hz	5 – 0 = 5	No
4000 Hz	10 – 5 = 5	No
Left Ear	**AB Gap$_T$**	**AB Gap$_T$ ≥15 dB?**
250 Hz	50 – 0 = 50	Yes
500 Hz	50 – 5 = 45	Yes
1000 Hz	40 – 5 = 35	Yes
2000 Hz	45 – 0 = 45	Yes
4000 Hz	40 – 5 = 35	Yes

D. How Much Masking: Pure-Tone Bone-Conduction Audiometry

We have decided that contralateral masking will be required at all frequencies when measuring bone-conduction thresholds in the left ear. We again will use the plateau procedure for establishing masked pure-tone thresholds. Initial minimum masking levels will be calculated using Martin's (1967, 1974) recommendation. Recall that initial minimum masking level (M_{min}) during bone-conduction audiometry is simply equal to the air-conduction threshold of the nontest ear (AC_{NT}) plus compensation for the occlusion effect (OE) plus a safety factor of 10 dB:

$$M_{min} = AC_{NT} + OE + 10\ dB$$

Recall that patients with either normal hearing or a sensorineural hearing loss will exhibit an occlusion effect. The right ear will be covered (i.e., occluded) when contralateral masking is introduced during measurement of masked bone-conduction thresholds in the left ear. Because this patient exhibits normal hearing (and no evidence of significant air-bone gaps) in the masked (i.e., occluded) ear, she theoretically will exhibit an occlusion effect. In this particular example, we will use *average* values when compensating for the occlusion effect: 30 dB at 250 Hz, 20 dB at 500 Hz, 10 dB at 1000 Hz, and 0 dB at frequencies above 1000 Hz.

$$M_{min} = AC_{NT} + OE + 10 \text{ dB}$$

Left Ear (Test Ear)		How Much Masking (Nontest Ear)?
250 Hz	10 dB HL + 30 dB + 10 dB	50 dB EM
500 Hz	15 dB HL + 20 dB + 10 dB	45 dB EM
1000 Hz	10 dB HL + 10 dB + 10 dB	30 dB EM
2000 Hz	5 dB HL + 0 dB + 10 dB	15 dB EM
4000 Hz	10 dB HL + 0 dB + 10 dB	20 dB EM

We will introduce masking during the plateau procedure using the levels calculated above.

Case 5-EF

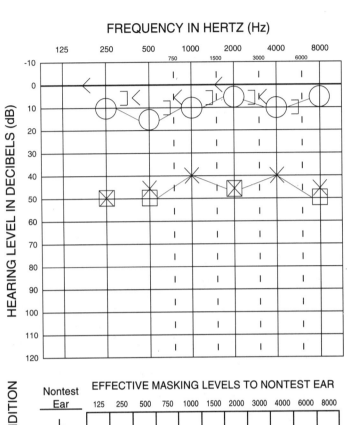

FREQUENCY IN HERTZ (Hz)

HEARING LEVEL IN DECIBELS (dB)

RESPONSE			
	Ear		
Modality	Left	Unspecified	Right
Air Conduction Earphones			
Unmasked	X		O
Masked	□		△
Bone Conduction Mastoid			
Unmasked	>	∧	<
Masked	⊐		⊏

NO RESPONSE			
	Ear		
Modality	Left	Unspecified	Right
Air Conduction Earphones			
Unmasked	X		O
Masked	□		△
Bone Conduction Mastoid			
Unmasked	>	∧	<
Masked	⊐	∨	⊏

TEST CONDITION

EFFECTIVE MASKING LEVELS TO NONTEST EAR

Nontest Ear		125	250	500	750	1000	1500	2000	3000	4000	6000	8000
AC	L											
	R		35	40				30				35
BC	L											
	R		65	60		45		35		45		

ABBREVIATIONS	
AC	Air Conduction
BC	Bone Conduction
CNT	Could Not Test
DNT	Did Not Test
EM	Effective Masking
FA	Fletcher Average
LDL	Loudness Discomfort Level
MCL	Most Comfortable Loudness
NR	No Response
PTA	Pure-Tone Average
SDT	Speech Detection Threshold
SL	Sensation Level
SRT	Speech Recognition Threshold

SPEECH AUDIOMETRY

	PTA	SRT	SDT	MCL / LDL	Speech Recognition	
					Test:	
					SL / %	SL / %
Right Ear	10	?10				
Effective Masking in Left Ear		dB EM	dB EM		dB EM	dB EM
Left Ear	45	?45				
Effective Masking in Right Ear		dB EM	dB EM		dB EM	dB EM

COMMENTS:

_____

_____

_____

_____

_____

_____

_____

_____

E. When to Mask: Threshold Speech Audiometry

Masked bone-conduction thresholds have been obtained in the left ear using the plateau procedure and are presented on the adjacent audiogram. The final masking level used to obtain masked threshold at each frequency is also reported for the nontest (i.e., right) ear. (See Commentary 1 below.)

Is contralateral masking required when obtaining speech recognition threshold in either ear?

Based on the pure-tone averages, it is predicted that SRTs will be measured at approximately 10 dB HL and 45 dB HL for the right and left ears respectively. Prior to measurement of SRTs, we can determine whether contralateral masking will likely be required:

$$\text{Presentation level}_T - IA \geq \text{Best BC}_{NT}$$

Recall from Chapter 4 that there are two approaches to selecting interaural attenuation values during speech audiometry. In the first approach, we can use 45 dB as the estimate of interaural attenuation for spondaic words (i.e., SRT) and the more conservative value of 35 dB for suprathreshold speech measures. In the second approach, we can use a single interaural attenuation value of 40 dB for *all* threshold and suprathreshold speech measures. *For this particular case study, we will use a single value of 40 dB as our estimate of interaural attenuation for all speech audiometric measures.*

Before we determine whether contralateral masking will be required, we need to briefly discuss presentation level. Although the estimated SRT can be used to represent Presentation level$_T$, the procedure that is used to measure SRT must also be considered. Assume that we will be using ASHA's (1988) recommended procedure for measuring the SRT. Recall from Chapter 4 that the test phase involves presenting spondaic words initially at hearing levels approximately 10 dB higher than the calculated SRT. *Patient responses at these higher presentation levels contribute to the calculated SRT. These higher levels must be considered when determining the need for masking.* Consequently, we will add 10 dB to the predicted SRTs of 10 dB HL and 45 dB HL when calculating Presentation level$_T$.

$$\text{Presentation level}_T - IA \geq \text{Best BC}_{NT}$$

Right Ear	20 dB HL – 40 dB ≥ 5 dB HL?	
	–20 dB HL ≥ 5 dB HL?	*No*
Left Ear	55 dB HL – 40 dB ≥ 0 dB HL?	
	15 dB HL ≥ 0 dB HL?	*Yes*

When measuring SRT in the left ear, the predicted cross-hearing level of the speech signal reaching the nontest (i.e., right) ear is 15 dB HL. Because the best bone-conduction threshold in the nontest ear is 0 dB HL, theoretically cross hearing will occur. Therefore, it will be necessary to use contralateral masking when measuring the SRT in the left ear.

There will be no need for contralateral masking, however, when measuring SRT in the right ear. The predicted level of the cross-hearing signal (i.e., –20 dB HL) is considerably lower than the best bone-conduction threshold in the nontest ear (i.e., 5 dB HL).

Commentary

1. There was the possibility of overmasking during the measurement of masked bone-conduction thresholds in this particular case, particularly in the low frequencies. First, bone-conduction sensitivity in the test ear is good; masked bone-conduction thresholds range from 5 to 10 dB HL. Consequently, the risk of overmasking is increased. Recall the equation for calculation of maximum masking (M$_{max}$):

$$M_{max} = BC_T + IA - 5 \text{ dB}$$

It should be evident that M_{max} is proportional to BC_T; that is, the effect of good bone-conduction sensitivity in the test ear is a decrease in M_{max}. Second, high initial masking levels were required in the low frequencies because of the correction factor for the occlusion effect. Yet, overmasking did not occur.

Consider the results obtained at 250 Hz. Contralateral masking levels as high as 65 dB EM were used in the right ear. Overmasking would have occurred *if certain assumptions proved correct*. Let us calculate M_{max} at 250 Hz:

$$M_{max} = BC_T + IA - 5 \text{ dB}$$
$$= 5 \text{ dB HL} + 50 \text{ dB} - 5 \text{ dB}$$
$$= 50 \text{ dB EM}$$

The masked bone-conduction threshold in the left ear is 5 dB HL and represents BC_T. We will use 50 dB as our estimate of interaural attenuation (IA). This is estimated by comparing the unmasked bone-conduction threshold (i.e., 0 dB HL) to the unmasked air-conduction threshold in the left ear (i.e., 50 dB HL). Pure-tone results suggest that interaural attenuation for air-conducted sound at 250 Hz is equal to 50 dB or greater; a value of 50 dB is considered a more accurate estimate of interaural attenuation at this frequency than the standard value of 40 dB. Given this assumption about interaural attenuation, overmasking would occur when contralateral masking exceeds 50 dB EM (i.e., M_{max}). Yet a masking plateau was achieved using masking levels (i.e., 65 dB EM) that *exceeded* the estimated M_{max}. Thus, we can assume that the actual interaural attenuation for this patient probably exceeded the estimated value of 50 dB. The ability to establish a masking plateau is strong evidence that overmasking is not occurring.

F. How Much Masking: Threshold Speech Audiometry

We have decided that contralateral masking will be required when measuring speech recognition threshold in the left ear. Recall from Chapter 6 that we can use either a psychoacoustic or acoustic approach when determining masking requirements during assessment of SRT. In this example, we will use an acoustic approach. That is, the required masking level is derived by calculating the estimated levels of the test and maker signals in the test and nontest ears. Specifically, we will calculate the mid-masking level:

$$M_{mid} = (M_{max} + M_{min}) / 2$$
$$\text{where}$$
$$M_{min} = \text{Presentation level}_T - IA + \text{Max AB Gap}_{NT}$$
$$M_{max} = \text{Best } BC_T + IA - 5 \text{ dB}$$

How much contralateral masking should be used when measuring speech recognition threshold in the left ear?

$$M_{min} = 55 \text{ dB HL} - 40 \text{ dB} + 10 \text{ dB (at 250, 500 Hz)}$$
$$= 25 \text{ dB EM}$$
$$M_{max} = 5 \text{ dB HL} + 40 \text{ dB} - 5 \text{ dB}$$
$$= 40 \text{ dB EM}$$
$$M_{mid} = (40 \text{ dB} + 25 \text{ dB}) / 2$$
$$= 32.5 \text{ dB EM}$$

The mid-masking level is calculated as 32.5 dB EM. A masking level of 35 dB EM is recommended. In addition to falling approximately at midplateau, a value of 35 dB EM is at least 10 dB above the minimum masking level required (i.e., 10 dB safety factor), and it does not exceed the estimated maximum.

Case 5-GH

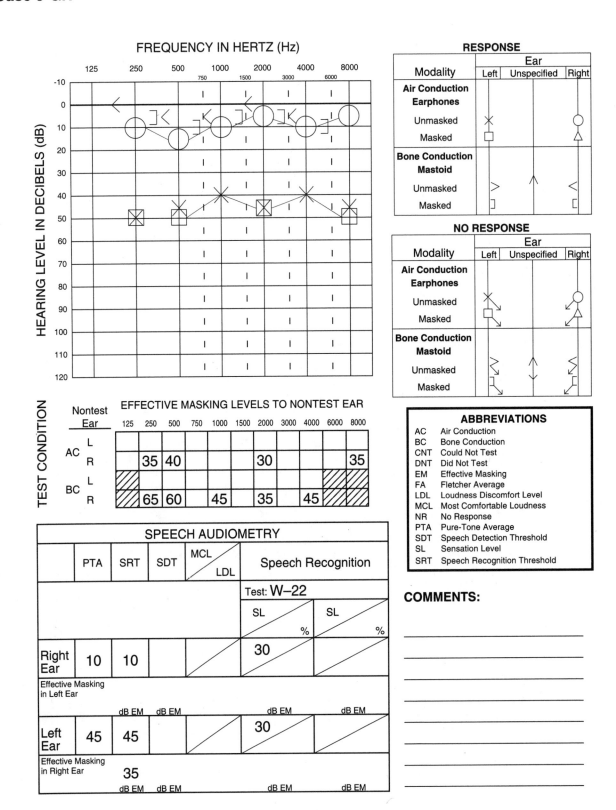

FREQUENCY IN HERTZ (Hz)

HEARING LEVEL IN DECIBELS (dB)

EFFECTIVE MASKING LEVELS TO NONTEST EAR

TEST CONDITION

Nontest Ear		125	250	500	750	1000	1500	2000	3000	4000	6000	8000
AC	L											
	R		35	40				30				35
BC	L											
	R		65	60		45		35		45		

RESPONSE

Modality	Ear		
	Left	Unspecified	Right
Air Conduction Earphones			
Unmasked	✕		◯
Masked	☐		△
Bone Conduction Mastoid			
Unmasked	>	∧	<
Masked	⊐		⊏

NO RESPONSE

Modality	Ear		
	Left	Unspecified	Right
Air Conduction Earphones			
Unmasked	✕		◯
Masked	☐		△
Bone Conduction Mastoid			
Unmasked	>	∧	<
Masked	⊐		⊏

ABBREVIATIONS

AC	Air Conduction
BC	Bone Conduction
CNT	Could Not Test
DNT	Did Not Test
EM	Effective Masking
FA	Fletcher Average
LDL	Loudness Discomfort Level
MCL	Most Comfortable Loudness
NR	No Response
PTA	Pure-Tone Average
SDT	Speech Detection Threshold
SL	Sensation Level
SRT	Speech Recognition Threshold

SPEECH AUDIOMETRY

	PTA	SRT	SDT	MCL / LDL	Speech Recognition
					Test: W–22
					SL ___ % / SL ___ %
Right Ear	10	10			30
Effective Masking in Left Ear					
		dB EM	dB EM		dB EM / dB EM
Left Ear	45	45			30
Effective Masking in Right Ear	35				
		dB EM	dB EM		dB EM / dB EM

COMMENTS:

_____

_____

_____

_____

_____

_____

_____

_____

_____

G. When to Mask: Suprathreshold Speech Audiometry

Suprathreshold speech recognition will be assessed using a traditional, open-set monosyllabic word test: CID W-22 (Auditec recording). In this particular case, we will present the test words at 30 dB SL re: SRT. Speech recognition thresholds were measured at 10 dB HL and 45 dB HL in the right and left ears, respectively. The patient reported that speech was comfortably loud when presented at 30 dB SL.

Is contralateral masking required when assessing suprathreshold speech recognition ability at 30 dB SL?
Recall our rule for when to mask during speech audiometry:

$$\text{Presentation level}_T - IA \geq \text{Best BC}_{NT}$$

The presentation level during suprathreshold speech audiometry is determined by simply adding the selected sensation level (e.g., 30 dB SL) to the test ear SRT.

Right Ear   Presentation level = 10 dB HL + 30 dB SL = 40 dB HL
Left Ear   Presentation level = 45 dB HL + 30 dB SL = 75 dB HL

Recall that in this example we will use a value of 40 dB as our estimate of interaural attenuation for suprathreshold speech. Because the *Auditec recordings* of W-22 are being used to evaluate suprathreshold speech recognition, it probably is not necessary to use a more conservative estimate of interaural attenuation than that used when measuring the SRT (see Chapter 4 for further discussion). Is contralateral masking required in either ear?

Right Ear   40 dB HL – 40 dB ≥ 5 dB HL?
            0 dB HL ≥ 5 dB HL?   *No*
Left Ear   75 dB HL – 40 dB ≥ 0 dB HL?
            35 dB HL ≥ 0 dB HL?   *Yes*

Contralateral masking will be required when assessing suprathreshold speech recognition ability in the left ear. This is not unexpected because contralateral masking was required during *threshold* testing in that ear. Contralateral masking is not required, however, when testing the right ear; the predicted cross-hearing signal of 0 dB HL does not equal or exceed the best bone-conduction threshold of 5 dB HL in the nontest (i.e., left) ear.

Commentary

1. The goal of traditional suprathreshold speech recognition testing under earphones is to evaluate the patient's maximum ability to recognize speech. The highest performance that can be achieved for phonetically/phonemically balanced (PB) monosyllabic words (in percent correct), regardless of intensity level, is called the PB Max. Assuming that the patient has normal hearing, a sensation level of at least 30 dB SL should prove adequate when estimating PB Max using traditional phonetically/phonemically balanced monosyllabic word lists (i.e., W-22, NU-6) (Beattie, Edgerton, & Svihovec, 1977). Remember that the majority of audiologists evaluate suprathreshold speech recognition ability using a sensation level of typically 40 dB (Martin et al., 1994). We selected a sensation level of 30 dB in this particular case to avoid the use of contralateral masking when measuring speech recognition ability in the right ear, a situation that may have resulted in overmasking.

Assume that we had decided to use a sensation level of 40 dB (i.e., a presentation level of 50 dB HL). Contralateral masking would have been required when testing the right ear.

$$\text{Presentation level}_T - IA \geq \text{Best BC}_{NT}$$
Right Ear   50 dB HL – 40 dB ≥ 5 dB HL?
                 10 dB HL ≥ 5 dB HL?   *Yes*

A masking dilemma would have resulted: Estimated M_{min} would exceed M_{max}. How much contralateral masking should be used when assessing suprathreshold speech recognition ability in the right ear?

$$M_{min} = \text{Presentation level}_T - IA + \text{Max AB gap}_{NT}$$
$$M_{max} = \text{Best BC}_T + IA - 5 \text{ dB}$$

Right Ear $M_{min} = 50 \text{ dB HL} - 40 \text{ dB} + 45 \text{ dB (at 250 Hz)}$
$$= 55 \text{ dB EM}$$
$$M_{max} = 5 \text{ dB HL} + 40 \text{ dB} - 5 \text{ dB}$$
$$= 40 \text{ dB EM}$$

The estimated M_{min} of 55 dB EM exceeds M_{max} by 15 dB. The use of a lower sensation level of 30 dB has eliminated the need for contralateral masking when testing the right ear *and* has avoided potential overmasking.

H. How Much Masking: Suprathreshold Speech Audiometry

Ideally, the selected masking level should be placed at approximately the middle of the masking plateau (i.e., midplateau). Recall that the mid-masking level (M_{mid}) is the midpoint between the minimum (M_{min}) and maximum (M_{max}) masking levels. The mid-masking level can be calculated as follows:

$$M_{mid} = (M_{max} + M_{min}) / 2$$
where
$$M_{min} = \text{Presentation level}_T - IA + \text{Max AB Gap}_{NT}$$
$$M_{max} = \text{Best BC}_T + IA - 5 \text{ dB}$$

Remember that bone-conduction sensitivity is always considered at frequencies from 250 through 4000 Hz.

How much contralateral masking should be used when assessing suprathreshold speech recognition ability at 30 dB SL in the left ear?

Left Ear $M_{min} = 75 \text{ dB HL} - 40 \text{ dB} + 10 \text{ dB (at 250, 500 Hz)}$
$$= 45 \text{ dB EM}$$
$$M_{max} = 5 \text{ dB HL} + 40 \text{ dB} - 5 \text{ dB}$$
$$= 40 \text{ dB EM}$$
$$M_{mid} = \text{Cannot be determined } (M_{min} \geq M_{max})$$

A masking dilemma has occurred: M_{min} exceeds M_{max}. One approach to managing this masking dilemma would involve substituting the supra-aural earphones for 3A insert tubephones. Although contralateral masking would still be required when testing the left ear using insert earphones, the masking dilemma would be eliminated (see Commentary 2).

Let us assume, however, that insert earphones are not available. How can we address a potential masking dilemma? Basically, we need to consider the possible effects of overmasking on suprathreshold speech recognition testing. Although overmasking is predicted, it may not actually occur. Our prediction of overmasking is based on the assumption that interaural attenuation for speech is only 40 dB; remember that this is a very conservative estimate that reflects the smallest interaural attenuation value reported in the literature. There is some probability, however, that the actual interaural attenuation for this patient will be greater than the conservative estimate of only 40 dB. If such is the case, M_{max} will be raised, and thus, we may be able to introduce adequate contralateral masking without the risk of overmasking.

If crossover of the masking stimulus to the test ear has in fact occurred, the effects of overmasking should be evaluated. It is important to keep in mind that we are testing *suprathreshold* speech recognition. If the masking stimulus has crossed over to the test ear, what effect, if any, would this have on suprathreshold speech recognition performance?

We can conceptualize the effect of masking noise that has crossed over to the test ear in two ways. First, the masking noise will reduce hearing sensitivity for speech in the test ear; therefore, the effective sensation level of the speech signal will be reduced. Second, the presence of the masking noise in the test ear will reduce the effective signal-to-noise ratio. There is a plethora of research documenting the adverse effects of background noise on suprathreshold speech recognition ability, particularly in sensorineural hearing-impaired listeners (see Nábělek & Nábělek, 1994, for a review). Therefore, the presence of masking noise that has crossed over to the test ear has the potential to reduce suprathreshold speech recognition ability. It is important to keep in mind, however, that the goal of traditional suprathreshold speech recognition testing is to estimate PB Max, that is, the maximum ability to recognize phonetically/phonemically balanced (PB) monosyllabic words. *If your patient exhibits normal suprathreshold speech recognition ability (i.e., 90 to 100 percent correct) in the presence of contralateral masking, there is no evidence that there has been a significant effect of overmasking.* You have met the goal of your suprathreshold speech recognition testing. Conversely, if the patient exhibits reduced speech recognition performance (i.e., less than 90 percent correct), then the possibility of overmasking must be considered.

Let us again consider the current case study. M_{min} and M_{max} are estimated as 45 dB EM and 40 dB EM, respectively. If we use a masking level that is a minimum of 10 dB greater than M_{min} (i.e., 45 dB EM), then theoretically the selected level of 55 dB EM will exceed M_{max} by 15 dB (i.e., M_{min} of 45 dB EM + 10 = 55 dB EM, M_{max} = 45 dB EM). Although overmasking is clearly a possibility, we will proceed and present contralateral masking at 55 dB EM. Remember, there is the *possibility* that interaural attenuation for air-conducted sound will be greater for this particular patient. In addition, an adequate signal-to-noise ratio may be maintained in the test ear, even though cross hearing for the masking stimulus may be occurring. *If the patient obtains a percent correct score within the normal range (i.e., 90 to 100 percent), then it can be concluded that a valid measure of suprathreshold speech recognition has been obtained.* Although cross hearing of the masking noise may be occurring, there is no indication of a detrimental effect on suprathreshold speech recognition in the test ear. Conversely, if the patient exhibits reduced speech recognition performance (e.g., 80 percent), the possibility of overmasking cannot be ruled out. Is reduced performance the result of reduced speech recognition ability, overmasking, or both? Ideally, cross hearing of the masking stimulus should not occur during suprathreshold speech audiometry. It can be tolerated in some clinical situations, however, *if significant effects of overmasking can be ruled out* (i.e., the patient exhibits normal speech recognition ability).

Commentary

1. The short-cut an approach for selecting appropriate level of masking during suprathreshold speech audiometry can be used *provided that the following two conditions are met*: (a) There are no *significant* air-bone gaps in either ear; (b) suprathreshold speech recognition is evaluated at a *moderate* sensation level (i.e., approximately 40 dB SL). The short-cut procedure is not appropriate in this particular example because one of the required conditions has not been met. Although suprathreshold speech recognition is being evaluated at a relatively moderate sensation level (i.e., 30 dB SL), there are significant air-bone gaps in the left ear. Therefore, the use of the short-cut approach would result in the selection of an inappropriate masking level.

Recall the equation for calculating effective masking level using the short-cut approach:

$$dB\ EM = PL_T - 20\ dB$$

In this case study, contralateral masking is required when assessing suprathreshold speech recognition in the left ear. The effective masking level in the nontest (i.e., right) ear would be calculated as follows using the short-cut approach:

$$75\ dB\ HL - 20\ dB = 55\ dB\ EM$$

Recall our earlier calculations using the midplateau procedure:

$$M_{min} = 45 \text{ dB EM}$$
$$M_{max} = 40 \text{ dB EM}$$
$$M_{mid} = \text{Cannot be determined } (M_{min} \geq M_{max})$$

It should be apparent that the masking level of 55 dB EM calculated using the short-cut approach theoretically could result in overmasking (i.e., the selected masking level is 10 dB greater than M_{max}). A masking dilemma also occurred when using the midplateau procedure. However, a major advantage of the midplateau approach is that information is available about minimum and maximum masking levels *and* the possible occurrence of overmasking. Subsequently, the audiologist can make a well-informed decision when selecting appropriate masking levels.

2. Recall from Chapter 8 that interaural attenuation for speech is increased by 20 dB when using 3A insert earphones rather than the traditional supra-aural configuration. If a value of 40 dB is used as our estimate of interaural attenuation for speech when using supra-aural earphones, then a value of 60 dB can be substituted when using the 3A insert earphones. In this particular case, contralateral masking would still be required when measuring suprathreshold speech recognition in the left ear using the insert transducer.

$$\text{Presentation level}_T - IA \geq \text{Best } BC_{NT}?$$
$$75 \text{ dB HL} - 60 \text{ dB} \geq 0 \text{ dB HL}?$$
$$15 \text{ dB HL} \geq 0 \text{ dB HL}? \qquad \textit{Yes}$$

However, a masking dilemma would be avoided. How much contralateral masking should be used when assessing suprathreshold speech recognition in the left ear?

$$M_{mid} = (M_{max} + M_{min}) / 2$$
$$\text{where}$$
$$M_{min} = \text{Presentation Level}_T - IA + \text{Max AB Gap}_{NT}$$
$$M_{max} = \text{Best } BC_T + IA - 5 \text{ dB}$$

Left Ear $\quad M_{min} = 75 \text{ dB HL} - 60 \text{ dB} + 10 \text{ dB (at 250, 500 Hz)}$
$$= 25 \text{ dB EM}$$
$$M_{max} = 5 \text{ dB HL} + 60 \text{ dB} - 5 \text{ dB}$$
$$= 60 \text{ dB EM}$$
$$M_{mid} = (60 \text{ dB} + 25 \text{ dB}) / 2$$
$$= 42.5 \text{ dB EM}$$

The recommended masking level of either 40 or 45 dB EM falls at midplateau, occurs at least 10 dB above M_{min} (i.e., the 10-dB safety factor), *and* will not result in overmasking.

Case 5-J

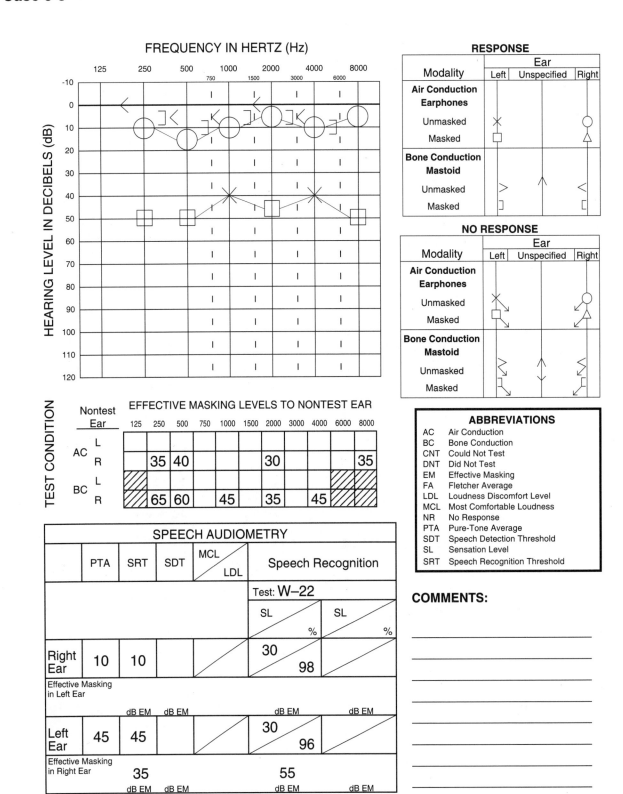

FREQUENCY IN HERTZ (Hz)

HEARING LEVEL IN DECIBELS (dB)

RESPONSE

Modality	Ear		
	Left	Unspecified	Right
Air Conduction Earphones			
Unmasked	×		○
Masked	□		△
Bone Conduction Mastoid			
Unmasked	>	∧	<
Masked	⊐		⊏

NO RESPONSE

Modality	Ear		
	Left	Unspecified	Right
Air Conduction Earphones			
Unmasked	×		○
Masked	□		△
Bone Conduction Mastoid			
Unmasked	>	∨	<
Masked	⊐		⊏

TEST CONDITION

EFFECTIVE MASKING LEVELS TO NONTEST EAR

Nontest Ear		125	250	500	750	1000	1500	2000	3000	4000	6000	8000
AC	L											
	R		35	40				30				35
BC	L											
	R		65	60		45		35		45		

ABBREVIATIONS

AC	Air Conduction
BC	Bone Conduction
CNT	Could Not Test
DNT	Did Not Test
EM	Effective Masking
FA	Fletcher Average
LDL	Loudness Discomfort Level
MCL	Most Comfortable Loudness
NR	No Response
PTA	Pure-Tone Average
SDT	Speech Detection Threshold
SL	Sensation Level
SRT	Speech Recognition Threshold

SPEECH AUDIOMETRY

	PTA	SRT	SDT	MCL / LDL	Speech Recognition
					Test: W–22
					SL / %	SL / %
Right Ear	10	10			30 / 98	
Effective Masking in Left Ear		dB EM	dB EM		dB EM	dB EM
Left Ear	45	45			30 / 96	
Effective Masking in Right Ear		35 dB EM	dB EM		55 dB EM	dB EM

COMMENTS:

_____
_____
_____
_____
_____
_____
_____
_____

J. Audiogram Interpretation

Pure-tone testing revealed normal hearing in the right ear. There is a moderate, conductive hearing loss of flat configuration in the left ear. Speech recognition thresholds confirmed the pure-tone findings. Suprathreshold word recognition ability assessed using traditional monosyllabic words was excellent bilaterally.

Tympanometry revealed normal admittance and peak pressure in the right ear; there was reduced admittance with normal peak pressure in the left ear. Equivalent ear canal volume was normal in both ears. Contralateral acoustic reflexes were absent bilaterally. Ipsilateral acoustic reflexes were present at normal hearing levels in the right ear and were absent in the left ear. The results of acoustic immittance measurements suggest normal middle ear function in the right ear and conductive pathology in the left ear.

Commentary

1. Although the possibility of overmasking was of concern when evaluating suprathreshold speech recognition ability in the left ear, the patient achieved percent correct scores within the normal range. Consequently, *significant* effects of overmasking have been ruled out. If the patient had exhibited reduced speech recognition performance, the possibility of overmasking should be addressed in the audiological report.

Case 6

History

Your patient is a 22-year-old woman who reports a unilateral "total" hearing loss in her left ear of unknown etiology since childhood. She has noted increasing hearing difficulty, however, over the past two weeks following an upper respiratory infection. The results of a recent otologic examination suggested the presence of acute otitis media with effusion in the right ear. The patient also reports two prior occurrences of otitis media in her right ear during the past two years. Other medical history is negative.

Acoustic Immittance Measurements

	Right Ear	Left Ear
Tympanometry		
Static acoustic immittance (mmho)	0.1	1.2
Tympanometric peak pressure (daPa)	—	–5
Equivalent ear canal volume (mmho)	0.8	0.9
Contralateral Acoustic Reflexes (dB HL)		
500 Hz	NR	NR
1000 Hz	NR	NR
2000 Hz	NR	NR
Ipsilateral Acoustic Reflexes (dB HL)		
500 Hz	NR	NR
1000 Hz	NR	NR
2000 Hz	NR	NR

Tympanometry revealed no point of maximum admittance in the right ear (i.e., a "flat" tympanogram) and normal admittance (Van Camp et al., 1986) and peak pressure (Silman & Silverman, 1991) in the left ear. Measures of ear-canal acoustic admittance were within the normal range bilaterally (Margolis & Heller, 1987). Contralateral and ipsilateral acoustic reflexes were absent bilaterally. In summary, the preliminary results of acoustic immittance measurements *suggest the presence of significant conductive pathology in the right ear.*

Case 6-AB

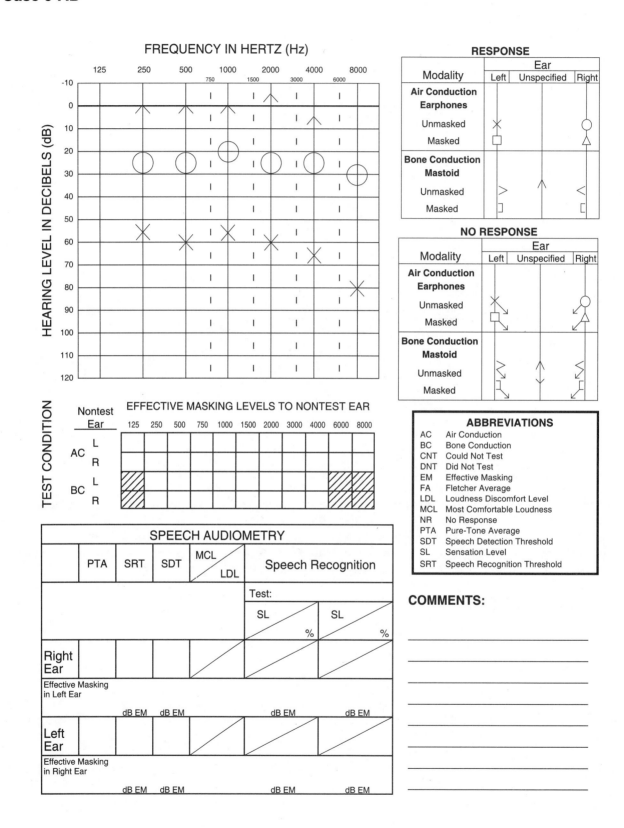

FREQUENCY IN HERTZ (Hz)

RESPONSE

Modality	Ear		
	Left	Unspecified	Right
Air Conduction Earphones			
Unmasked	✕		◯
Masked	⊡		△
Bone Conduction Mastoid			
Unmasked	>	∧	<
Masked	⊐		⊏

NO RESPONSE

Modality	Ear		
	Left	Unspecified	Right
Air Conduction Earphones			
Unmasked	✕↘		◯↙
Masked	⊡↘		↙△↘
Bone Conduction Mastoid			
Unmasked	>↙	∨	<↘
Masked	⊐↙	∨	⊏↙

ABBREVIATIONS

AC	Air Conduction
BC	Bone Conduction
CNT	Could Not Test
DNT	Did Not Test
EM	Effective Masking
FA	Fletcher Average
LDL	Loudness Discomfort Level
MCL	Most Comfortable Loudness
NR	No Response
PTA	Pure-Tone Average
SDT	Speech Detection Threshold
SL	Sensation Level
SRT	Speech Recognition Threshold

EFFECTIVE MASKING LEVELS TO NONTEST EAR

TEST CONDITION

Nontest Ear

		125	250	500	750	1000	1500	2000	3000	4000	6000	8000
AC	L											
	R											
BC	L											
	R											

SPEECH AUDIOMETRY

	PTA	SRT	SDT	MCL / LDL	Speech Recognition	
					Test:	
					SL / %	SL / %
Right Ear						
Effective Masking in Left Ear		dB EM	dB EM		dB EM	dB EM
Left Ear						
Effective Masking in Right Ear		dB EM	dB EM		dB EM	dB EM

COMMENTS:

_____
_____
_____
_____
_____
_____
_____
_____

A. When to Mask: Pure-Tone Air-Conduction Audiometry

Is contralateral masking required when measuring air-conduction thresholds in either ear?
We will use the following equation when making a decision about the need for masking:

$$AC_T - BC_{NT} \geq 40 \text{ dB}$$

Right Ear (Test Ear)		Masking Needed?
250 Hz	25 − 0 ≥ 40?	No
500 Hz	25 − 0 ≥ 40?	No
1000 Hz	20 − 0 ≥ 40?	No
2000 Hz	25 − (−5) ≥ 40?	No
4000 Hz	25 − 5 ≥ 40?	No
8000 Hz	30 − 0* ≥ 40?	No

Left Ear (Test Ear)		Masking Needed?
250 Hz	55 − 0 ≥ 40?	Yes
500 Hz	60 − 0 ≥ 40?	Yes
1000 Hz	55 − 0 ≥ 40?	Yes
2000 Hz	60 − (−5) ≥ 40?	Yes
4000 Hz	65 − 5 ≥ 40?	Yes
8000 Hz	80 − 0* ≥ 40?	Yes

*Estimated bone-conduction threshold

Contralateral masking is not required when measuring air-conduction thresholds in the right ear: Measured air-conduction threshold does not exceed or equal bone-conduction threshold in the nontest ear (i.e., unmasked bone-conduction threshold) by the amount of interaural attenuation (i.e., 40 dB). However, contralateral masking will be required when measuring air-conduction thresholds *at all frequencies* in the left ear.

Commentary

1. Because bone-conduction thresholds cannot be measured at 8000 Hz, we again will make some assumptions about bone-conduction sensitivity. All unmasked bone-conduction thresholds were measured at −5 to 5 dB HL. Thus, it is predicted that unmasked bone-conduction threshold would also occur at approximately 0 dB HL.

2. Although information about bone-conduction sensitivity theoretically is required, we often can make a correct decision about the need to mask during pure-tone air-conduction audiometry by considering only the *air-conduction thresholds* in the two ears:

$$AC_T - AC_{NT} \geq IA$$

Specifically, contralateral masking is required when measuring air-conduction threshold in the poorer ear if the difference between the *unmasked* air-conduction thresholds in the two ears equals or exceeds interaural attenuation (i.e., 40 dB). In this particular case, there exists a difference of 40 dB or greater between the unmasked air-conduction thresholds only at 4000 and 8000 Hz: There already is evidence that contralateral masking will be required when testing the *poorer* ear without consideration of unmasked bone-conduction thresholds. Conversely, the need for contralateral masking when measuring air-conduction thresholds at 250, 500, 1000, and 2000 Hz would not become apparent until unmasked bone-conduction thresholds were obtained: Comparison of *unmasked air-conduction thresholds* between ears does not suggest the need for contralateral masking when testing the poorer ear.

B. How Much Masking: Pure-Tone Air-Conduction Audiometry

We have decided that contralateral masking will be required when measuring air-conduction thresholds at all frequencies in the left ear. We will use the plateau procedure for establishing masked pure-tone thresholds. The initial minimum masking levels will be calculated using Martin's (1967, 1974) recommendation. Recall that the initial minimum masking level (M_{min}) is simply equal to the air-conduction threshold of the nontest ear (AC_{NT}) plus a safety factor of 10 dB to account for intersubject variability with respect to effectiveness of masking levels:

$$M_{min} = AC_{NT} + 10 \text{ dB}$$

Left Ear (Test Ear)		How Much Masking (Nontest Ear)?
250 Hz	25 dB HL + 10 dB	35 dB EM
500 Hz	25 dB HL + 10 dB	35 dB EM
1000 Hz	20 dB HL + 10 dB	30 dB EM
2000 Hz	25 dB HL + 10 dB	35 dB EM
4000 Hz	25 dB HL + 10 dB	35 dB EM
8000 Hz	30 dB HL + 10 dB	40 dB EM

We will introduce masking during the plateau procedure using the levels calculated above.

Case 6-CD

FREQUENCY IN HERTZ (Hz)

EFFECTIVE MASKING LEVELS TO NONTEST EAR

Nontest Ear		125	250	500	750	1000	1500	2000	3000	4000	6000	8000
AC	L											
	R		75	90		95		90		90		65
BC	L											
	R											

RESPONSE

Modality	Ear		
	Left	Unspecified	Right
Air Conduction Earphones			
Unmasked	X		O
Masked	□		△
Bone Conduction Mastoid			
Unmasked	>	∧	<
Masked	⊏		⊐

NO RESPONSE

Modality	Ear		
	Left	Unspecified	Right
Air Conduction Earphones			
Unmasked	X↘		O↓
Masked	□↘		△
Bone Conduction Mastoid			
Unmasked	>↘	∧↓	<↘
Masked	⊏↘		⊐↘

ABBREVIATIONS

AC	Air Conduction
BC	Bone Conduction
CNT	Could Not Test
DNT	Did Not Test
EM	Effective Masking
FA	Fletcher Average
LDL	Loudness Discomfort Level
MCL	Most Comfortable Loudness
NR	No Response
PTA	Pure-Tone Average
SDT	Speech Detection Threshold
SL	Sensation Level
SRT	Speech Recognition Threshold

SPEECH AUDIOMETRY

	PTA	SRT	SDT	MCL / LDL	Speech Recognition		
					Test:		
					SL		SL
						%	%
Right Ear	23						
Effective Masking in Left Ear		dB EM	dB EM		dB EM		dB EM
Left Ear	FA= 108						
Effective Masking in Right Ear		dB EM	dB EM		dB EM		dB EM

COMMENTS:

_____

_____

_____

_____

_____

_____

_____

_____

_____

C. When to Mask: Pure-Tone Bone-Conduction Audiometry

Masked air-conduction thresholds have been obtained in the left ear using the plateau procedure and are presented on the adjacent audiogram. The final masking level used to obtain masked threshold at each frequency is also reported for the nontest (i.e., right) ear. Masked pure-tone audiometry reveals a profound hearing impairment of fragmentary configuration in the left ear. The unmasked air-conduction thresholds in the left ear reflect cross-hearing responses from the right ear.

Is contralateral masking required when measuring bone-conduction thresholds in either ear?

When comparing unmasked bone-conduction thresholds to the air-conduction thresholds, it is important to remember that *masked* air-conduction thresholds are always considered because they represent the true thresholds for that ear. For example, contralateral masking was required at all frequencies when measuring air-conduction thresholds in the left ear. Thus, we must consider the *masked* air-conduction thresholds in the left ear when making a decision about the need for contralateral masking during bone-conduction audiometry in that ear. Remember that contralateral masking is required during bone-conduction audiometry whenever comparison of the unmasked bone-conduction threshold (Unmasked BC) and the air-conduction threshold in the test ear (AC_T) at that frequency reveals a potential air-bone gap (AB Gap$_T$) of 15 dB or greater:

$$AB\ Gap_T \geq 15\ dB?$$
$$AC_T - Unmasked\ BC \geq 15\ dB?$$

Right Ear	AB Gap$_T$	AB Gap$_T$ ≥15 dB?
250 Hz	25 – 0 = 25	Yes
500 Hz	25 – 0 = 25	Yes
1000 Hz	20 – 0 = 20	Yes
2000 Hz	25 – (–5) = 30	Yes
4000 Hz	25 – 5 = 20	Yes
Left Ear	**AB Gap$_T$**	**AB Gap$_T$ ≥15 dB?**
250 Hz	85 – 0 = 80	Yes
500 Hz	100 – 0 = 100	Yes
1000 Hz	115 – 0 = 115	Yes
2000 Hz	120↓ – (–5) > 125	Yes
4000 Hz	120↓ – 5 > 115	Yes

D. How Much Masking: Pure-Tone Bone-Conduction Audiometry

Theoretically, masked bone-conduction thresholds are required in both ears. Yet it is predicted that masked bone-conduction thresholds will only be required in the left ear. It is important to remember that the *maximum* conductive hearing loss will result in air-bone gaps that do not exceed approximately 60 dB. Potential air-bone gaps in the right ear range from 20 to 30 dB. Yet there are potential air-bone gaps in the left ear that are considerably greater than the theoretical maximum of 60 dB (e.g., 80 dB to greater than 125 dB). It is improbable that the unmasked bone-conduction thresholds of –5 dB to 5 dB HL are originating from the left ear. Our knowledge of maximum conductive hearing impairment allows us to rule out this possibility. It is far more likely that the unmasked bone-conduction thresholds are originating from the right ear, a prediction that is also consistent with the results of tympanometry that suggest significant conductive involvement. Therefore, initially we will calculate required masking levels when measuring masked bone-conduction thresholds in the left ear only.

We again will use the plateau procedure to establish masked pure-tone thresholds. The initial minimum masking levels will be calculated using Martin's (1967, 1974) recommendation. Recall that the initial minimum masking level (M_{min}) during bone-conduction audiometry is equal to air-conduction threshold of the nontest ear (AC_{NT}) plus compensation for the occlusion effect (OE) plus a safety factor of 10 dB:

$$M_{min} = AC_{NT} + OE + 10 \text{ dB}$$

Recall that patients with either normal hearing or a sensorineural hearing loss will exhibit an occlusion effect at frequencies of 1000 Hz and below. The right ear will be covered (i.e., occluded) when contralateral masking is introduced during measurement of masked bone-conduction thresholds in the left ear. Because this patient exhibits potentially significant air-bone gaps in the masked (i.e., occluded) ear, she theoretically will not exhibit the occlusion effect. The flat tympanogram (with normal equivalent ear canal volume) also suggests probable conductive involvement in the right (i.e., masked) ear. Thus, there is no indication that the occlusion effect should be compensated for when estimating M_{min}.

$$M_{min} = AC_{NT} + OE + 10 \text{ dB}$$

Left Ear (Test Ear)		How Much Masking (Nontest Ear)?
250 Hz	25 dB HL + OE + 10 dB	35 dB EM
500 Hz	25 dB HL + OE + 10 dB	35 dB EM
1000 Hz	20 dB HL + OE + 10 dB	30 dB EM
2000 Hz	25 dB HL + 10 dB	35 dB EM
4000 Hz	25 dB HL + 10 dB	35 dB EM

We will introduce masking during the plateau procedure using the levels calculated above.

Case 6-EF

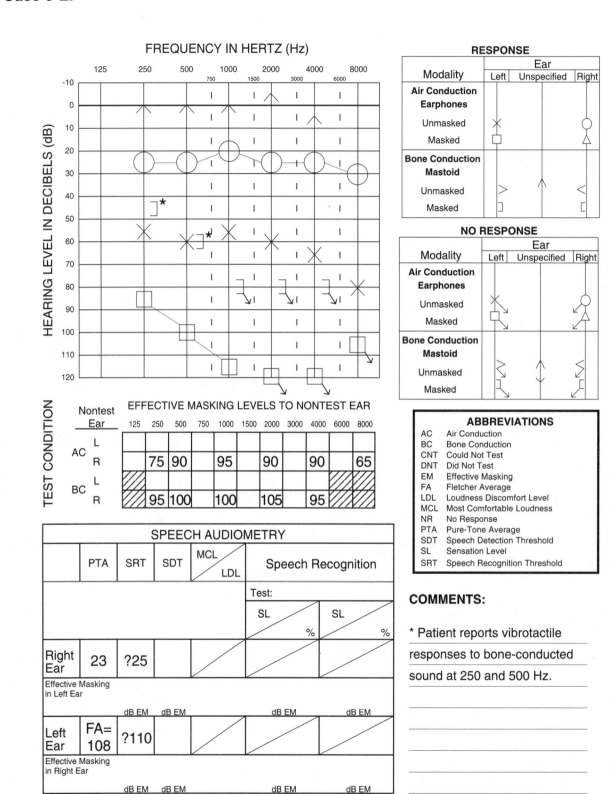

FREQUENCY IN HERTZ (Hz)

EFFECTIVE MASKING LEVELS TO NONTEST EAR

Nontest Ear		125	250	500	750	1000	1500	2000	3000	4000	6000	8000
AC	L											
	R		75	90		95		90		90		65
BC	L											
	R		95	100		100		105		95		

RESPONSE

Modality	Ear		
	Left	Unspecified	Right
Air Conduction Earphones			
Unmasked	✕		◯
Masked	☐		△
Bone Conduction Mastoid			
Unmasked	>	∧	<
Masked	⊐		⊏

NO RESPONSE

Modality	Ear		
	Left	Unspecified	Right
Air Conduction Earphones			
Unmasked	✕↘		◯↙
Masked	☐↘		△↙
Bone Conduction Mastoid			
Unmasked	>↘	↕	<↙
Masked	⊐↘		⊏↙

ABBREVIATIONS

AC	Air Conduction
BC	Bone Conduction
CNT	Could Not Test
DNT	Did Not Test
EM	Effective Masking
FA	Fletcher Average
LDL	Loudness Discomfort Level
MCL	Most Comfortable Loudness
NR	No Response
PTA	Pure-Tone Average
SDT	Speech Detection Threshold
SL	Sensation Level
SRT	Speech Recognition Threshold

SPEECH AUDIOMETRY

	PTA	SRT	SDT	MCL / LDL	Speech Recognition			
					Test:			
					SL	%	SL	%
Right Ear	23	?25						
Effective Masking in Left Ear					dB EM	dB EM	dB EM	dB EM
Left Ear	FA= 108	?110						
Effective Masking in Right Ear					dB EM	dB EM	dB EM	dB EM

COMMENTS:

* Patient reports vibrotactile responses to bone-conducted sound at 250 and 500 Hz.

E. When to Mask: Threshold Speech Audiometry

Masked bone-conduction thresholds have been obtained in the left ear using the plateau procedure and are presented on the adjacent audiogram. The final masking level used to obtain the masked threshold at each frequency is also reported for the nontest (i.e., right) ear.

Masked bone-conduction thresholds were not required when testing the right ear. Masked bone-conduction audiometry revealed bone-conduction responses in the left ear that were significantly poorer than the unmasked responses. In fact, no responses to bone-conducted sound were obtained at equipment limits from 1000 through 4000 Hz. *We have confirmed through the use of contralateral masking that the unmasked bone-conduction responses were not originating from the left ear.* Thus, we can conclude that the unmasked bone-conduction thresholds reflect responses from the right ear. The presence of air-bone gaps in the right ear is supported by the results of tympanometry (i.e., a flat tympanogram) and acoustic reflex tests (i.e., absent ipsilateral acoustic reflex thresholds in the right ear).

Is contralateral masking required when obtaining speech recognition threshold in either ear?

Based on the pure-tone averages, it is predicted that SRTs will be measured at approximately 25 dB HL and 110 dB HL for the right and left ears, respectively. Prior to measurement of speech recognition thresholds, we can determine whether contralateral masking will likely be required:

$$\text{Presentation level}_T - IA \geq \text{Best BC}_{NT}$$

In this example, we will use a value of 45 dB as our estimate of interaural attenuation for spondaic words.

Right Ear	25 dB HL – 45 dB ≥ 85 dB HL?	
	–20 dB HL ≥ 85 dB HL?	*No*
Left Ear	110 dB HL – 45 dB ≥ –5 dB HL?	
	65 dB HL ≥ –5 dB HL?	*Yes*

There will be no need for contralateral masking when measuring the SRT in the right ear. The predicted level of the cross-hearing signal (i.e., –20 dB HL) is considerably lower than the estimated best bone-conduction threshold in the nontest ear (i.e., 85 dB HL at 250 Hz) (see Commentary 3 below for a discussion of the estimate of best bone-conduction threshold). Because of the predicted SRT at a very low intensity level in the right ear and the poor bone-conduction sensitivity in the nontest ear, contralateral masking will not be required.

When measuring SRT in the left ear, however, the predicted cross-hearing level of the speech signal reaching the nontest (i.e., right) ear is 65 dB HL. Because the best bone-conduction threshold in the nontest ear is –5 dB HL, cross hearing theoretically will occur. Therefore, it will be necessary to use contralateral masking when measuring the SRT in the left ear.

Commentary

1. There were no responses to bone-conducted sound at equipment limits at frequencies from 1000 through 4000 Hz in the left ear. Because masked bone-conduction audiometry did not reveal the presence of air-bone gaps in the left ear, it is conventional to assume that the loss is sensorineural in nature. This assumption is consistent with the results of normal tympanometry in the left ear.

2. Bone-conduction responses of 45 dB and 60 dB HL were obtained at 250 and 500 Hz, respectively, in the left ear with contralateral masking. The patient reported, however, that the responses were "vibrotactile" rather than auditory in nature. It has long been documented that high intensity air- and bone-conducted sound can be perceived through the sense of touch (e.g., Boothroyd & Cawkwell, 1970; Nober, 1964, 1970). Boothroyd and Cawkwell (1970) emphasize the importance of noting the intensity levels at which vibrotactile responses can be expected when testing profoundly hearing-impaired subjects. Incorrect interpretation of vibrotactile responses as true auditory thresholds can lead to misdiagnosis of degree (e.g., misinterpreted air-conduction thresholds)

and type (e.g., misinterpreted bone-conducted thresholds) of hearing impairment. Vibrotactile responses are most typical in the low frequencies (i.e., 250 and 500 Hz). For example, the reporting of vibrotactile bone-conduction responses as true auditory thresholds in an individual with a profound hearing impairment (e.g., "false" or "artifactual" air-bone gaps) can lead to the misdiagnosis of a conductive component.

Nober (1964) has demonstrated that vibrotactile bone-conduction thresholds can be differentiated from auditory responses through the use of high-intensity contralateral masking. This procedure is based on the assumption that the high-intensity masking stimulus will shift an auditory threshold, yet will have no effect on a vibrotactile response. Stated differently, the inability to overmask a bone-conduction threshold can suggest that the response is vibrotactile rather than auditory (Rudmin, 1983). Boothroyd and Cawkwell (1970) reported, however, that subjects with unilateral, profound hearing impairment can consistently distinguish vibrotactile from auditory sensations, although there is considerably intersubject variability in vibrotactile sensitivity. Boothroyd and Cawkwell (1970) provide an excellent discussion of vibrotactile thresholds in pure-tone audiometry.

3. We assumed that the best bone-conduction threshold in the left ear was equal to the best air-conduction threshold when making a decision about the need for contralateral masking. It should be noted that vibrotactile responses to bone-conducted sound were obtained at 250 and 500 Hz in the left ear. In addition, there were no responses to bone-conducted sound (at equipment limits) at frequencies of 500 through 4000 Hz. Because of the absence of measured air-bone gaps in the left ear, it is assumed that the hearing impairment is sensorineural. In addition, the results of tympanometry suggest normal middle ear function. Thus, we can assume that bone-conduction thresholds in the left ear would be approximately equal to the air-conduction responses. Because the best air-conduction threshold in the left ear is 85 dB HL at 250 Hz, we are predicting that the best bone-conduction threshold would also be approximately 85 dB HL.

F. How Much Masking: Threshold Speech Audiometry

We have decided that contralateral masking will be required when measuring speech recognition threshold in the left ear. Recall from Chapter 6 that we can use either a psychoacoustic or acoustic approach when determining masking requirements during assessment of SRT. In this example, we will use an acoustic approach. That is, the required masking level is derived by calculating the estimated levels of the test and masker signals in the test and nontest ears. Specifically, we will calculate the mid-masking level:

$$M_{mid} = (M_{max} + M_{min}) / 2$$

where

$$M_{min} = \text{Presentation level}_T - IA + \text{Max AB Gap}_{NT}$$

$$M_{max} = \text{Best BC}_T + IA - 5 \text{ dB}$$

How much contralateral masking should be used when measuring speech recognition threshold in the left ear?

$$M_{min} = 110 \text{ dB HL} - 45 \text{ dB} + 30 \text{ dB (at 2000 Hz)}$$
$$= 95 \text{ dB EM}$$
$$M_{max} = 85 \text{ dB HL (at 250 Hz)} + 45 \text{ dB} - 5 \text{ dB}$$
$$= 125 \text{ dB EM}$$
$$M_{mid} = (125 \text{ dB} + 95 \text{ dB}) / 2$$
$$= 110 \text{ dB EM}$$

The mid-masking level was calculated as 110 dB EM. Because the output limit for speech spectrum noise for our particular audiometer is 105 dB EM, we will present the contralateral masking at 105 dB. This value is considered appropriate because it falls within the vicinity of midplateau. In addition, it takes into account a safety factor of at least 10 dB above the calculated M_{min}.

Prior to establishing the SRT in the left ear, it will be necessary to first familiarize the patient with the spondees. Because the patient exhibits a profound, sensorineural hearing loss, it is expected that she will probably experience difficulty recognizing speech. Only those spondees that the patient can recognize at suprathreshold intensity levels should be included in the set of words used for establishing the SRT. Any spondaic word that the patient cannot recognize should be eliminated from the test list (ASHA, 1988).

We will familiarize the patient with the spondees at 115 dB HL (i.e., the output limit for our particular audiometer), a level only 5 dB above the estimated SRT. In addition, we will present contralateral masking at 105 dB EM, our estimated mid-masking level for establishing the SRT. This masking level should prove adequate because the presentation level of speech during familiarization is only 5 dB greater than the estimated SRT. In addition, the selected masking level of 105 dB EM included a safety factor of 10 dB. (Also keep in mind that 105 dB EM is the greatest output that our audiometer will produce. A higher masking level cannot be used.).

The standard list of thirty-six spondees (CID W-1) was presented using monitored live voice to the left ear at 115 dB HL with 105 dB EM of contralateral masking. The patient was able to correctly recognize only two of the thirty-six spondees (i.e., approximately 6 percent performance). Because a valid SRT cannot be obtained when using a set size of only two spondees (see Commentary 1 below), the speech detection threshold (SDT) will be measured in the left ear. Recall that the SDT is the minimum hearing level for speech at which the patient can just "discern" (i.e., detect) the presence of speech 50 percent of the time (ASHA, 1988).

It is not unexpected that contralateral masking will be required when measuring speech detection threshold in the left ear: There is normal bone-conduction hearing sensitivity in the nontest (i.e., right) ear and a profound hearing impairment in the test (i.e., left ear). Recall that the SDT typically will require 8 to 9 dB less intensity (on the average) than the SRT. If we assume that the estimated SRT would occur at approximately 110 dB HL in the left ear, then it is predicted that the SDT will occur at about 100 dB HL. Recall from Chapter 4 that there is some evidence that a more conservative estimate of interaural attenuation should be used when making decisions about masking requirements during measurement of the SDT. Specifically, a 10-dB more conservative estimate of interaural attenuation is recommended in cases in which the SDT in the poorer ear is being compared to the SRT (or bone-conduction thresholds predictive of the SRT) in the better ear. Consequently, *35 dB will be used as our estimate of interaural attenuation during measurement of the SDT in this particular example.* Recall the rule for when to mask during speech audiometry:

$$\text{Presentation level}_T - \text{IA} \geq \text{Best BC}_{NT}$$

Left Ear	$100 \text{ dB HL} - 35 \text{ dB} \geq -5 \text{ dB HL}?$
	$65 \text{ dB HL} \geq -5 \text{ dB HL}?$ *Yes*

How much contralateral masking should be used when measuring speech detection threshold in the left ear?

We can use either a psychoacoustic or acoustic approach when determining masking requirements during assessment of SDT. In this example, both approaches will be described.

Acoustic Approach   Recall that the required masking level is derived by calculating the estimated levels of the test and maker signals in the test and nontest ears. Mid-masking level can be calculated as follows:

$$M_{min} = 100 \text{ dB HL} - 35 \text{ dB} + 30 \text{ dB (at 2000 Hz)}$$
$$= 95 \text{ dB EM}$$
$$M_{max} = 85 \text{ dB HL (at 250 Hz)} + 35 \text{ dB} - 5 \text{ dB}$$
$$= 115 \text{ dB EM}$$
$$M_{mid} = (115 \text{ dB} + 95 \text{ dB}) / 2$$
$$= 105 \text{ dB EM}$$

The mid-masking level is calculated as 105 dB EM. This value is comparable to the estimated mid-masking level considered appropriate for measuring the SRT. A major advantage of the midplateau approach is that the estimated value of interaural attenuation will not affect the calculated mid-masking level. The value of interaural attenuation will have an equal yet opposite effect on M_{min} and M_{max}, thus, the estimate of M_{mid} is unaltered. We could easily justify using our original mid-masking level for the SRT when estimating the SDT. The SDT will probably occur at a slightly lower intensity level. Therefore, a masking level of 105 dB EM would prove adequate for both the SRT and SDT. Depending on the assumptions about expected SDT and estimated interaural attenuation, it should be apparent that the mid-masking levels for SDT and SRT will typically be very similar.

Psychoacoustic Approach   Psychoacoustic procedures rely on observations of measured threshold shifts in the test ear as a function of masker effective levels in the nontest ear. The plateau procedure can be used during measurement of the SDT. This procedure is described in greater detail in Chapter 6. Very simply, an initial masking level is introduced to the nontest ear. Speech detection threshold is re-established for a series of 10-dB increments in masker level until a plateau of at 20 to 30 dB is reached. Initial masking level for the SDT is calculated as follows:

$$M_{min} = SRT_{NT} + 10 \text{ dB correction factor} + 10 \text{ dB safety factor}$$
$$= SRT_{NT} + 20 \text{ dB}$$

Let us assume that we already have established the SRT in the nontest (i.e., right) ear. We obtained an SRT of 25 dB HL, a finding consistent with the pure-tone findings. The initial masking level is calculated as follows:

$$M_{min} = SRT_{NT} + 20 \text{ dB}$$
$$= 25 \text{ dB HL} + 20 \text{ dB}$$
$$= 45 \text{ dB EM}$$

Use of either the acoustic or psychoacoustic approach will yield a valid estimate of the SDT.

Commentary

1. Punch and Howard (1985) evaluated the effect of set size on the speech recognition threshold. Theoretically, human performance is related to uncertainty of the test stimuli. Performance should improve when the subject is knowledgeable of the possible stimuli. The standard list of spondees, CID Auditory Test W-1, contains thirty-six test items. Punch and Howard measured the SRT in normal-hearing listeners using set sizes ranging from only three to thirty-six spondees (i.e., full list). There was a systematic decrease in the intensity level required for the SRT as the set size used to establish the speech threshold decreased. It was reported, however, that SRTs measured using set sizes of nine words or greater (i.e., nine, eighteen, twenty-seven, and thirty-six spondees) did not differ significantly. This latter finding suggests that a minimum set size of approximately nine spondees is required to obtain a valid measure of the speech recognition threshold.

It is interesting to note that the range in intensity level for the SRT established with the full list of thirty-six spondees versus only three stimuli was *7 dB* (i.e., 19.1 dB SPL for thirty-six spondees versus 12.2 dB SPL for only three spondees). Recall that speech can be detected at a lower intensity than that required to reach the speech recognition threshold; specifically, the SRT requires an average of *8 to 9-dB* greater intensity than the SDT. It appears that the measured SRT approaches the speech detection threshold when only three spondees are used in threshold measurement. If the patient can correctly recognize only a few spondees at suprathreshold levels (as is often the case in an individual with a profound, sensorineural hearing loss), then the SDT will be the more appropriate measure of speech threshold.

Case 6-G

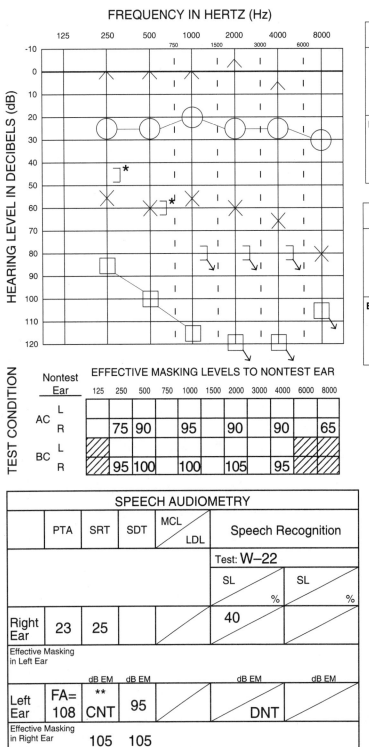

RESPONSE

Modality	Ear		
	Left	Unspecified	Right
Air Conduction Earphones			
Unmasked	✕		○
Masked	☐		△
Bone Conduction Mastoid			
Unmasked	>	∧	<
Masked	☐		☐

NO RESPONSE

Modality	Ear		
	Left	Unspecified	Right
Air Conduction Earphones			
Unmasked	✕↘		○↙
Masked	☐↘		△↙
Bone Conduction Mastoid			
Unmasked	>↘	∧↓	<↙
Masked	☐↘		☐↙

ABBREVIATIONS

AC	Air Conduction
BC	Bone Conduction
CNT	Could Not Test
DNT	Did Not Test
EM	Effective Masking
FA	Fletcher Average
LDL	Loudness Discomfort Level
MCL	Most Comfortable Loudness
NR	No Response
PTA	Pure-Tone Average
SDT	Speech Detection Threshold
SL	Sensation Level
SRT	Speech Recognition Threshold

EFFECTIVE MASKING LEVELS TO NONTEST EAR

Nontest Ear		125	250	500	750	1000	1500	2000	3000	4000	6000	8000
AC	L											
	R		75	90		95		90		90		65
BC	L	▨									▨	
	R	▨	95	100		100		105		95	▨	

SPEECH AUDIOMETRY

	PTA	SRT	SDT	MCL / LDL	Speech Recognition
					Test: W–22
					SL / %	SL / %
Right Ear	23	25			40	
Effective Masking in Left Ear						
		dB EM	dB EM		dB EM	dB EM
Left Ear	FA= 108	** CNT	95		DNT	
Effective Masking in Right Ear	105	105				
	dB EM	dB EM			dB EM	dB EM

COMMENTS:

* Patient reports vibrotactile responses to bone-conducted sound at 250 and 500 Hz.

** Patient was able to correctly recognize 2 of 36 spondees (CID W-1) presented at 115 dB HL.

G. When to Mask: Suprathreshold Speech Audiometry

Speech thresholds were obtained in both ears. An SRT of 25 dB HL was measured in the right ear; the SDT was 95 dB HL in the left ear. Suprathreshold speech recognition will be assessed in the right ear using a live-voice presentation of a traditional, open-set monosyllabic word test: CID W-22. In this particular case, we will present the test words at 40 dB SL re: SRT. The patient reported that speech presented at 40 dB SL was comfortably loud.

Is contralateral masking required when assessing suprathreshold speech recognition ability in the right ear at 40 dB SL?

Recall our rule for when to mask during speech audiometry:

$$\text{Presentation level}_T - IA \geq \text{Best BC}_{NT}$$

The presentation level during suprathreshold speech audiometry is determined simply by adding the selected sensation level (e.g., 40 dB SL) to the test ear SRT.

$$\text{Right Ear} \quad \text{Presentation level} = 25 \text{ dB HL} + 40 \text{ dB SL} = 65 \text{ dB HL}$$

In this example, we will use the very conservative value of 35 dB as our estimate of interaural attenuation for suprathreshold speech (i.e., IA of 45 dB for spondaic words minus a correction factor of 10 dB). Is contralateral masking required?

$$65 \text{ dB HL} - 35 \text{ dB} \geq 85 \text{ dB HL}?$$

$$30 \text{ dB HL} \geq 85 \text{ dB HL}? \quad \textit{No}$$

Contralateral masking will not be required when assessing suprathreshold speech recognition ability in the right ear. This is not unexpected given the profound sensorineural hearing impairment in the left ear. Again, we have used the best air-conduction threshold in the left ear (85 dB HL at 250 Hz) as our estimate of best bone-conduction threshold when determining the need for contralateral masking.

We will not evaluate suprathreshold speech recognition ability using traditional materials (e.g., NU-6, W-22) in the left ear. Recall that the patient earlier was familiarized with spondaic words at suprathreshold in the left ear. The thirty-six spondees of CID W-1 were presented at 115 dB HL; the patient was able to correctly recognize only two of the thirty-six spondees, resulting in percent correct performance of approximately 6 percent. It is known that individuals with profound sensorineural hearing impairment perform more poorly on suprathreshold speech tests using monosyllabic rather than spondaic words (Owens, Kessler, Witte-Raggio, & Schubert, 1985). We already have determined that suprathreshold speech recognition ability using spondaic words is very poor in the left ear. The evaluation of suprathreshold speech recognition using traditional monosyllabic words would not provide additional information about speech recognition ability in this patient. However, we can address this patient's suprathreshold speech recognition ability as assessed with spondaic words in our audiologic report (see Section J, Audiometric Interpretation).

Commentary

1. Many individuals with profound sensorineural hearing impairment will achieve scores of approximately zero percent on standard suprathreshold speech recognition tests (e.g., NU-6, CID W-22). In fact, it is not uncommon for some audiologists to not even attempt measurement of the SRT because of the assumption that speech recognition ability is severely limited or absent. An SDT is often the only speech audiometric measurement obtained. However, there is a wide range of speech perception cues that enable a hearing-impaired individual to derive meaning from a speech signal. There are now a battery of tests available to evaluate the speech perception capabilities of individuals with profound sensorineural hearing impairment. Examples of such tests are the Minimal Auditory Capabilities Battery (MAC) (Owens et al., 1981; Owens et al., 1985) and the Iowa Cochlear Implant Test Battery (Tyler et al., 1985). These test batteries can provide very useful information when evaluating individuals with profound hearing impairment for hearing aid use and when determining aural rehabilitative needs.

Case 6-J

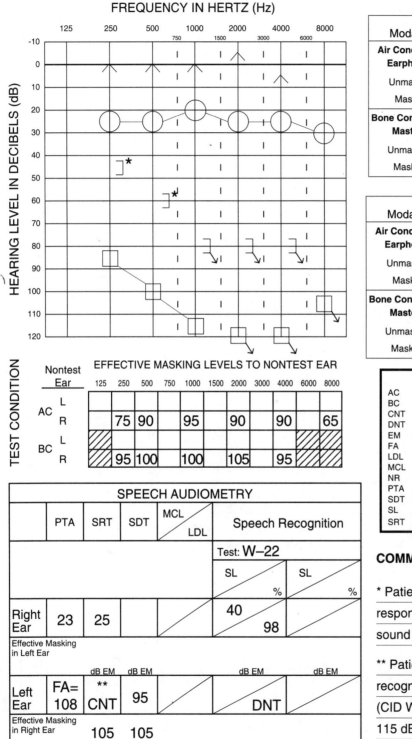

FREQUENCY IN HERTZ (Hz)

EFFECTIVE MASKING LEVELS TO NONTEST EAR

Nontest Ear		125	250	500	750	1000	1500	2000	3000	4000	6000	8000
AC	L											
	R		75	90		95		90		90		65
BC	L											
	R		95	100		100		105		95		

SPEECH AUDIOMETRY

	PTA	SRT	SDT	MCL / LDL	Speech Recognition	
					Test: W–22	
					SL / %	SL / %
Right Ear	23	25			40 / 98	
Effective Masking in Left Ear			dB EM	dB EM	dB EM	dB EM
Left Ear	FA= 108	** CNT	95		DNT	
Effective Masking in Right Ear		105	105			
		dB EM	dB EM		dB EM	dB EM

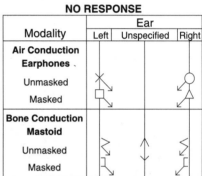

RESPONSE

Modality	Ear		
	Left	Unspecified	Right
Air Conduction Earphones			
Unmasked	×		○
Masked	□		△
Bone Conduction Mastoid			
Unmasked	>	∧	<
Masked	]		[

NO RESPONSE

Modality	Ear		
	Left	Unspecified	Right
Air Conduction Earphones			
Unmasked	×		○
Masked	□		○
Bone Conduction Mastoid			
Unmasked	>	∧	<
Masked	]		[

ABBREVIATIONS

AC	Air Conduction
BC	Bone Conduction
CNT	Could Not Test
DNT	Did Not Test
EM	Effective Masking
FA	Fletcher Average
LDL	Loudness Discomfort Level
MCL	Most Comfortable Loudness
NR	No Response
PTA	Pure-Tone Average
SDT	Speech Detection Threshold
SL	Sensation Level
SRT	Speech Recognition Threshold

COMMENTS:

* Patient reports vibrotactile responses to bone-conducted sound at 250 and 500 Hz.

** Patient was able to correctly recognize 2 of 36 spondees (CID W-1) presented at 115 dB HL.

J. Audiogram Interpretation

Pure-tone testing revealed a mild, conductive hearing loss of flat configuration in the right ear; air-bone gaps ranged from 20 to 30 dB. There is a profound, sensorineural hearing loss of fragmentary configuration in the right ear. According to the patient's observations, the bone-conduction thresholds obtained at 250 and 500 Hz in the left ear reflected vibrotactile rather than auditory responses to sound. Speech thresholds confirmed the pure-tone findings bilaterally. Suprathreshold word recognition ability assessed using traditional monosyllabic words was excellent in the right ear. The patient was able to recognize only two of thirty-six spondaic words (6 percent correct) presented at 115 dB HL in the left ear, a finding that suggests very poor speech recognition ability.

Tympanometry revealed normal admittance and peak pressure in the left ear. The flat tympanogram with normal equivalent ear canal volume in the right ear is consistent with the medical diagnosis of middle ear effusion. Contralateral and ipsilateral acoustic reflexes were absent bilaterally, a finding consistent with the presence of conductive hearing impairment in the right ear and profound, sensorineural hearing impairment in the left ear.

Case 7

History

Your patient is a 44-year-old woman who reports a bilateral "nerve" hearing loss since early childhood. Hearing impairment was gradual in onset and was first identified through a school hearing screening. The patient reports that hearing is better in her left ear. She currently wears an in-the-ear (ITE) hearing aid full-time in her left ear and generally reports little communicative difficulty. She indicates, however, that she continues to encounter difficulty understanding speech in noisy situations. She has noted a slight deterioration in her hearing over the past several years, particularly in her right ear. The results of a recent otologic evaluation were within normal limits. Hereditary hearing loss is the suspected etiology because of the patient's report of a mother and brother with hearing impairment. There is no history of middle ear disorders; other medical history is negative.

Acoustic Immittance Measurements

	Right Ear	Left Ear
Tympanometry		
Static acoustic immittance (mmho)	0.6	0.8
Tympanometric peak pressure (daPa)	0	–5
Equivalent ear canal volume (mmho)	0.9	1.1
Contralateral Acoustic Reflexes (dB HL)		
500 Hz	105	90
1000 Hz	110	90
2000 Hz	115	90

Tympanometry revealed normal admittance (Van Camp et al., 1986), peak pressure (Silman & Silverman, 1991), and equivalent ear canal volume (Margolis & Heller, 1987) in both ears. Contralateral acoustic reflexes were elicited at normal hearing levels in the left ear; reflexes were elevated in the right ear (Wiley et al., 1987). In summary, the preliminary results of acoustic immittance measurements *do not suggest the presence of significant conductive pathology in either ear.*

Case 7-AB

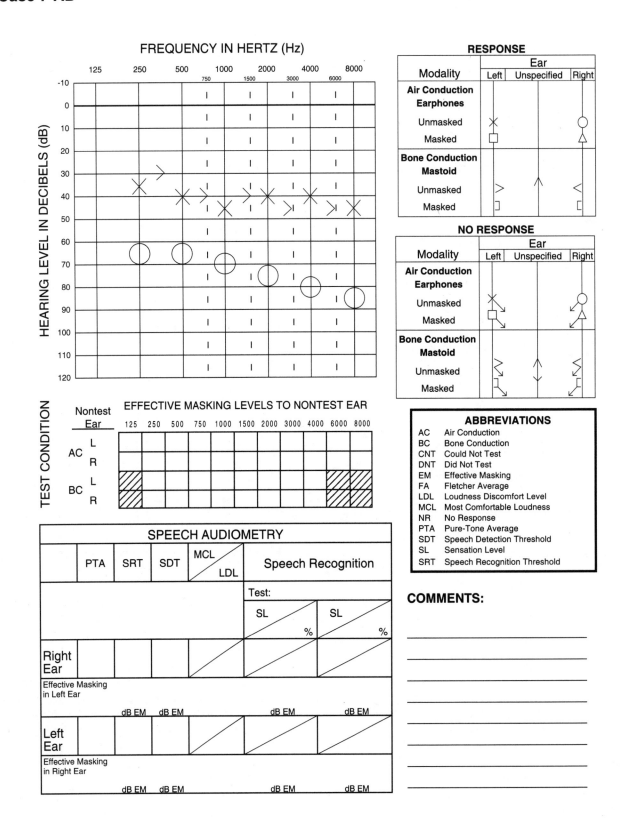

A. When to Mask: Pure-Tone Air-Conduction Audiometry

Is contralateral masking required when measuring air-conduction thresholds in either ear?

Contralateral masking is not required when measuring air-conduction thresholds in the left ear: Measured air-conduction threshold does not equal or exceed bone-conduction threshold in the nontest ear (i.e., unmasked bone-conduction threshold) by the amount of interaural attenuation (i.e., 40 dB). However, contralateral masking will be required when measuring air-conduction thresholds in the right ear. We will use the following equation when making a decision about the need for contralateral masking:

$$AC_T - BC_{NT} \geq 40 \text{ dB}$$

Right Ear (Test Ear)		Masking Needed?
250 Hz	$65 - 30 \geq 40$?	No
500 Hz	$65 - 40 \geq 40$?	No
1000 Hz	$70 - 40 \geq 40$?	No
2000 Hz	$75 - 40^* \geq 40$?	No
4000 Hz	$80 - 40^* \geq 40$?	Yes
8000 Hz	$85 - 45^{**} \geq 40$?	Yes

Left Ear (Test Ear)		Masking Needed?
250 Hz	$35 - 30 \geq 40$?	No
500 Hz	$40 - 40 \geq 40$?	No
1000 Hz	$45 - 40 \geq 40$?	No
2000 Hz	$40 - 40^* \geq 40$?	No
4000 Hz	$40 - 40^* \geq 40$?	No
8000 Hz	$45 - 45^{**} \geq 20$?	No

*See Commentary 1

**Estimated bone-conduction threshold

Commentary

1. It should be noted that the unmasked bone-conduction thresholds at 2000 and 4000 Hz are poorer by 5 dB than the unmasked air-conduction thresholds in the better (i.e., left) ear. Theoretically, this should not occur because a sensitivity loss in part of the auditory system (i.e., a bone-conduction threshold) cannot exceed the loss in the whole system (i.e., an air-conduction threshold). Clinically, however, bone-conduction thresholds that are poorer than air-conduction thresholds are not unexpected. In fact, the current standard for calibration of pure-tone bone-conduction audiometers states that "exact equivalence of air- and bone-conduction thresholds for any individual cannot be expected" (ANSI S3.43-1992, p. 1). Studebaker (1967b) noted that bone-conduction thresholds should exceed air-conduction thresholds in a predictable percentage of patients with normal middle ears because of the variability associated with measurement of pure-tone thresholds. The average difference between air- and bone-conduction thresholds should be 0 dB when a conductive component does not exist. Assuming a normal distribution of differences between air- and bone-conduction thresholds, however, Studebaker states that approximately 87 percent of air- and bone-conduction measurements should fall ±5 dB; about 13 percent of the two measurements would fall ±10 dB of each other. Other factors that may affect the relationship between measured air- and bone-conduction thresholds include variable contributions of the external and middle ears to the bone-conduction response (ANSI S3.43-1992) (see Dirks, 1994, for an excellent review of variables associated with bone-conduction testing). For the purpose of decision-making about the need for clinical masking, it is conventional to assume that the true bone-conduction threshold is not poorer than the air-conduction threshold. In

cases in which the bone-conduction threshold is poorer, the bone-conduction threshold is considered equal to the air-conduction response.

2. Because bone-conduction thresholds cannot be measured at 8000 Hz, it will be necessary to make some assumptions about bone-conduction sensitivity. Unmasked bone-conduction thresholds interweave (i.e., occur ± 10 dB) with air-conduction thresholds in the better (i.e., left) ear and do not suggest the presence of a significant air-bone gap in that ear. Therefore, it is reasonable to assume that bone-conduction sensitivity at 8000 Hz is approximately equal to the air-conduction threshold of the better ear (i.e., 45 dB HL).

B. How Much Masking: Pure-Tone Air-Conduction Audiometry

We have decided that contralateral masking will be required when measuring air-conduction thresholds at 4000 and 8000 Hz in the right ear. We will use the plateau procedure for establishing masked pure-tone thresholds. We will calculate initial minimum masking levels using Martin's (1967, 1974) recommendation. Recall that the initial minimum masking level (M_{min}) is simply equal to the air-conduction threshold of the nontest ear (AC_{NT}) plus a safety factor of 10 dB to account for intersubject variability in the effectiveness of masking levels:

$$M_{min} = AC_{NT} + 10 \text{ dB}$$

Right Ear (Test Ear)		How Much Masking (Nontest Ear)?
4000 Hz	40 dB HL + 10 dB	50 dB EM
8000 Hz	45 dB HL + 10 dB	55 dB EM

We will introduce masking during the plateau procedure using the levels calculated above.

Case 7-CD

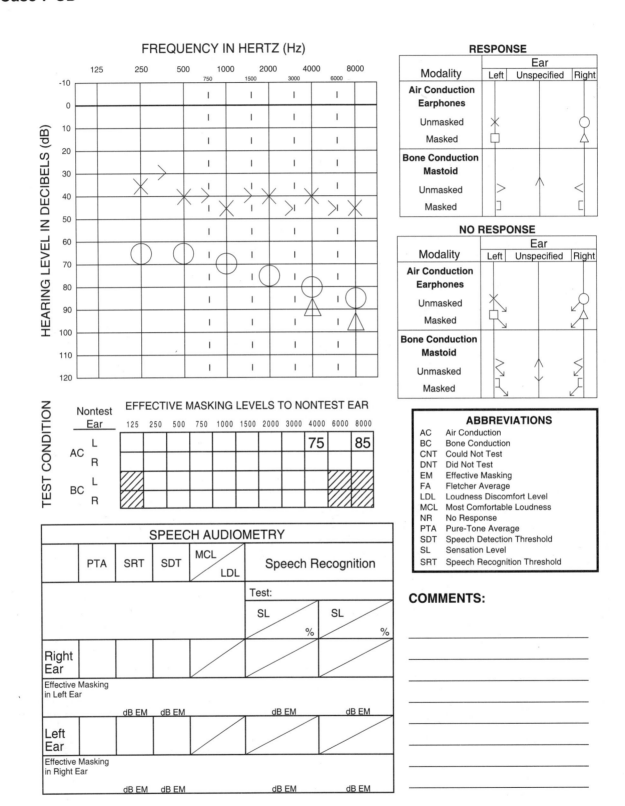

FREQUENCY IN HERTZ (Hz)

RESPONSE

Modality	Ear		
	Left	Unspecified	Right
Air Conduction Earphones			
Unmasked	✕		○
Masked	▢		△
Bone Conduction Mastoid			
Unmasked	>	∧	<
Masked	�		⊏

NO RESPONSE

Modality	Ear		
	Left	Unspecified	Right
Air Conduction Earphones			
Unmasked	✕		○
Masked	▢		○
Bone Conduction Mastoid			
Unmasked	>	∧	<
Masked			

EFFECTIVE MASKING LEVELS TO NONTEST EAR

Nontest Ear	125	250	500	750	1000	1500	2000	3000	4000	6000	8000
AC L										75	85
AC R											
BC L	▨									▨	▨
BC R	▨									▨	▨

ABBREVIATIONS

AC	Air Conduction
BC	Bone Conduction
CNT	Could Not Test
DNT	Did Not Test
EM	Effective Masking
FA	Fletcher Average
LDL	Loudness Discomfort Level
MCL	Most Comfortable Loudness
NR	No Response
PTA	Pure-Tone Average
SDT	Speech Detection Threshold
SL	Sensation Level
SRT	Speech Recognition Threshold

SPEECH AUDIOMETRY

	PTA	SRT	SDT	MCL / LDL	Speech Recognition	
					Test:	
					SL %	SL %
Right Ear						
Effective Masking in Left Ear		dB EM	dB EM		dB EM	dB EM
Left Ear						
Effective Masking in Right Ear		dB EM	dB EM		dB EM	dB EM

COMMENTS:

_____
_____
_____
_____
_____
_____
_____
_____
_____

C. When to Mask: Pure-Tone Bone-Conduction Audiometry

Masked air-conduction thresholds have been obtained in the right ear at 4000 and 8000 Hz using the plateau procedure and are presented on the adjacent audiogram. The final masking level used to obtain masked threshold at each frequency is also reported for the nontest (i.e., left) ear.

Is contralateral masking required when measuring bone-conduction thresholds in either ear?

When comparing unmasked bone-conduction thresholds to the air-conduction thresholds, it is important to remember that *masked* air-conduction thresholds are always considered because they represent the true thresholds for that ear. For example, contralateral masking was required at 4000 and 8000 Hz when measuring air-conduction thresholds in the right ear. Consequently, we must consider the *masked* air-conduction thresholds in the right ear when making a decision about the need for contralateral masking during bone-conduction audiometry in that ear. Remember that contralateral masking is required during bone-conduction audiometry whenever comparison of the unmasked bone-conduction threshold (Unmasked BC) and the air-conduction threshold in the test ear (AC_T) at that frequency reveals a potential air-bone gap (AB Gap_T) of 15 dB or greater:

$$AB\ Gap_T \geq 15\ dB?$$
$$AC_T - Unmasked\ BC \geq 15\ dB?$$

Right Ear	AB Gap_T	AB $Gap_T \geq$15 dB?
250 Hz	65 – 30 = 35	Yes
500 Hz	65 – 40 = 25	Yes
1000 Hz	70 – 40 = 30	Yes
2000 Hz	75 – 45[*] = 30	Yes
4000 Hz	90 – 45[*] = 45	Yes

Left Ear	AB Gap_T	AB $Gap_T \geq$15 dB?
250 Hz	35 – 30 = 5	No
500 Hz	40 – 40 = 0	No
1000 Hz	45 – 40 = 5	No
2000 Hz	40 – 45[*] = –5	No
4000 Hz	40 – 45[*] = –5	No

[*]See Commentary 1

Commentary

1. Recall that the unmasked bone-conduction thresholds at 2000 and 4000 Hz were poorer by 5 dB than the air-conduction thresholds in the better (i.e., left) ear. Because our goal is to identify significant air-bone gaps (i.e., ≥ 15 dB), it is appropriate to use the *measured* unmasked bone-conduction thresholds at 2000 and 4000 Hz when making a decision about the need for masking during bone-conduction audiometry. The negative air-bone gaps (i.e., –5 dB) at 2000 and 4000 Hz in the left ear do not suggest the presence of a significant conductive component in that ear; consequently, contralateral masking is not required. Remember that "negative" air-bone gaps do occur clinically because of the variability associated with measurement of air- and bone-conduction thresholds (Barry, 1994; Studebaker, 1967b).

D. How Much Masking: Pure-Tone Bone-Conduction Audiometry

We have decided that contralateral masking will be required at all frequencies when measuring bone-conduction thresholds in the right ear. We again will use the plateau procedure for establishing masked pure-tone thresholds.

The initial minimum masking levels will be calculated using Martin's (1967, 1974) recommendation. The initial minimum masking level (M_{min}) during bone-conduction audiometry is simply equal to the air-conduction threshold of the nontest ear (AC_{NT}) plus compensation for the occlusion effect (OE) plus a safety factor of 10 dB:

$$M_{min} = AC_{NT} + OE + 10 \text{ dB}$$

Remember that patients with either normal hearing or a sensorineural hearing loss will exhibit an occlusion effect. The left ear will be covered (i.e., occluded) when contralateral masking is introduced during measurement of masked bone-conduction thresholds in the right ear. Because this patient exhibits a sensorineural hearing loss (and no evidence of significant air-bone gaps) in the masked (i.e., occluded) ear, she theoretically will exhibit an occlusion effect. Recall from Chapter 5 that there are two approaches to correcting for the occlusion effect. First, *average* values can be used when compensating for the occlusion effect: 30 dB at 250 Hz, 20 dB at 500 Hz, 10 dB at 1000 Hz, and 0 dB at frequencies above 1000 Hz. Second, *individual* occlusion effects can be determined for each patient. Specifically, the patient's unoccluded bone-conduction thresholds are measured initially at 250, 500, and 1000 Hz. Occluded thresholds are remeasured by placing the supra-aural earphone over the nontest ear *without* masking noise present. The patient's occlusion effect in the nontest ear is determined by subtracting the occluded threshold at each frequency from the unoccluded threshold. This value is then added to the initial masking level (Martin et al., 1974). In this case study, we will use the second approach when compensating for the occlusion effect. Unmasked bone-conduction thresholds with the bone vibrator placed at the left mastoid have already been measured. We only need to redetermine unmasked bone-conduction threshold with the earphone (without masking) placed over the left (i.e., nontest) ear.

	250 Hz	500 Hz	1000 Hz
Unoccluded BC	30 dB HL	40 dB HL	40 dB HL
Occluded BC	10 dB HL	25 dB HL	30 dB HL
Occlusion Effect	20 dB	15 dB	10 dB

Minimum masking level is calculated as follows:

$$M_{min} = AC_{NT} + OE + 10 \text{ dB}$$

Right Ear (Test Ear)		How Much Masking (Nontest Ear)?
250 Hz	35 dB HL + 20 dB + 10 dB	65 dB EM
500 Hz	40 dB HL + 15 dB + 10 dB	65 dB EM
1000 Hz	45 dB HL + 10 dB + 10 dB	65 dB EM
2000 Hz	40 dB HL + 0 dB + 10 dB	50 dB EM
4000 Hz	40 dB HL + 0 dB + 10 dB	50 dB EM

We will introduce masking during the plateau procedure using the levels calculated above.

Case 7-EF

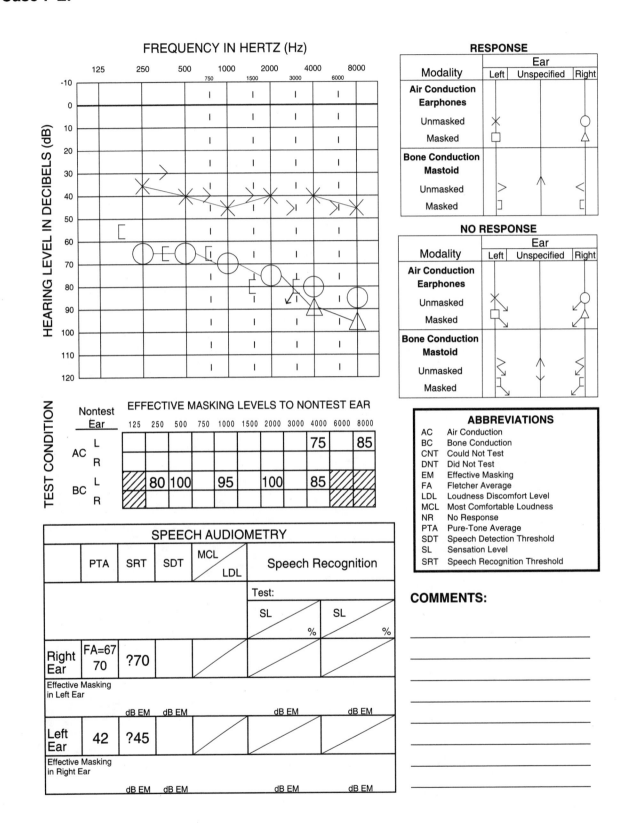

FREQUENCY IN HERTZ (Hz)

| | 125 | 250 | 500 | 750 | 1000 | 1500 | 2000 | 3000 | 4000 | 6000 | 8000 |

RESPONSE

Modality	Ear		
	Left	Unspecified	Right
Air Conduction Earphones			
Unmasked	✕		○
Masked	☐		△
Bone Conduction Mastoid			
Unmasked	>	∧	<
Masked	⊐		⊏

NO RESPONSE

Modality	Ear		
	Left	Unspecified	Right
Air Conduction Earphones			
Unmasked	✕↘		○↙
Masked	☐↘		
Bone Conduction Mastoid			
Unmasked	>↙	∧↓	<↙
Masked	⊐↙		⊏↙

ABBREVIATIONS

AC	Air Conduction
BC	Bone Conduction
CNT	Could Not Test
DNT	Did Not Test
EM	Effective Masking
FA	Fletcher Average
LDL	Loudness Discomfort Level
MCL	Most Comfortable Loudness
NR	No Response
PTA	Pure-Tone Average
SDT	Speech Detection Threshold
SL	Sensation Level
SRT	Speech Recognition Threshold

TEST CONDITION — EFFECTIVE MASKING LEVELS TO NONTEST EAR

Nontest Ear		125	250	500	750	1000	1500	2000	3000	4000	6000	8000
AC	L									75		85
	R											
BC	L		80	100		95		100		85		
	R											

SPEECH AUDIOMETRY

	PTA	SRT	SDT	MCL / LDL	Speech Recognition			
					Test:			
					SL	%	SL	%
Right Ear	FA=67 / 70	?70						
Effective Masking in Left Ear		dB EM	dB EM			dB EM		dB EM
Left Ear	42	?45						
Effective Masking in Right Ear		dB EM	dB EM			dB EM		dB EM

COMMENTS:

_____
_____
_____
_____
_____
_____
_____
_____

E. When to Mask: Threshold Speech Audiometry

Masked bone-conduction thresholds have been obtained in the right ear using the plateau procedure and are presented on the adjacent audiogram. The final masking level used to obtain the masked threshold at each frequency is also reported for the nontest (i.e., left) ear.

Is contralateral masking required when obtaining speech recognition threshold in either ear?

Based on the pure-tone averages, it is predicted that SRTs will be measured at approximately 70 dB HL and 45 dB HL for the right and left ears, respectively. Prior to measurement of speech recognition thresholds, we can determine whether contralateral masking will likely be required:

$$\text{Presentation level}_T - \text{IA} \geq \text{Best BC}_{NT}$$

In this case study, we will use a single value of 40 dB as our estimate of interaural attenuation for all measurements during speech audiometry (i.e. threshold and suprathreshold).

Right Ear	70 dB HL – 40 dB ≥ 30 dB HL?	
	30 dB HL ≥ 30 dB HL?	*Yes*
Left Ear	45 dB HL – 40 dB ≥ 55 dB HL?	
	5 dB HL ≥ 55 dB HL?	*No*

When measuring SRT in the right ear, the predicted cross-hearing level of the speech signal reaching the nontest (i.e., left) ear is 30 dB HL. Because the best bone-conduction threshold in the nontest ear is also 30 dB HL, theoretically cross hearing will occur. Therefore, it will be necessary to use contralateral masking when measuring the SRT in the right ear.

There will be no need for contralateral masking, however, when measuring SRT in the left ear. The predicted level of the cross-hearing signal (i.e., 5 dB HL) is considerably lower than the best bone-conduction threshold in the nontest ear (i.e., 55 dB HL at 250 Hz).

F. How Much Masking: Threshold Speech Audiometry

We have decided that contralateral masking will be required when measuring speech recognition threshold in the right ear. Recall from Chapter 6 that we can use either a psychoacoustic or acoustic approach when determining masking requirements during assessment of SRT. In this example, we will use an acoustic approach. That is, the required masking level will be derived by calculating the estimated levels of the test and maker signals in the test and nontest ears. Specifically, we will calculate the mid-masking level:

$$M_{mid} = (M_{max} + M_{min}) / 2$$
$$\text{where}$$
$$M_{min} = \text{Presentation level}_T - \text{IA} + \text{Max AB Gap}_{NT}$$
$$M_{max} = \text{Best BC}_T + \text{IA} - 5 \text{ dB}$$

How much contralateral masking should be used when measuring speech recognition threshold in the right ear?

$$M_{min} = 70 \text{ dB HL} - 40 \text{ dB} + 5 \text{ dB}$$
$$= 35 \text{ dB EM}$$
$$M_{max} = 55 \text{ dB HL (at 250 Hz)} + 40 \text{ dB} - 5 \text{ dB}$$
$$= 90 \text{ dB EM}$$
$$M_{mid} = (90 \text{ dB} + 35 \text{ dB}) / 2$$
$$= 62.5 \text{ dB EM}$$

The mid-masking level is calculated as 62.5 dB EM; a masking level of 60 dB EM will be used. In addition to falling at midplateau, a value of 60 dB EM is 25 dB above the minimum masking level required. Thus, there is "reserve" masking available should speech be presented at levels higher than the predicted SRT of 70 dB HL. It is important to consider your SRT procedure when evaluating the appropriateness of the selected masking level.

Case 7-GH

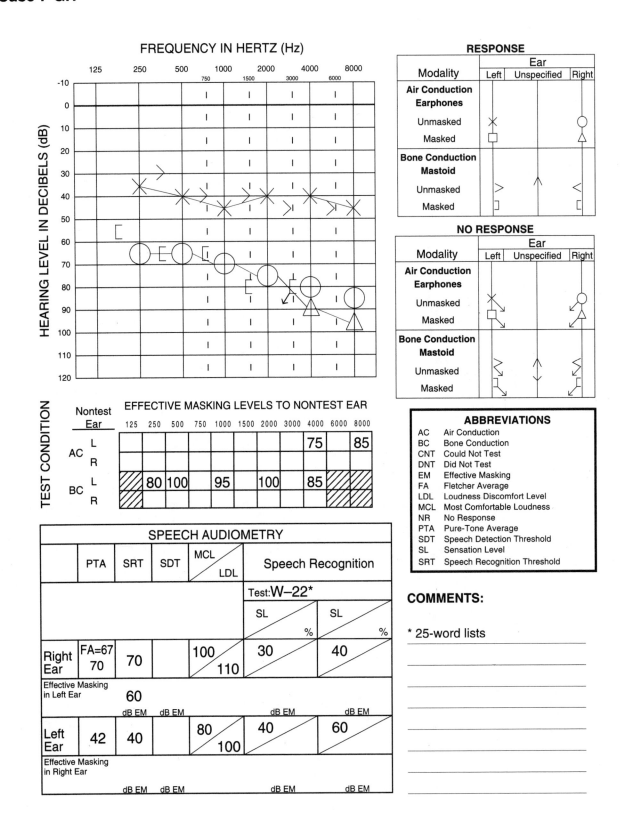

FREQUENCY IN HERTZ (Hz)

RESPONSE

Modality	Ear		
	Left	Unspecified	Right
Air Conduction Earphones			
Unmasked	X		O
Masked	□		△
Bone Conduction Mastoid			
Unmasked	>	∧	<
Masked	⊏		⊐

NO RESPONSE

Modality	Ear		
	Left	Unspecified	Right
Air Conduction Earphones			
Unmasked	X↘		O↙
Masked	□↘		△↙
Bone Conduction Mastoid			
Unmasked	⟩↘	↑	⟨↘
Masked	⊏↘		⊐↘

EFFECTIVE MASKING LEVELS TO NONTEST EAR

Nontest Ear		125	250	500	750	1000	1500	2000	3000	4000	6000	8000
AC	L									75		85
	R											
BC	L	▨	80	100		95		100		85	▨	▨
	R	▨									▨	▨

ABBREVIATIONS

AC — Air Conduction
BC — Bone Conduction
CNT — Could Not Test
DNT — Did Not Test
EM — Effective Masking
FA — Fletcher Average
LDL — Loudness Discomfort Level
MCL — Most Comfortable Loudness
NR — No Response
PTA — Pure-Tone Average
SDT — Speech Detection Threshold
SL — Sensation Level
SRT — Speech Recognition Threshold

SPEECH AUDIOMETRY

	PTA	SRT	SDT	MCL / LDL	Speech Recognition	
					Test: W−22*	
					SL	SL
					%	%
Right Ear	FA=67 / 70	70		100 / 110	30	40
Effective Masking in Left Ear		60				
	dB EM	dB EM			dB EM	dB EM
Left Ear	42	40		80 / 100	40	60
Effective Masking in Right Ear						
	dB EM	dB EM			dB EM	dB EM

COMMENTS:

* 25-word lists

G. When to Mask: Suprathreshold Speech Audiometry

Suprathreshold speech recognition will be assessed using a traditional, open-set monosyllabic word test: CID W-22 (Auditec recording). Although it is generally agreed that suprathreshold speech recognition should be assessed at more than one intensity level (e.g., Beattie & Raffin, 1985; Beattie & Zipp, 1990; Bess, 1983; Olsen & Matkin, 1991), the majority of audiologists evaluate speech recognition at only one presentation level (Martin et al., 1994; Martin & Morris, 1989). Recall that the goal of traditional suprathreshold speech recognition testing under earphones is to present phonetically/phonemically balanced (PB) monosyllabic words at an intensity level that will permit the patient to achieve maximum performance (i.e., PB Max). There is considerable evidence to suggest that presenting a single list of words at the most comfortable loudness (MCL) will not necessarily result in maximum performance in sensorineural hearing-impaired listeners (see Bess, 1983, and Olsen & Matkin, 1991, for a review of procedural variables affecting suprathreshold speech recognition performance). In fact, recent research by Beattie and Zipp (1990) suggests that assessing speech recognition at the loudness discomfort level (LDL) is more likely to provide an accurate estimate of PB Max than testing at MCL. Although construction of a performance-intensity (PI) function is recognized as a valid approach to measuring maximum speech recognition performance, it is very time-consuming. This approach involves presenting different lists of monosyllabic words at successively higher presentation levels (approximately five to six intensity levels). In this particular case study, we will assess suprathreshold speech recognition using a test protocol first described by Beattie and Raffin (1985).

Beattie and Raffin (1985) described a test protocol that is empirically based on data obtained using Auditec recordings of CID W-22 with a sensorineural hearing-impaired population. Essentially, the procedure is a compromise between presenting speech at only one intensity level and constructing an entire performance-intensity function. They recommend that at least two twenty-five-word lists be presented, one at the patient's LDL and another at a level judged to yield PB Max (usually 20 to 60 dB SL). If both scores are within 8 percent (i.e., ± two words), they are averaged to represent a stable estimate of PB Max. If the two word lists do not yield a plateau (i.e., two scores that are ± 8 percent), additional lists are presented in 5 to 20 dB steps until the plateau is obtained. (The reader is referred to the article by Beattie and Raffin for a more complete description of the test protocol's development.)

Is contralateral masking required when assessing suprathreshold speech recognition ability?

Twenty-five word lists of the Auditec recordings of CID W-22 will be presented to each ear at two intensity levels: Loudness discomfort level (LDL) and a fixed sensation level referenced to SRT that ideally will yield PB Max. The loudness discomfort level is the sound level *above which* an individual reports that speech is uncomfortably loud (Dirks & Morgan, 1983) (see Dirks & Morgan, 1983, for an excellent review of measurement of loudness discomfort and most comfortable loudness). For example, if speech is reported to be uncomfortably loud at 110 dB HL, then the LDL is recorded as 105 dB HL.

Initially, the sensation levels of 30 dB and 40 dB were selected for the right and left ears, respectively; the patient reported that speech was comfortably loud at these presentation levels (i.e., 100 dB HL in the right ear; 80 dB HL in the left ear). The patient reported that speech was uncomfortably loud at 115 dB HL in the right ear and at 105 dB HL in the left ear. Therefore, LDLs were reported as 110 dB HL and 100 dB HL in the right and left ears, respectively (i.e., SLs of 40 dB and 60 dB). In summary, suprathreshold speech recognition will be measured at two presentation levels in each ear:

Right Ear	100 dB HL (SRT of 70 dB HL + 30 dB SL)
	110 dB HL (or 40 dB SL) (LDL)
Left Ear	80 dB HL (SRT of 40 dB HL + 40 dB SL)
	100 dB HL (or 60 dB SL) (LDL)

Recall our rule for when to mask during speech audiometry:

$$\text{Presentation level}_T - IA \geq \text{Best BC}_{NT}$$

We are using a single value of 40 dB as our estimate of interaural attenuation for all measurements during speech audiometry (i.e., threshold and suprathreshold). Because the *Auditec recordings* of W-22 are being used to evaluate suprathreshold speech recognition, it probably is not necessary to use a more conservative estimate of interaural attenuation than that used when measuring the SRT (see Chapter 4 for further discussion). Is contralateral masking required in either ear?

Right Ear	100 dB HL – 40 dB ≥ 30 dB HL?	
	60 dB HL ≥ 30 dB HL?	*Yes*
	110 dB HL – 40 dB ≥ 30 dB HL?	
	70 dB HL ≥ 30 dB HL?	*Yes*
Left Ear	80 dB HL – 40 dB ≥ 55 dB HL?	
	40 dB HL ≥ 55 dB HL?	*No*
	100 dB HL – 40 dB ≥ 55 dB HL?	
	60 dB HL ≥ 55 dB HL?	*Yes*

Contralateral masking will be required when assessing suprathreshold speech recognition ability at both presentation levels in the right ear. However, contralateral masking will be required only when measuring speech recognition at the higher presentation level (i.e., 100 dB HL) in the left ear.

Commentary

1. There are two reasons for assessing suprathreshold speech recognition at LDL. First, as already mentioned, testing at LDL is more likely to yield PB Max than when presenting speech at MCL. Second, testing at LDL evaluates for the possibility of "rollover" (i.e., progressive deterioration in speech recognition ability with increasing speech intensity) (Beattie & Zipp, 1990). Bess (1983) and Olsen & Matkin (1991) provide excellent discussions of the diagnostic implications of speech recognition tests.

2. Although cross hearing can occur during the measurement of MCL and LDL, contralateral masking is typically not used. Generally, the inclusion of the nontest ear during these suprathreshold speech measurements does not affect the test results or interpretation (Martin, 1994).

H. How Much Masking: Suprathreshold Speech Audiometry

We will use the mid-masking method for selecting an appropriate masking level during assessment of suprathreshold speech recognition. Recall that mid-masking level (M_{mid}) is the midpoint between the minimum (M_{min}) and maximum (M_{max}) masking levels. The mid-masking level can be calculated as follows:

$$M_{mid} = (M_{max} + M_{min}) / 2$$

where

$$M_{min} = \text{Presentation level}_T - IA + \text{Max AB Gap}_{NT}$$
$$M_{max} = \text{Best BC}_T + IA - 5 \text{ dB}$$

Remember that bone-conduction sensitivity is always considered at frequencies from 250 through 4000 Hz.

How much contralateral masking should be used when assessing suprathreshold speech recognition ability in the right ear?

Keep in mind that only M_{min} will vary for each of the two presentation levels in the same ear; M_{max} remains constant.

Right Ear   Presentation level = 100 dB HL

$$M_{min} = 100 \text{ dB HL} - 40 \text{ dB} + 5 \text{ dB (at 250 Hz)}$$
$$= 65 \text{ dB EM}$$
$$M_{max} = 55 \text{ dB HL (at 250 Hz)} + 40 \text{ dB} - 5 \text{ dB}$$
$$= 90 \text{ dB EM}$$
$$M_{mid} = (90 \text{ dB} + 65 \text{ dB}) / 2$$
$$= 77.5 \text{ dB EM or 80 dB EM}$$

Presentation level = 110 dB HL

$$M_{min} = 110 \text{ dB HL} - 40 \text{ dB} + 5 \text{ dB (at 250 Hz)}$$
$$= 75 \text{ dB EM}$$
$$M_{max} = 55 \text{ dB HL (at 250 Hz)} + 40 \text{ dB} - 5 \text{ dB}$$
$$= 90 \text{ dB EM}$$
$$M_{mid} = (90 \text{ dB} + 65 \text{ dB}) / 2$$
$$= 82.5 \text{ dB EM or 85 dB EM}$$

Masking levels of 80 dB EM and 85 dB EM will be used when measuring speech recognition at 100 dB HL and 110 dB HL in the right ear. The selected masking levels are considered appropriate because they occur at mid-plateau. In addition, they also take into account a 10-dB safety factor (i.e., . M_{min} + 10 dB) and do not exceed the estimated maximum levels.

How much contralateral masking should be used when assessing suprathreshold speech recognition ability in the left ear?

Left Ear   Presentation level = 100 dB HL

$$M_{min} = 100 \text{ dB HL} - 40 \text{ dB} + 5 \text{ dB (at 250 Hz)}$$
$$= 65 \text{ dB EM}$$
$$M_{max} = 30 \text{ dB HL (at 250 Hz)} + 40 \text{ dB} - 5 \text{ dB}$$
$$= 65 \text{ dB EM}$$
$$M_{mid} = \text{Cannot be established } (M_{max} > M_{min})$$

A masking dilemma has occurred when measuring suprathreshold speech recognition at 100 dB HL in the left ear: M_{min} equals M_{max}. Remember that ideally the selected masking level should fall at least 10 dB above M_{min} in order to account for intersubject variability in effective masking. However, a masking level of 75 dB EM (i.e., M_{min} of 65 dB EM + 10 dB) exceeds M_{max} by 10 dB. Remember that M_{max} is equal to 65 dB EM; theoretically, over-masking would occur once contralateral masking reaches 70 dB EM. Assuming that interaural attenuation is equal to our conservative estimate of 40 dB, then speech-spectrum noise of 75 dB EM theoretically would reach the test ear at an effective level (i.e., 5 dB above the level of 70 dB EM that produces overmasking). Because the speech signal is being presented to the test ear at a high sensation level (i.e., 60 dB SL), the low level of masking noise that has crossed over *may not* have a significant effect on suprathreshold speech recognition. Although this clearly is not an ideal situation, an adequate signal-to-noise ratio in the test ear may be still be maintained to ensure maximum performance. Obviously, overmasking will be reduced or eliminated if the patient's actual interaural attenuation is greater than our conservative estimate of 40 dB.

There is no easy solution to the masking dilemma that has resulted in the left ear. We could present the contralateral masking at 75 dB EM (i.e., M_{min} + 10 dB safety factor). However, overmasking is a possibility. An alternative approach involves presenting the masker at a slightly lower intensity level in order to reduce the potential for overmasking. For example, masking could be presented at either 65 dB EM (i.e., M_{min} + 0 dB safety factor) or 70 dB EM (i.e., M_{min} + 5 dB safety factor). However, *undermasking* could occur (in a small percentage of cases) because of the use of an inadequate safety factor (i.e., < 10 dB). In addition, overmasking could theoretically still occur at 70 dB EM *if* interaural attenuation for this patient is as small as 40 dB. Although there is no correct answer to our masking dilemma, we will present contralateral masking at 75 dB EM (i.e., M_{min} + 10 dB safety factor) and subsequently evaluate *very carefully* the suprathreshold speech recognition test results in the left ear.

Commentary

1. It will be necessary to evaluate the results of the suprathreshold speech recognition test presented at 100 dB HL in the left ear because of the risk of overmasking. If the two speech recognition scores obtained at 80 dB HL and 100 dB HL are within 8 percent, then we have obtained a stable estimate of PB Max. If the masking stimulus *did* in fact cross over to the test (i.e., left) ear, it apparently did not have a significant effect on speech recognition performance. Conversely, if speech recognition performance deteriorates at 100 dB HL, it will be difficult to determine if overmasking was a contributing factor. A major advantage of the midplateau masking procedure is that it allows the audiologist to make a well-informed decision about selected masking levels.

2. An alternative solution to the masking dilemma in the left ear would be to substitute supra-aural earphones with 3A insert earphones because of their significantly increased interaural attenuation for speech. This case study was presented *assuming that insert earphones were not available*.

3. We can consider the use of the short-cut approach when selecting masking levels during suprathreshold speech audiometry. It will become apparent, however, that this approach will prove effective only when evaluating the right ear.

Recall that suprathreshold speech recognition will be evaluated at two intensity levels. Contralateral masking is required when evaluating the right ear at both presentation levels of 100 dB HL and 110 dB HL (or sensation levels of 30 dB and 40 dB). However, contralateral masking will be required only when measuring speech recognition at the higher presentation level (i.e., 100 dB HL) in the left ear.

When evaluating suprathreshold speech recognition in the right ear, the short-cut approach for selecting masking levels can be used because both required conditions have been met: a) There are no *significant* air-bone gaps in either ear and b) the suprathreshold speech recognition is assessed at moderate sensation levels (i.e., 30 dB and 40 dB SL). Effective masking levels are calculated as follows when using the short-cut approach:

$$dB\ EM = PL_T - 20\ dB$$

Right Ear   Presentation level = 100 dB HL
$$dB\ EM = 100\ dB\ HL - 20\ dB$$
$$= 80\ dB$$
Presentation level = 110 dB HL
$$dB\ EM = 110\ dB\ HL - 20\ dB$$
$$= 90\ dB$$

It should be noted that the effective masking levels calculated using the short-cut approach are similar to those values calculated using the midplateau procedure:

Right Ear   Presentation level = 100 dB HL
$$M_{min} = 65\ dB\ EM$$
$$M_{max} = 90\ dB\ EM$$
$$M_{mid} = 77.5\ dB\ EM\ or\ 80\ dB\ EM$$
Presentation level = 110 dB HL
$$M_{min} = 75\ dB\ EM$$
$$M_{max} = 90\ dB\ EM$$
$$M_{mid} = 82.5\ dB\ EM\ or\ 85\ dB\ EM$$

The use of the short-cut procedure would result in appropriate masking levels when evaluating the right ear: The selected masking levels fall at least 10 dB above M_{min}, yet they do not exceed M_{max}.

When assessing suprathreshold speech recognition at 100 dB HL in the left ear, the short-cut procedure will not prove effective. One of the prerequisite conditions of the procedure has not been met: Suprathreshold speech recognition is being evaluated at a higher sensation level (i.e., 60 dB SL). The effective masking level is calculated as follows when using the short-cut approach:

$$dB\ EM = PL_T - 20\ dB$$

Left Ear   Presentation level = 100 dB HL
$$dB\ EM = 100\ dB\ HL - 20\ dB$$
$$= 80\ dB$$

It should be noted that the effective masking level calculated using the short-cut approach exceeds M_{max} by 15 dB: Recall our earlier calculations using the midplateau procedure:

$$M_{min} = 65\ dB\ EM$$
$$M_{max} = 65\ dB\ EM$$
$$M_{mid} = \text{Cannot be determined } (M_{min} > M_{max})$$

When using the short-cut approach, the audiologist would not be aware that the selected masking level was potentially producing overmasking. Recall from Chapter 6 that the use of the short-cut procedure is not recommended when assessing suprathreshold speech recognition at higher sensation levels (i.e., greater than approximately 50 dB SL) because of the increased likelihood of overmasking. A major advantage of the midplateau procedure is that the audiologist has information about the characteristics of the masking plateau and subsequently can make a more well-informed decision when selecting masking levels.

Case 7-J

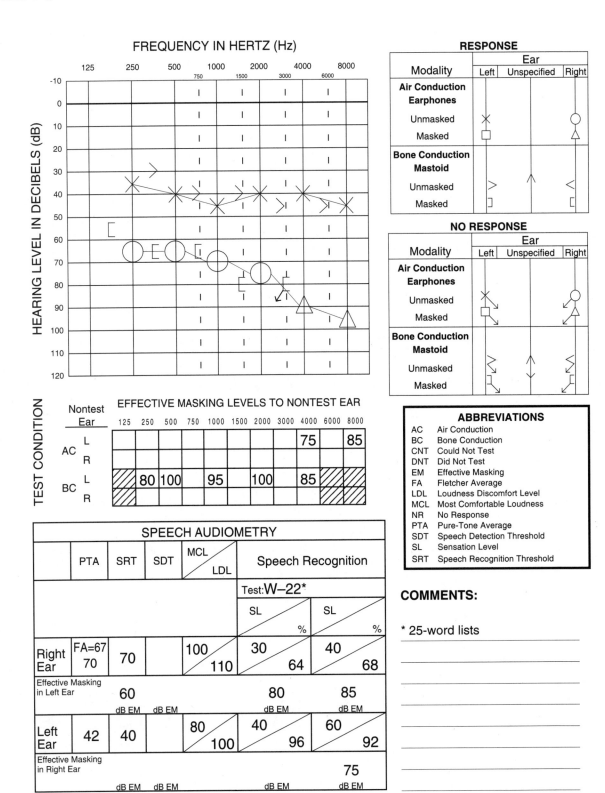

RESPONSE

Modality	Ear		
	Left	Unspecified	Right
Air Conduction Earphones			
Unmasked	X		O
Masked	☐		△
Bone Conduction Mastoid			
Unmasked	>	∧	<
Masked	⅃		⊏

NO RESPONSE

Modality	Ear		
	Left	Unspecified	Right
Air Conduction Earphones			
Unmasked	X↓		O↓
Masked	☐↓		△↓
Bone Conduction Mastoid			
Unmasked	>↓	∧↓	<↓
Masked	⅃↓		⊏↓

FREQUENCY IN HERTZ (Hz)

HEARING LEVEL IN DECIBELS (dB)

EFFECTIVE MASKING LEVELS TO NONTEST EAR

TEST CONDITION

Nontest Ear		125	250	500	750	1000	1500	2000	3000	4000	6000	8000
AC	L									75		85
	R											
BC	L	▨	80	100		95		100		85	▨	▨
	R	▨										▨

ABBREVIATIONS

AC	Air Conduction
BC	Bone Conduction
CNT	Could Not Test
DNT	Did Not Test
EM	Effective Masking
FA	Fletcher Average
LDL	Loudness Discomfort Level
MCL	Most Comfortable Loudness
NR	No Response
PTA	Pure-Tone Average
SDT	Speech Detection Threshold
SL	Sensation Level
SRT	Speech Recognition Threshold

SPEECH AUDIOMETRY

	PTA	SRT	SDT	MCL / LDL	Speech Recognition	
					Test: W–22*	
					SL / %	SL / %
Right Ear	FA=67 / 70	70		100 / 110	30 / 64	40 / 68
Effective Masking in Left Ear	60 dB EM	dB EM			80 dB EM	85 dB EM
Left Ear	42	40		80 / 100	40 / 96	60 / 92
Effective Masking in Right Ear	dB EM	dB EM			75 dB EM	dB EM

COMMENTS:

* 25-word lists

J. Audiogram Interpretation

Pure-tone testing revealed a severe-to-profound, sensorineural hearing loss of sloping configuration in the right ear . There is a mild-to-moderate, sensorineural hearing impairment of flat configuration in the left ear. Speech recognition thresholds confirmed the pure-tone findings. Suprathreshold word recognition ability assessed using monosyllabic words was fair in the right ear and excellent in the left ear.

Tympanometry revealed normal admittance and peak pressure in both ears. Contralateral acoustic reflex thresholds were elicited at hearing levels consistent with the presence of cochlear pathology bilaterally (Gelfand et al., 1990).

Commentary

1. It should be noted that both speech recognition scores in each ear are within 8 percent; thus, the average represents a stable estimate of PB Max for that ear (i.e., 66 percent in the right ear and 94 percent in the left ear).

2. The two speech recognition scores obtained in the left ear are within 8 percent. Although overmasking was a possibility when assessing speech recognition at a presentation level of 100 dB HL (with 75 dB EM in the contralateral ear), there was no observed deterioration in performance when compared to the results obtained at 80 dB HL. In addition, speech recognition performance remains within the normal range (i.e., 90 to 100 percent correct). Consequently, there is no evidence that overmasking has occurred (i.e., no significant effect on suprathreshold speech recognition performance).

Case 8

History

Your patient is an 8-year-old boy with a history of allergies and serous otitis media. Drug therapy consisting of decongestant-antihistamine combinations has proven successful until recently. The results of a current otologic examination suggested the presence of otitis media with effusion bilaterally. The patient reports hearing difficulty for the past four weeks. The parents also report that the child frequently experiences difficulty understanding conversational speech, an observation also supported by the classroom teacher. The results of audiological testing conducted six months previously revealed normal hearing sensitivity; suprathreshold word recognition ability was excellent bilaterally. The results of acoustic immittance measurements suggested normal middle ear function in both ears. The otologist is considering surgical intervention consisting of bilateral myringotomies with insertion of pressure-equalizing (PE) tubes.

Acoustic Immittance Measurements

	Right Ear	**Left Ear**
Tympanometry		
Static acoustic admittance (mmho)	0.1	0.1
Tympanometric peak pressure (daPa)	—	—
Equivalent ear canal volume (mmho)	0.8	0.7
Contralateral Acoustic Reflexes (dB HL)		
500 Hz	NR	NR
1000 Hz	NR	NR
2000 Hz	NR	NR
Ipsilateral Acoustic Reflexes (dB HL)		
500 Hz	NR	NR
1000 Hz	NR	NR
2000 Hz	NR	NR

NR = no response

Tympanometry revealed no point of maximum admittance with changes in air pressure (i.e., flat tympanograms) in both ears. Measures of ear-canal acoustic admittance were within the normal range bilaterally (Margolis & Heller, 1987). Contralateral and ipsilateral acoustic reflexes were absent bilaterally. In summary, the preliminary results of acoustic immittance measurements *are consistent with the presence of conductive pathology bilaterally.*

Case 8-AI

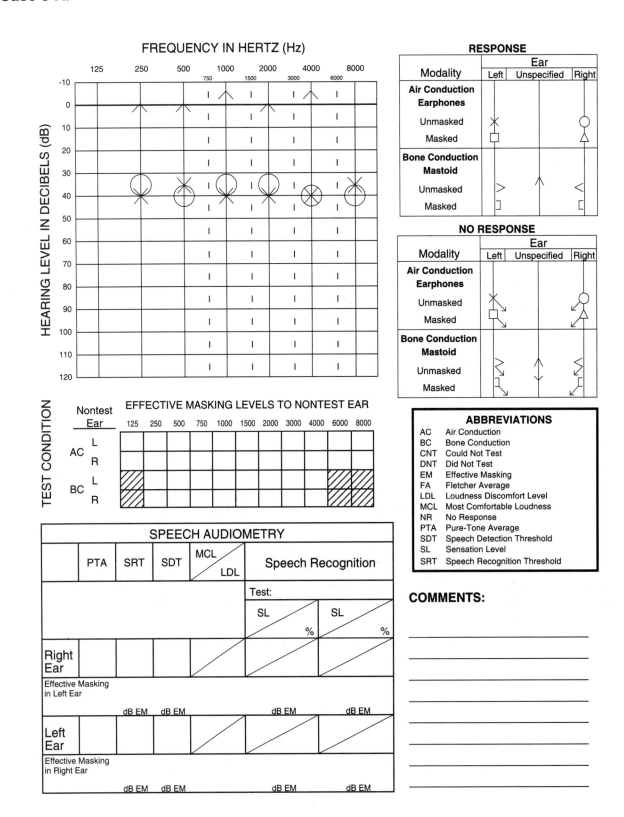

A. When to Mask: Pure-Tone Air-Conduction Audiometry

I. Use of Insert Earphones

Given the patient's case history information, the current otologic report, and the current results of acoustic immittance measurements, there is a strong possibility that the patient will exhibit a bilateral conductive hearing loss. *To avoid a possible masking dilemma, we will use 3A insert earphones during all audiological testing.* Recall from Chapter 8 that interaural attenuation for air-conducted sound is increased when using an insert receiver. The use of an earphone with increased interaural attenuation provides two major advantages. First, the need for contralateral masking is significantly reduced during air-conduction testing. Second, the range between minimum and maximum masking levels is increased, thereby *increasing* the width of the masking plateau and the range of permissible masking levels (Studebaker, 1962). Consequently, the risk of overmasking is significantly reduced. The use of insert earphones will also prove advantageous during masked bone-conduction audiometry because of increased interaural attenuation of the masking stimulus, thereby increasing maximum masking levels.

Is contralateral masking required when measuring air-conduction thresholds in either ear?

Contralateral masking is not required when measuring air-conduction thresholds in either ear: Measured air-conduction thresholds do not equal or exceed bone-conduction thresholds in the nontest ear (i.e., unmasked bone-conduction threshold) by the amount of interaural attenuation. Based on currently available data, conservative estimates of interaural attenuation for the 3A insert earphone are *75 dB at 1000 Hz and below* and *50 dB at frequencies above 1000 Hz* (see Chapter 8). We will use the following equation when making a decision about the need for contralateral masking:

$$AC_T - BC_{NT} \geq IA$$

Right Ear (Test Ear)			Masking Needed?
250 Hz	35 − 0	≥ 75?	No
500 Hz	40 − 0	≥ 75?	No
1000 Hz	35 − (−5)	≥ 75?	No
2000 Hz	35 − 0	≥ 50?	No
4000 Hz	40 − (−5)	≥ 50?	No
8000 Hz	40 − (−5*)	≥ 50?	No

Left Ear (Test Ear)			Masking Needed?
250 Hz	40 − 0	≥ 75?	No
500 Hz	35 − 0	≥ 75?	No
1000 Hz	40 − (−5)	≥ 75?	No
2000 Hz	40 − 0	≥ 50?	No
4000 Hz	40 − (−5)	≥ 50?	No
8000 Hz	35 − (−5*)	≥ 50?	No

*Estimated bone-conduction threshold

Commentary

1. Because an unmasked bone-conduction threshold is unavailable at 8000 Hz, it will be necessary to estimate a probable threshold at that frequency. It should be noted that unmasked bone-conduction thresholds at 250 through 4000 Hz occur at either −5 or 0 dB HL, suggesting substantial air-bone gaps in at least one ear. Consequently, it is reasonable to conclude that an unmasked bone-conduction threshold at 8000 Hz would probably occur at approximately −5 or 0 dB HL.

2. Because we used an air-conduction receiver with increased interaural attenuation, the need for contralateral masking was completely eliminated. If conventional supra-aural earphones had been used, however, masking would have been required when measuring air-conduction thresholds at 500, 1000, 4000, and 8000 Hz in the right ear and 250, 1000, 2000, 4000, and 8000 Hz in the left ear.

$$AC_T - BC_{NT} \geq IA$$

Right Ear (Test Ear)		Masking Needed?
250 Hz	$35 - 0 \geq 40?$	No
500 Hz	$40 - 0 \geq 40?$	Yes
1000 Hz	$35 - (-5) \geq 40?$	Yes
2000 Hz	$35 - 0 \geq 40?$	No
4000 Hz	$40 - (-5) \geq 40?$	Yes
8000 Hz	$40 - (-5^*) \geq 40?$	Yes

Left Ear (Test Ear)		Masking Needed?
250 Hz	$40 - 0 \geq 40?$	Yes
500 Hz	$35 - 0 \geq 40?$	No
1000 Hz	$40 - (-5) \geq 40?$	Yes
2000 Hz	$40 - 0 \geq 40?$	Yes
4000 Hz	$40 - (-5) \geq 40?$	Yes
8000 Hz	$35 - (-5^*) \geq 40?$	Yes

*Estimated bone-conduction threshold

Because of reduced interaural attenuation for the supra-aural earphone, the probability of cross hearing is increased. Contralateral masking is now required. Given the presence of a bilateral conductive hearing loss, the risk of overmasking would be greatly increased.

Case 8-CDI

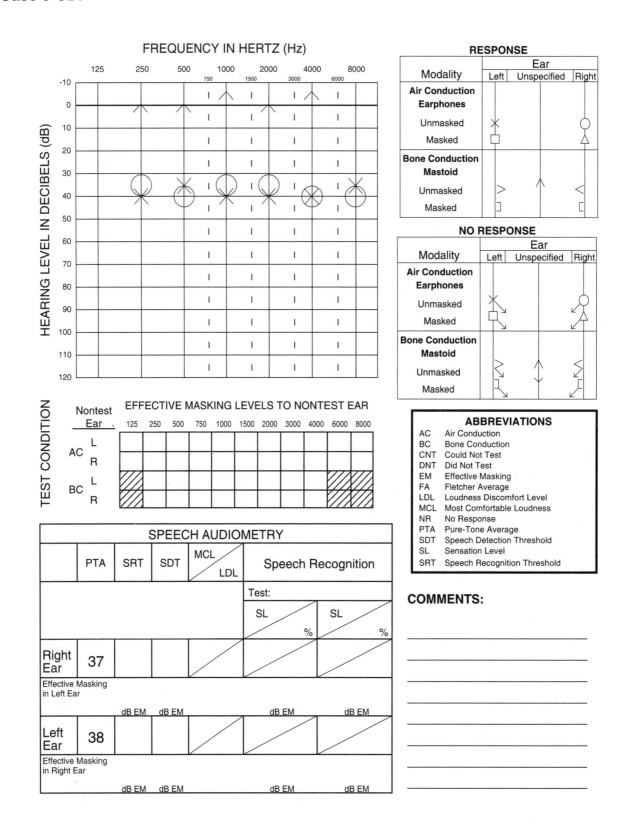

RESPONSE

Modality	Ear		
	Left	Unspecified	Right
Air Conduction Earphones			
Unmasked	×		○
Masked	□		△
Bone Conduction Mastoid			
Unmasked	>	∧	<
Masked	⊐		⊏

NO RESPONSE

Modality	Ear		
	Left	Unspecified	Right
Air Conduction Earphones			
Unmasked	×		○
Masked	□		△
Bone Conduction Mastoid			
Unmasked	>	∧	<
Masked	⊐		⊏

ABBREVIATIONS

AC	Air Conduction
BC	Bone Conduction
CNT	Could Not Test
DNT	Did Not Test
EM	Effective Masking
FA	Fletcher Average
LDL	Loudness Discomfort Level
MCL	Most Comfortable Loudness
NR	No Response
PTA	Pure-Tone Average
SDT	Speech Detection Threshold
SL	Sensation Level
SRT	Speech Recognition Threshold

SPEECH AUDIOMETRY

	PTA	SRT	SDT	MCL / LDL	Speech Recognition
					Test:
					SL / %	SL / %
Right Ear	37					
Effective Masking in Left Ear		dB EM	dB EM		dB EM	dB EM
Left Ear	38					
Effective Masking in Right Ear		dB EM	dB EM		dB EM	dB EM

COMMENTS:

_____
_____
_____
_____
_____
_____
_____
_____
_____

C. When to Mask: Pure-Tone Bone-Conduction Audiometry

Is contralateral masking required when measuring bone-conduction thresholds in either ear?

Contralateral masking is required during bone-conduction audiometry whenever comparison of the unmasked bone-conduction threshold (Unmasked BC) and the air-conduction threshold in the test ear (AC_T) at that frequency reveals a potential air-bone gap (AB Gap_T) of 15 dB or greater:

$$AB\ Gap_T \geq 15\ dB?$$
$$AC_T - Unmasked\ BC \geq 15\ dB?$$

Right Ear	AB Gap_T	AB Gap_T ≥15 dB?
250 Hz	35 – 0 = 35	Yes
500 Hz	40 – 0 = 40	Yes
1000 Hz	35 – (–5) = 40	Yes
2000 Hz	35 – 0 = 35	Yes
4000 Hz	40 – (–5) = 45	Yes
Left Ear	**AB Gap_T**	**AB Gap_T ≥15 dB?**
250 Hz	40 – 0 = 40	Yes
500 Hz	35 – 0 = 35	Yes
1000 Hz	40 – (–5) = 45	Yes
2000 Hz	40 – 0 = 40	Yes
4000 Hz	40 – (–5) = 45	Yes

Unmasked bone-conduction threshold audiometry revealed the presence of a significant conductive hearing impairment *in at least one ear*. Masked bone-conduction thresholds will be required bilaterally in order to determine if one or both ears exhibit the conductive impairment.

D. How Much Masking: Pure-Tone Bone Conduction Audiometry

I. Use of Insert Earphones

We have decided that contralateral masking will be required at all frequencies when measuring bone-conduction thresholds bilaterally. We again will use the plateau procedure to establish masked pure-tone thresholds. The initial minimum masking levels will be calculated using Martin's (1967, 1974) recommendation.

$$M_{min} = AC_{NT} + OE + 10\ dB$$

Average values when compensating for the occlusion effect with 3A insert earphones are as follows: 10 dB at 250 Hz and 0 dB at frequencies of 500 Hz and higher. Recall that only patients with either normal hearing or a sensorineural hearing loss will exhibit an occlusion effect; individuals with significant conductive pathology will not demonstrate the occlusion effect. Unmasked bone-conduction thresholds suggest the presence of a significant conductive hearing impairment in at least one ear. There is additional evidence that the conductive pathology is bilateral (e.g., otologic report, acoustic immittance measurements). Consequently, there is sufficient evidence to conclude that this patient will not exhibit the occlusion effect. It will not be necessary to compensate for this effect when calculating the minimum masking level (M_{min}).

$$M_{min} = AC_{NT} + OE + 10 \text{ dB}$$

Right Ear (Test Ear)			**How Much Masking (Nontest Ear)?**
250 Hz	40 dB HL + 10 dB + 10 dB		50 dB EM
500 Hz	35 dB HL	+ 10 dB	45 dB EM
1000 Hz	40 dB HL	+ 10 dB	50 dB EM
2000 Hz	40 dB HL	+ 10 dB	50 dB EM
4000 Hz	40 dB HL	+ 10 dB	50 dB EM

Left Ear (Test Ear)			**How Much Masking (Nontest Ear)?**
250 Hz	35 dB HL + 10 dB + 10 dB		45 dB EM
500 Hz	40 dB HL	+ 10 dB	50 dB EM
1000 Hz	35 dB HL	+ 10 dB	45 dB EM
2000 Hz	35 dB HL	+ 10 dB	45 dB EM
4000 Hz	40 dB HL	+ 10 dB	50 dB EM

We will introduce masking during the plateau procedure using the levels calculated above.

Commentary

1. It should be noted that the calculated minimum masking levels during bone-conduction audiometry would have been the same if supra-aural earphones had been used to deliver contralateral masking. Because of evidence of a bilateral conductive hearing impairment, it was not necessary to compensate for the occlusion effect. The magnitude of the occlusion effect is the only difference in the calculated minimum masking levels for 3A insert and supra-aural earphones. In this particular example, the major advantage of delivering contralateral masking through an insert earphone is an increase in the maximum permissible masking (i.e., maximum masking level), particularly in the lower frequencies (i.e., ≤ 1000 Hz).

2. Although the maximum masking level (i.e., M_{max}) is calculated in the same way when using an insert earphone, the estimated value should be greater because of increased interaural attenuation. Recall the equation for calculating M_{max}:

$$M_{max} \text{ (in dB EM)} = B_T + IA - 5 \text{ dB}$$

Let us calculate the estimated M_{max} when using 3A insert and supra-aural earphones. Remember that the unmasked bone-conduction threshold is used as our estimate of B_T.

	3A Insert Earphone	**Supra-aural Earphone**
250 Hz	0 dB + 75 dB – 5 = 70 dB	0 dB + 40 dB – 5 = 35 dB
500 Hz	0 dB + 75 dB – 5 = 70 dB	0 dB + 40 dB – 5 = 35 dB
1000 Hz	–5 dB + 75 dB – 5 = 65 dB	–5 dB + 40 dB – 5 = 30 dB
2000 Hz	0 dB + 50 dB – 5 = 45 dB	0 dB + 40 dB – 5 = 35 dB
4000 Hz	–5 dB + 50 dB – 5 = 40 dB	–5 dB + 40 dB – 5 = 30 dB

The advantage of using insert earphones to deliver contralateral masking should be apparent: Maximum masking levels are significantly increased, particularly in the lower frequencies. Consequently, the risk of overmasking is reduced.

3. Comparison of calculated minimum and maximum masking levels reveals that overmasking is a very strong possibility during masked bone-conduction threshold audiometry when using supra-aural earphones to deliver contralateral masking: M_{min} exceeds M_{max} at all frequencies.

The risk of overmasking is greatly reduced, however, when delivering contralateral masking through insert earphones, particularly in the lower frequencies. It should be noted that for both ears M_{max} exceeds M_{min} at frequencies of 250 through 1000 Hz by 15 to 25 dB. This range should allow the establishment of an adequate masking plateau. In fact, this range may even be greater if the patient's actual interaural attenuation is greater than the conservative estimate of 75 dB. Overmasking is still a possibility, however, at 2000 and 4000 Hz because of smaller interaural attenuation (i.e., 50 dB): M_{min} equals or slightly exceeds M_{max} in both ears. It will be necessary to carefully evaluate the patient's masked pure-tone responses at these frequencies. A major advantage of the plateau procedure is that observations about the relationship between the masker level in the nontest ear and the measured threshold in the test ear can rule out the occurrence of overmasking. Specifically, if a masking plateau can be established, it then can be concluded that overmasking has not occurred. Although overmasking may be predicted in a particular case, in many instances a masking plateau can be established because the patient's actual interaural attenuation is greater than the conservative value used when calculating M_{max}.

4. Recall from Chapter 5 that when using the plateau procedure, masker level can be increased using either 5-dB or 10-dB step sizes. This becomes an important consideration when overmasking is a possibility. Because the width of the masking plateau may be very narrow in cases of bilateral conductive hearing loss, it is recommended that 5-dB masker increments be used. The use of a 10-dB step size may be too large to precisely measure a masking plateau that is very narrow (i.e., 10 to 15 dB).

Case 8-EI

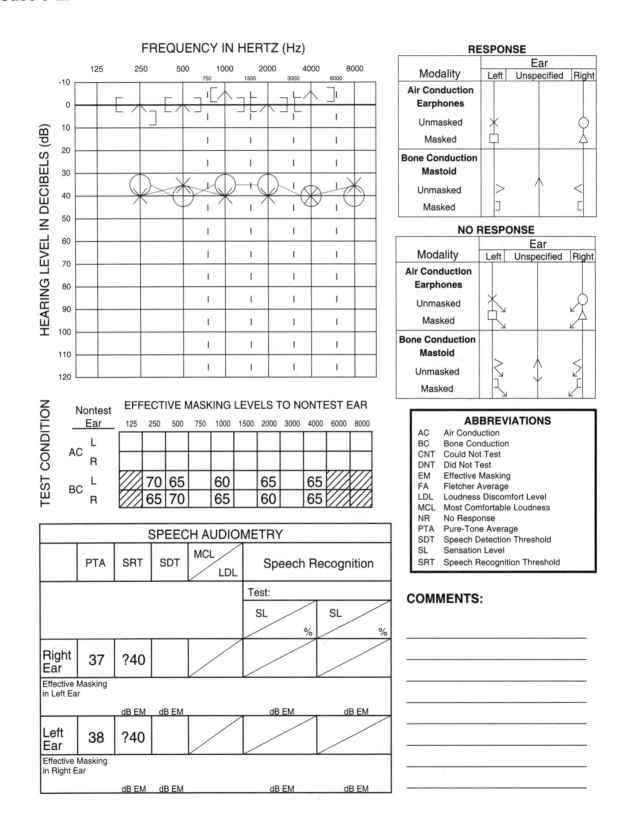

FREQUENCY IN HERTZ (Hz)

HEARING LEVEL IN DECIBELS (dB)

RESPONSE

Modality	Ear		
	Left	Unspecified	Right
Air Conduction Earphones			
Unmasked	×		○
Masked	□		△
Bone Conduction Mastoid			
Unmasked	>	∧	<
Masked	⊐		⊏

NO RESPONSE

Modality	Ear		
	Left	Unspecified	Right
Air Conduction Earphones			
Unmasked	×		○
Masked	□		△
Bone Conduction Mastoid			
Unmasked	>	∧	<
Masked	⊐		⊏

ABBREVIATIONS

AC	Air Conduction
BC	Bone Conduction
CNT	Could Not Test
DNT	Did Not Test
EM	Effective Masking
FA	Fletcher Average
LDL	Loudness Discomfort Level
MCL	Most Comfortable Loudness
NR	No Response
PTA	Pure-Tone Average
SDT	Speech Detection Threshold
SL	Sensation Level
SRT	Speech Recognition Threshold

TEST CONDITION

EFFECTIVE MASKING LEVELS TO NONTEST EAR

Nontest Ear	125	250	500	750	1000	1500	2000	3000	4000	6000	8000
AC L											
AC R											
BC L		70	65		60		65		65		
BC R		65	70		65		60		65		

SPEECH AUDIOMETRY

	PTA	SRT	SDT	MCL / LDL	Speech Recognition	
					Test:	
					SL %	SL %
Right Ear	37	?40				
Effective Masking in Left Ear			dB EM	dB EM	dB EM	dB EM
Left Ear	38	?40				
Effective Masking in Right Ear			dB EM	dB EM	dB EM	dB EM

COMMENTS:

_____

_____

_____

_____

_____

_____

_____

_____

_____

E. When to Mask: Threshold Speech Audiometry

I. Use of Insert Earphones

Masked bone-conduction thresholds have been obtained in both ears using the plateau procedure and are presented on the adjacent audiogram (see Commentary 1 below). The final masking level used to obtain masked threshold at each frequency is also reported for the nontest ear. The results of masked bone-conduction audiometry suggest the presence of conductive hearing impairment bilaterally.

Is contralateral masking required when obtaining speech recognition threshold in either ear?

Based on the pure-tone averages, it is predicted that SRTs will be measured at approximately 40 dB HL in both ears. Prior to measurement of speech recognition thresholds, we can predict whether contralateral masking will be required:

$$\text{Presentation level}_T - \text{IA} \geq \text{Best BC}_{NT}$$

Because we are using 3A insert earphones, there will be increased interaural attenuation for speech. Recall from Chapter 8 that 65 dB is *a conservative estimate of interaural attenuation for spondaic words*. We have increased interaural attenuation by 20 dB by using insert earphones rather than the conventional supra-aural configuration.

Right Ear	40 dB HL – 65 dB ≥ –5 dB HL (4000 Hz)?	
	–25 dB HL ≥ –5 dB HL?	*No*
Left Ear	40 dB HL – 65 dB ≥ –5 dB HL (1000 Hz)?	
	–25 dB HL ≥ –5 dB HL?	*No*

There will be no need for contralateral masking when measuring the SRT in either ear. The predicted level of the cross-hearing signal is lower than the best bone-conduction threshold in the nontest ear.

Commentary

1. Although overmasking was a possibility during measurement of bone-conduction thresholds, particularly above 1000 Hz, masking plateaus were established. Thus, it was possible to establish valid masked bone-conduction thresholds in both ears.

2. The need for contralateral masking was eliminated during measurement of speech recognition thresholds because of the use of 3A insert earphones. A different situation would have resulted if traditional supra-aural earphones were used. We will use a value of 45 dB as our conservative estimate of interaural attenuation when making a decision about the need for contralateral masking when measuring the SRT:

Right Ear	40 dB HL – 45 dB ≥ –5 dB HL (4000 Hz)?	
	–5 dB HL ≥ –5 dB HL?	*Yes*
Left Ear	40 dB HL – 45 dB ≥ –5 dB HL (1000 Hz)?	
	–5 dB HL ≥ –5 dB HL?	*Yes*

If supra-aural earphones had been used, contralateral masking would have been required when measuring the SRT in both ears. Because of increased interaural attenuation of 3A insert earphones, however, the need for contralateral masking was eliminated.

Case 8-GHI

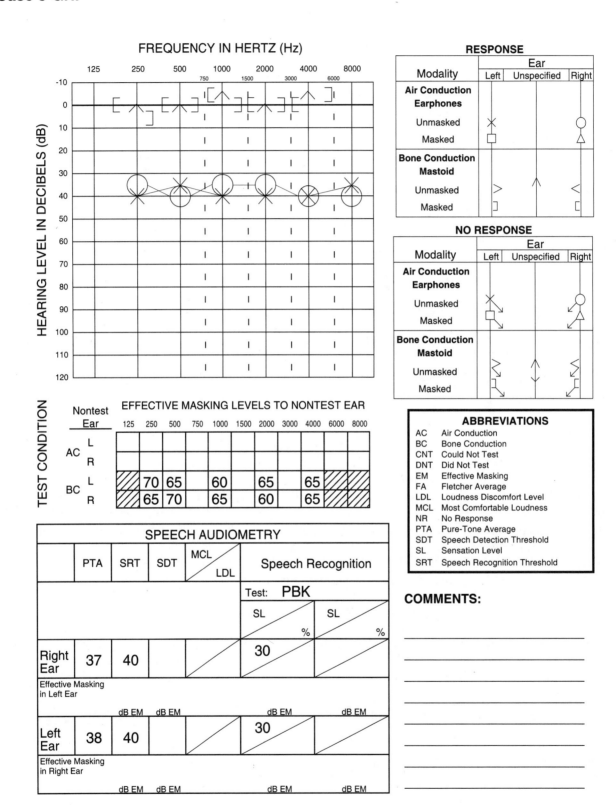

FREQUENCY IN HERTZ (Hz)

HEARING LEVEL IN DECIBELS (dB)

TEST CONDITION

EFFECTIVE MASKING LEVELS TO NONTEST EAR

Nontest Ear		125	250	500	750	1000	1500	2000	3000	4000	6000	8000
AC	L											
	R											
BC	L		70	65		60		65		65		
	R		65	70		65		60		65		

SPEECH AUDIOMETRY

	PTA	SRT	SDT	MCL / LDL	Speech Recognition			
					Test: **PBK**			
					SL	%	SL	%
Right Ear	37	40			30			
Effective Masking in Left Ear		dB EM	dB EM		dB EM		dB EM	
Left Ear	38	40			30			
Effective Masking in Right Ear		dB EM	dB EM		dB EM		dB EM	

RESPONSE

Modality	Ear		
	Left	Unspecified	Right
Air Conduction Earphones			
Unmasked	×		○
Masked	□		△
Bone Conduction Mastoid			
Unmasked	>	∧	<
Masked	]		[

NO RESPONSE

Modality	Ear		
	Left	Unspecified	Right
Air Conduction Earphones			
Unmasked	×		○
Masked	□		
Bone Conduction Mastoid			
Unmasked	>	∨	<
Masked	]		[

ABBREVIATIONS

AC   Air Conduction
BC   Bone Conduction
CNT   Could Not Test
DNT   Did Not Test
EM   Effective Masking
FA   Fletcher Average
LDL   Loudness Discomfort Level
MCL   Most Comfortable Loudness
NR   No Response
PTA   Pure-Tone Average
SDT   Speech Detection Threshold
SL   Sensation Level
SRT   Speech Recognition Threshold

COMMENTS:

G. When to Mask: Suprathreshold Speech Audiometry

I. Use of Insert Earphones

Speech recognition thresholds were obtained at 40 dB HL in both ears. Suprathreshold speech recognition will be assessed using a traditional, open-set monosyllabic word test for children: PBK-50. These lists of phonetically balanced words were developed by Haskins in 1949 and are considered appropriate for children (with normal speech and language) approximately of five and a half years and older (Sanderson-Leepa & Rintelmann, 1976). Materials will be presented using monitored live voice. In this particular case, we will present the test words at 30 dB SL re: SRT. The patient reported that speech was comfortably loud when presented at 30 dB SL (i.e., 70 dB HL).

Is contralateral masking required when assessing suprathreshold speech recognition ability at 30 dB SL? Recall our rule for when to mask during speech audiometry:

$$\text{Presentation level}_T - IA \geq \text{Best BC}_{NT}$$

Presentation level during suprathreshold speech audiometry is determined by simply adding the selected sensation level (i.e., 30 dB SL) to the SRT of the test ear:

Right Ear	Presentation level = 40 dB HL + 30 dB SL = 70 dB HL
Left Ear	Presentation level = 40 dB HL + 30 dB SL = 70 dB HL

In this example, we will use the very conservative value of 55 dB as our estimate of interaural attenuation for suprathreshold speech. Recall from Chapter 8 that there is some evidence that a more conservative estimate of interaural attenuation should be used when measuring suprathreshold speech recognition (i.e., a 10-dB more conservative value than that used for the SRT—65 dB). Is contralateral masking required in either ear?

Right Ear	70 dB HL – 55 dB ≥ –5 dB HL?	
	15 dB HL ≥ –5 dB HL?	*Yes*
Left Ear	70 dB HL – 55 dB ≥ –5 dB HL?	
	15 dB HL ≥ –5 dB HL?	*Yes*

Contralateral masking will be required when assessing suprathreshold speech recognition ability in both ears. This is not unexpected given the relatively high presentation level (i.e., 70 dB HL) and the presence of normal hearing sensitivity by bone conduction.

Commentary

1. It should be noted that contralateral masking would also have been required when assessing suprathreshold speech recognition ability *if traditional supra-aural earphones had been used*. However, the probability of overmasking would be greatly increased when using traditional earphones because of their decreased interaural attenuation. The use of 3A insert earphones will reduce the probability of overmasking in cases of bilateral, conductive hearing impairment.

H. How Much Masking: Suprathreshold Speech Audiometry

I. Use of Insert Earphones

How much contralateral masking should be used when assessing suprathreshold speech recognition ability in the left ear?

We will use the mid-masking method for selecting an appropriate masking level during assessment of suprathreshold speech recognition. Recall that mid-masking level (M_{mid}) is the midpoint between the minimum (M_{min}) and maximum (M_{max}) masking levels. Mid-masking level can be calculated as follows:

$$M_{mid} = (M_{max} + M_{min}) / 2$$

where

$$M_{min} = \text{Presentation level}_T - \text{IA} + \text{Max AB gap}_{NT}$$
$$M_{max} = \text{Best BC}_T + \text{IA} - 5 \text{ dB}$$

Bone-conduction sensitivity is always considered at frequencies from 250 through 4000 Hz.

Right Ear M_{min} = 70 dB HL – 55 dB + 45 dB (at 4000 Hz)
            = 60 dB EM

M_{max} = –5 dB HL (at 1000 Hz) + 55 dB – 5 dB
            = 45 dB EM

M_{mid} = Cannot be determined ($M_{min} \geq M_{max}$)

Left Ear M_{min} = 70 dB HL – 55 dB + 40 dB
            = 55 dB EM

M_{max} = –5 dB HL (at 4000 Hz) + 55 dB – 5 dB
            = 45 dB EM

M_{mid} = Cannot be determined ($M_{min} \geq M_{max}$)

The mid-masking level cannot be determined because M_{min} exceeds M_{max}. Although we are using insert earphones, a masking dilemma has resulted. Ideally, the selected masking level should be at least 10 dB above the minimum required (i.e., 10 dB safety factor). Using this rule (i.e., the "minimum noise method"), masking levels of 70 dB EM and 65 dB EM would be selected when testing the right and left ears respectively. Unfortunately, these levels could result in overmasking. How can we approach this masking dilemma?

First, we could proceed and present the masker at the originally selected levels. There is a possibility that overmasking *may not* occur. Remember that we are using a very conservative estimate of interaural attenuation. Yet, the range of interaural attenuation for speech is large (e.g., Snyder, 1973). If interaural attenuation for our patient is significantly greater than the minimum value reported in the literature, then overmasking may not occur. In addition, if some noise has in fact crossed over to the test ear, it is possible that an adequate signal-to-noise ratio may be maintained in the test ear when evaluating *suprathreshold* speech recognition. Although this is not the ideal situation, the patient may be still be able to achieve maximum word recognition performance.

Second, we may choose to use a lower level of contralateral masking. Although a 10-dB safety factor is desirable and recommended, the masker could be presented at a level that is 5 to 10 dB less in intensity. Of course, the contralateral masker should be presented at a level that is at least equal to M_{min}.

Third, we may decide *not to test* suprathreshold word recognition ability because of the risk of overmasking. In this particular case study, the patient was previously evaluated six months earlier. Results at that time revealed normal hearing sensitivity and suprathreshold word recognition ability in both ears. Consequently, it may not be critical to re-evaluate suprathreshold word recognition ability at this time. Information about hearing sensitivity is clearly more relevant to the physician because of the medical diagnosis of otitis media with effusion.

In this particular case, we will handle our masking dilemma using the last approach. Specifically, we will eliminate suprathreshold speech recognition testing from the current evaluation.

Commentary

1. Recall that the short-cut approach for selecting an appropriate level of masking during suprathreshold speech audiometry can be used *provided that the following two conditions are met*: a) There are no *significant* air-bone gaps in either ear; b) suprathreshold speech recognition is evaluated at a *moderate* sensation level (i.e., approximately 40 dB SL). The short-cut approach for selecting masking level during suprathreshold speech audiometry is not appropriate in this particular example because the first prerequisite has not been met. Examination of the pure-tone audiogram reveals significant air-bone gaps in both ears. Because overmasking is a potential problem in any case of bilateral, conductive hearing impairment, information about characteristics of the masking plateau (i.e., M_{min} and M_{max}) is critical when selecting masking levels. The midplateau procedure should always be used in such cases.

2. This case study clearly demonstrates that the use of insert earphones does not solve all masking dilemmas, particularly during suprathreshold testing.

Case 8-J

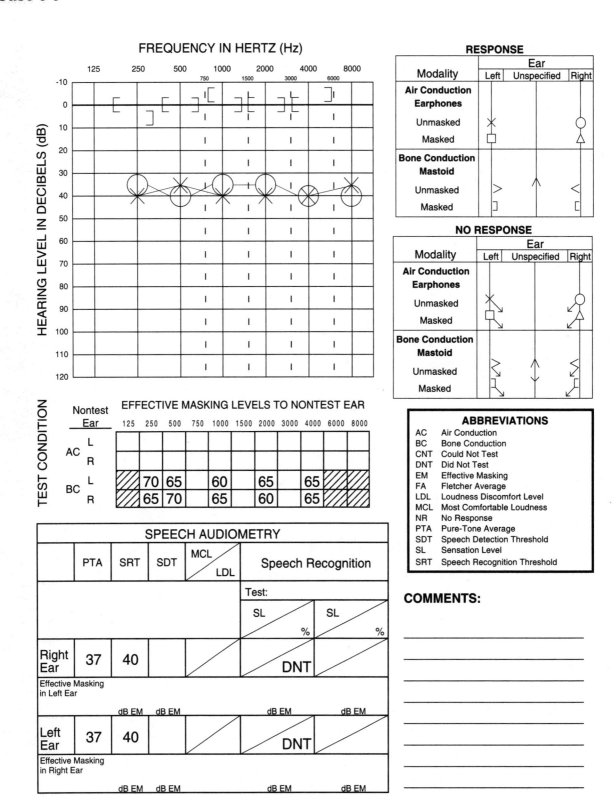

FREQUENCY IN HERTZ (Hz)

RESPONSE

Modality	Ear		
	Left	Unspecified	Right
Air Conduction Earphones			
Unmasked	×		○
Masked	☐		△
Bone Conduction Mastoid			
Unmasked	>	∧	<
Masked	]		[

NO RESPONSE

Modality	Ear		
	Left	Unspecified	Right
Air Conduction Earphones			
Unmasked	×		○
Masked	☐		△
Bone Conduction Mastoid			
Unmasked	>	∧	<
Masked	]		[

EFFECTIVE MASKING LEVELS TO NONTEST EAR

Nontest Ear	125	250	500	750	1000	1500	2000	3000	4000	6000	8000
AC L											
AC R											
BC L		70	65		60		65		65		
BC R		65	70		65		60		65		

ABBREVIATIONS

AC   Air Conduction
BC   Bone Conduction
CNT   Could Not Test
DNT   Did Not Test
EM   Effective Masking
FA   Fletcher Average
LDL   Loudness Discomfort Level
MCL   Most Comfortable Loudness
NR   No Response
PTA   Pure-Tone Average
SDT   Speech Detection Threshold
SL   Sensation Level
SRT   Speech Recognition Threshold

SPEECH AUDIOMETRY

	PTA	SRT	SDT	MCL / LDL	Speech Recognition	
					Test:	
					SL ____ %	SL ____ %
Right Ear	37	40				DNT
Effective Masking in Left Ear		dB EM	dB EM		dB EM	dB EM
Left Ear	37	40				DNT
Effective Masking in Right Ear		dB EM	dB EM		dB EM	dB EM

COMMENTS:

_____

_____

_____

_____

_____

_____

_____

_____

_____

J. Audiogram Interpretation

Pure-tone testing revealed a mild, conductive hearing impairment of flat configuration bilaterally. Speech recognition thresholds confirmed the pure-tone findings.

Tympanometry revealed no point of maximum admittance with changes in air pressure bilaterally. The flat tympanograms with normal equivalent ear canal volumes in both ears are consistent with the medical diagnosis of middle ear effusion. Contralateral and ipsilateral acoustic reflexes were absent bilaterally, a finding consistent with the presence of bilateral conductive hearing impairment.

Endnotes

1. It is beyond the scope of this book to review acoustic immittance measurements. Silman and Silverman (1991) provide an outstanding review of the clinical applications of acoustic immittance measurements.

Directory of Case Studies

A. When to Mask: Pure-Tone Air-Conduction Audiometry
   Cases 1–8

B. How Much Masking: Pure-Tone Air-Conduction Audiometry
   Cases 2, 3, 5, 6, 7

C. When to Mask: Pure-Tone Bone-Conduction Audiometry
   Cases 1–8

D. How Much Masking: Pure-Tone Bone-Conduction Audiometry
   Cases 2, 3, 4, 5, 6, 7, 8

E. When to Mask: Threshold Speech Audiometry
   Cases 1–8

F. How Much Masking: Threshold Speech Audiometry
   Cases 2, 5, 6, 7

G. When to Mask: Suprathreshold Speech Audiometry
   Cases 1–8

H. How Much Masking: Suprathreshold Speech Audiometry
   Cases 1, 2, 3, 4, 5, 7, 8

I. Use of Insert Earphones
   Cases 3, 8

J. Audiogram Interpretation
   Cases 1–8

References

American National Standards Institute. (1969). *Specification for audiometers* (ANSI S3.6-1969). New York: Author.

American National Standards Institute. (1989). *Specification for audiometers* (ANSI S3.6-1989). New York: Author.

American National Standards Institute. (1992). *Standard reference zero for the calibration of pure-tone bone-conduction audiometers* (ANSI S3.43-1992). New York: Author.

American Speech and Hearing Association. (1974). Guidelines for audiometric symbols. *ASHA, 16*, 260–264.

American Speech-Language-Hearing Association Committee. (1978). Guidelines for manual pure-tone threshold audiometry. *ASHA, 19*, 236–240.

American Speech-Language-Hearing Association. (1988). Guidelines for determining threshold level for speech. *ASHA, 30*, 85–89.

American Speech-Language-Hearing Association. (1990). Guidelines for audiometric symbols. *ASHA* (Suppl. 2), 25–30.

Barry, S.J. (1994). Can bone conduction thresholds really be poorer than air? *American Journal of Audiology, 3*, 21–22.

Beattie, R.C., Edgerton, B.J., & Svihovec, D.V. (1977). A comparison of the Auditec of St. Louis cassette recordings of NU-6 and CID W-22 on a normal hearing population. *Journal of Speech and Hearing Disorders, 42*, 60–64.

Beattie, R.C., & Raffin, M.J.M. (1985). Reliability of threshold, slope, and PB max for monosyllabic words. *Journal of Speech and Hearing Disorders, 50*, 166–178.

Beattie, R.C., Svihovec, D.V., & Edgerton, B.J. (1978). Comparison of speech detection and spondee thresholds for half- versus full-list intelligibility scores with MLV and taped presentations of NU-6. *Journal of the American Audiology Society, 3*, 267–272.

Beattie, R.C., & Zipp, J.A. (1990). Range of intensities yielding PB max and threshold for monosyllabic words for hearing impaired subjects. *Journal of Speech and Hearing Disorders, 55*, 417–426.

Beauchaine, K.A., Kaminski, J.R., & Gorga, M.P. (1987). Comparison of Beyer DT48 and Etymotic insert earphones: Auditory brain stem response measurements. *Ear and Hearing, 8*, 292–297.

Bekésy, G. v. (1948). Vibration of the head in a sound field and its role in hearing by bone conduction. *Journal of the Acoustical Society of America, 20*, 749–760.

Berger, E.H., & Kerivan, J.E. (1983). Influence of physiological noise and the occlusion effect on the measurement of real-ear attenuation at threshold. *Journal of the Acoustical Society of America, 74,* 81–94.

Berger, E.H., & Killion, M.C. (1989). Comparison of the noise attenuation of three audiometric earphones, with additional data on masking near threshold. *Journal of the Acoustical Society of America, 86,* 1392–1403.

Berrett, M.V. (1973). Some relations between interaural attenuation and the occlusion effect. Unpublished doctoral dissertation, University of Iowa, Iowa City.

Bess, F. H. (1983). Clinical assessment of speech recognition. In D.F. Konkle & W.F. Rintelmann (Eds.), *Principles of speech audiometry* (pp. 127–201). Baltimore: University Park Press.

Blackwell, K.L., Oyler, R.F., & Seyfried, D.N. (1991). A clinical comparison of Grason Stadler insert earphones and TDH-50P standard earphones. *Ear and Hearing, 12,* 361–362.

Boothroyd, A., & Cawkwell, S. (1970). Vibrotactile thresholds in pure tone audiometry. *Acta Otolaryngologica, 69,* 381–387.

Borton, T.E., Nolen, B.L., Luks, S.B., & Meline, N.C. (1989). Clinical applicability of insert earphones for audiometry. *Audiology, 28,* 61–70.

Cabot Safety Corporation, Auditory Systems Division (1990). Instructions for use of E-A-RTone™ 3A insert earphones. Cabot Safety Corporation, 5407 W. 79th Street, Indianapolis, IN 46268.

Carhart, R. (1957). Clinical determination of abnormal auditory adaptation. *Archives of Otolaryngology, 65,* 32–39.

Chaiklin, J.B. (1959). The relation among three selected auditory speech thresholds. *Journal of Speech and Hearing Research, 2,* 237–243.

Chaiklin, J.B. (1967). Interaural attenuation and cross-hearing in air-conduction audiometry. *Journal of Auditory Research, 7,* 413–424.

Chaiklin, J.B., & McClellan, M.E. (1971). Audiometric management of collapsible ear canals. *Archives of Otolaryngology, 93,* 397–407.

Clark, J.L., & Roeser, R.J. (1988). Three studies comparing performance of the ER-3A tubephone with the TDH-50P earphone. *Ear and Hearing, 9,* 268–274.

Clemis, J.D., Ballad, W.J., & Killion, M.C. (1986). Clinical use of an insert earphone. *Annals of Otology, Rhinology, and Laryngology, 95,* 520–524.

Coles, R.R.A., & Priede, V.M. (1970). On the misdiagnosis resulting from incorrect use of masking. *Journal of Laryngology and Otology, 84,* 41–63.

Coles, R.R.A., & Priede, V.M. (1975). Masking of the non-test ear in speech audiometry. *The Journal of Laryngology and Otology, 89,* 217–226.

Dirks, D.D. (1994). Bone-conduction threshold testing. In J. Katz (Ed.), *Handbook of clinical audiology* (4th ed.) (pp. 132–146). Baltimore: Williams & Wilkins.

Dirks, D.D., & Malmquist, C. (1964). Changes in bone-conduction thresholds produced by masking in the non-test ear. *Journal of Speech and Hearing Research, 7,* 271–278.

Dirks, D.D., & Morgan D.E. (1983). Measures of discomfort and most comfortable loudness. In D.F. Konkle & W.F. Rintelmann (Eds.), *Principles of speech audiometry* (pp. 203–229). Baltimore: University Park Press.

Dirks, D.D., & Swindeman, J.G. (1967). The variability of occluded and unoccluded bone-conduction thresholds. *Journal of Speech and Hearing Research, 10,* 232–249.

Dunn, H.K., & White, S.D. (1940). Statistical measurements on conversational speech. *Journal of the Acoustical Society of America, 11,* 278–288.

Elpern, B.S., & Naunton, R.F. (1963). The stability of the occlusion effect. *Archives of Otolaryngology, 77,* 376–382.

Etymotic Research (1991). ER-3A Tubephone™ insert earphone. Etymotic Research, 61 Martin Lane, Elk Grove Village, IL 60007.

Feldman, A.S. (1963). Maximum air-conduction hearing loss. *Journal of Speech and Hearing Disorders, 6,* 157–163.

Fletcher, H. (1940). Auditory patterns. *Review of Modern Physics, 12,* 47–65.

Frank, T., & Craig, C.H. (1984). Comparison of the Auditec and Rintelmann recordings of NU-6. *Journal of Speech and Hearing Disorders, 49,* 267–271.

Frank, T., & Vavrek, M.J. (1992). Reference threshold levels for an ER-3A insert earphone. *Journal of the American Academy of Audiology, 3,* 51–58.

Frank, T., & Wright, D.C. (1990). Attenuation provided by four different audiometric earphone systems. *Ear and Hearing, 11,* 70–78.

Franks, J.R., Engel, D.P., & Themann, C.L. (1992). Real ear attenuation at threshold for three audiometric headphone devices: Implications for maximum permissible ambient noise level standards. *Ear and Hearing, 13,* 2–10.

Gelfand, S.A., Schwander, R., & Silman, S. (1990). Acoustic reflex thresholds in normal and cochlear-impaired ears: Effects of no response rates on 90th percentiles in a large sample. *Journal of Speech and Hearing Disorders, 55,* 198–205.

Goldstein, D.P., & Hayes, C.S. (1965). The occlusion effect in bone-conduction hearing. *Journal of Speech and Hearing Research, 8,* 137–148.

Hall, J.W. (1991). Classic site-of-lesion tests: Foundation of diagnostic audiology. In W.F. Rintelmann (Ed.), *Hearing assessment* (2nd ed.) (pp. 653–677). Needham Heights, MA: Allyn & Bacon.

Hall, J.W. (1992). *Handbook of auditory evoked responses.* Needham Heights, MA: Allyn & Bacon.

Haskins, H. (1949). A phonetically balanced test of speech discrimination for children. Unpublished doctoral dissertation, Northwestern University, Evanston, Illinois.

Hawkins, J.E., & Stevens, S.S. (1950). Masking of pure tones and of speech by white noise. *Journal of the Acoustical Society of America, 22,* 6–13.

Hildyard, V.H., & Valentine, M.A. (1962). Collapse of the ear canal during audiometry. *Archives of Otolaryngology, 75,* 422–423.

Hodgson, W. (1980). *Basic audiologic evaluation.* Baltimore: Williams & Wilkins.

Hodgson, W., & Tillman, T. (1966). Reliability of bone conduction occlusion effects in normals. *Journal of Auditory Research, 6,* 141–151.

Hood, J.D. (1955). Auditory fatigue and adaptation in the differential diagnosis of end-organ disease. *Annals of Otology, Rhinology, and Laryngology, 64,* 507–518.

Hood, J.D. (1960). The principles and practice of bone-conduction audiometry. *Laryngoscope, 70,* 1211–1228.

Hosford-Dunn, H., Kuklinski, A.L., Raggio, M., & Haggerty, H.S. (1986). Solving audiometric masking dilemmas with an insert masker. *Archives of Otolaryngology, Head and Neck Surgery, 112,* 92–95.

Jerger, J., & Jerger, S. (1975). A simplified tone decay test. *Archives of Otolaryngology, 101,* 403–407.

Kaplan, H., Gladstone, V.S., & Lloyd, L.L. (1993). *Audiometric interpretation* (2nd ed.). Needham Heights, MA: Allyn & Bacon.

Killion, M.C. (1984). New insert earphones for audiometry. *Hearing Instruments, 35,* 28, 46.

Killion, M.C., & Villchur, E. (1989). Comments on "Earphones in audiometry" [Zwislocki et al., J. Acoust. Soc. Am. 83, 1688–1689)]. *Journal of the Acoustical Society of America, 85,* 1775–1778.

Killion, M.C., Wilber, L.A., & Gudmundsen, G.I. (1985). Insert earphones for more interaural attenuation. *Hearing Instruments, 36,* 34–36.

Konkle, D.F., & Berry, G.A. (1983). Masking in speech audiometry. In D.F. Konkle & W.F. Rintelmann (Eds.), *Principles of speech audiometry* (pp. 285–319). Baltimore: University Park Press.

Konkle, D.F., & Orchik, D.J. (1979). Auditory adaptation. In W.F. Rintelmann (Ed.), *Hearing assessment* (pp. 207–233). Baltimore: University Park Press.

Liden, G., Nilsson, G., & Anderson, H. (1959). Masking in clinical audiometry. *Acta Oto-Laryngologica, 50,* 125–136.

Lilly, D.J., & Purdy, J.K. (1993). On the routine use of Tubephone™ insert earphones. *American Journal of Audiology, 2,* 17–20.

Lindgren, F. (1990). A comparison of the variability in thresholds measured with insert and conventional supra-aural earphones. *Scandinavian Audiology, 19,* 19–23.

Littler, T.S., Knight, J.J., & Strange, P.H. (1952). Hearing by bone conduction and the use of bone-conduction hearing aids. *Proceedings of the Royal Society of Medicine, 45,* 783–790.

Margolis, R.H., & Heller, J.W. (1987). Screening tympanometry: Criteria for medical referral. *Audiology, 26,* 197–208.

Martin, F.N. (1966). Speech audiometry and clinical masking. *Journal of Auditory Research, 6,* 199–203.

Martin, F.N. (1967). A simplified method for clinical masking. *Journal of Auditory Research, 7,* 59–62.

Martin, F.N. (1974). Minimum effective masking levels in threshold audiometry. *Journal of Speech and Hearing Disorders, 39,* 280–285.

Martin, F.N. (1980). The masking plateau revisited. *Ear and Hearing, 1,* 112–116.

Martin, F.N. (1994). *Introduction to audiology* (5th ed.). Needham Heights, MA: Allyn & Bacon.

Martin, F.N., Armstrong, T.W., & Champlin, C.A. (1994). A survey of audiological practices in the United States in 1992. *American Journal of Audiology, 3,* 20–26.

Martin, F.N., Bailey, H.A.T., & Pappas, J.J. (1965). The effect of central masking on threshold for speech. *Journal of Auditory Research, 5,* 293–296.

Martin, F.N., & Blythe, M.E (1977). On the cross hearing of spondaic words. *Journal of Auditory Research, 17,* 221–224.

Martin, F.N., Butler, E.C., & Burns, P. (1974). Audiometric Bing test for determination of minimum masking levels for bone conduction tests. *Journal of Speech and Hearing Disorders, 39,* 148–152.

Martin, F.N., & DiGiovanni, D. (1979). Central masking effects on spondee threshold as a function of masker sensation level and masker sound pressure level. *Journal of the American Auditory Society, 4,* 141–146.

Martin, F.N., & Forbis, N.K. (1978). The present status audiometric practice: A follow-up study. *ASHA, 20,* 531–541.

Martin, F.N., & Morris, L.J. (1989). Current audiologic practices in the United States. *The Hearing Journal, 42,* 25–44.

Martin, F.N., & Pennington, C.D. (1971). Current trends in audiometric practice. *ASHA, 13,* 671–677.

Martin, F.N., Severance, G.K., & Thibodeau, L. (1991). Insert earphones for speech recognition testing. *Journal of the American Academy of Audiology, 2,* 55–58.

Martin, F.N., & Sides, D.G. (1985). Survey of current audiometric practices. *ASHA, 27,* 29–36.

Michael, P.L., & Bienvenue, G.R. (1980). A comparison of acoustical performance between a new one-piece cushion and the conventional two-piece MX-41/AR cushion. *Journal of the Acoustical Society of America, 67,* 693–698.

Michael, P.L., & Bienvenue, G.R. (1981). Noise attenuation characteristics for supra-aural audiometric headsets using the models MX-41/AR and 51 earphone cushions. *Journal of the Acoustical Society of America, 70,* 1235–1238.

Mueller, H.G., & Bright, K.E. (1994). Selection and verification of maximum output. In M. Valente (Ed.), *Strategies for selecting and verifying hearing aid fittings* (pp. 38–63). New York: Thieme Medical Publishers, Inc.

Nábělek, A.K., & Nábělek, I.V. (1994). Room acoustics and speech perception. In J. Katz (Ed.), *Handbook of clinical audiology* (4th ed.) (pp. 624–637). Baltimore: Williams & Wilkins.

Naunton, R.F. (1960). A masking dilemma in bilateral conduction deafness. *Archives of Otolaryngology, 72,* 753–757.

Nober, E.H. (1964). Pseudoauditory bone-conduction thresholds. *Journal of Speech and Hearing Disorders, 29,* 469–476.

Nober, E.H. (1970). Cutile air and bone conduction thresholds of the deaf. *Exceptional Children, 36,* 571–579.

Olsen, W.O., & Matkin, N.D. (1991). Speech audiometry. In W.R. Rintelmann (Ed.), *Hearing assessment* (pp. 39–140). Needham Heights, MA: Allyn & Bacon.

Olsen, W.O., & Noffsinger, P.D. (1974). Comparison of one new and three old tests of auditory adaptation. *Archives of Otolaryngology, 96,* 231–247.

Owens, E., Kessler, D.K., Telleen, C.C., & Schubert, E.D. (1981). The minimal auditory capabilities (MAC) battery. *Hearing Aid Journal, 34,* 9, 32, 34.

Owens, E., Kessler, D.K., Witte-Raggio, M., & Schubert, E.D. (1985). Analysis and revision of the minimal auditory capabilities (MAC) battery. *Ear and Hearing, 6,* 280–290.

Owens, E., & Schubert, E.D. (1977). Development of the California consonant test. *Journal of Speech and Hearing Research, 20,* 463–474.

Pennington, C.D., & Martin, F.N. (1972). Current trends in audiometric practices: Part II—Auditory tests for site of lesion. *ASHA, 14,* 199–203.

Punch, J.L., & Howard, M.T. (1985). Spondee recognition threshold as a function of set size. *Journal of Speech and Hearing Disorders, 50,* 120–125.

Rintelmann, W.F., & Associates. (1974). Six experiments on speech discrimination utilizing CNC monosyllables. *Journal of Auditory Research* (Suppl. 2), 1–30.

Rosenberg, P.E. (1958, November). *Rapid clinical measurement of tone decay*. Paper presented at the annual convention of the American Speech and Hearing Association, New York.

Rudmin, F. (1983). False air-bone gap. *Ear and Hearing, 4,* 106–107.

Sanders, J.W. (1972). Masking. In J. Katz (Ed.), *Handbook of clinical audiology* (pp. 111–142). Baltimore: Williams & Wilkins.

Sanders, J.W. (1978). Masking. In J. Katz (Ed.), *Handbook of clinical audiology* (2nd ed.) (pp. 124–140). Baltimore: Williams & Wilkins.

Sanders, J.W. (1991). Clinical masking. In W.F. Rintelmann (Ed.), *Hearing assessment* (2nd ed,) (pp. 141–178). Needham Heights, MA: Allyn & Bacon.

Sanders, F.W., & Rintelmann, W.F. (1964). Masking in audiometry. *Archives of Otolaryngology, 80,* 541–556.

Sanderson-Leepa, M.E., & Rintelmann, W.F. (1976). Articulation function and test-retest performance of normal-hearing children on three speech discrimination tests: WIPI, PBK-50, and NU auditory Test No. 6. *Journal of Speech and Hearing Disorders, 41,* 503–519.

Schow, R.L., & Goldbaum, D.E. (1980). Collapsed ear canals in the elderly nursing home population. *Journal of Speech and Hearing Disorders, 45,* 259–267.

Schwartz, D.M., & Surr, R. (1979). Three experiments on the California consonant test. *Journal of Speech and Hearing Disorders, 64,* 61–72.

Sher, A.E., & Owens, E. (1974). Consonant confusions associated with hearing loss above 2000 Hz. *Journal of Speech and Hearing Research, 17,* 669–680.

Silman, S., & Silverman, C.A. (1991). *Auditory diagnosis: Principles and applications*. San Diego: Academic Press.

Sklare, D.A., & Denenberg, L.J. (1987). Interaural attenuation for Tubephone insert earphones, *Ear and Hearing, 8,* 298–300.

Snyder, J.M. (1973). Interaural attenuation characteristics in audiometry. *Laryngoscope, 73,* 1847–1855.

Spencer, R., & Priede, V.M. (1974). The effects of contralateral masking on the intelligibility of speech. Unpublished manuscript, Institute of Sound and Vibration Research, Southampton. Cited in Coles, R.R.A., & Priede, V.M. (1975). Masking of the non-test ear in speech audiometry. *The Journal of Laryngology and Otology, 89,* 217–226.

Stuart, A., Stenstrom, R., Tompkins, C., & Vandenhoff, S. (1991). Test-retest variability in audiometric threshold with supra-aural and insert earphones among children and adults. *Audiology, 30,* 82–90.

Studebaker, G.A. (1962). On masking in bone-conduction testing. *Journal of Speech and Hearing Research, 5,* 215–227.

Studebaker, G.A. (1964). Clinical masking of air- and bone-conducted stimuli. *Journal of Speech and Hearing Disorders, 29,* 23–35.

Studebaker, G.A. (1967a). Clinical masking of the non-test ear. *Journal of Speech and Hearing Disorders, 32,* 360–371.

Studebaker, G.A. (1967b). Intertest variability and the air-bone gap. *Journal of Speech and Hearing Disorders, 32,* 82–86.

Studebaker, G.A. (1979). Clinical masking. In W.F. Rintelmann (Ed.), *Hearing assessment* (pp. 51–100). Baltimore: University Park Press.

Thurlow, W.R., Silverman, S.R., Davis, H., & Walsh, T.E. (1948). A statistical study of auditory tests in relation to the fenestration operation. *Laryngoscope, 58*, 43–66.

Tillman, T.W., & Carhart, R. (1966). An expanded test for speech discrimination utilizing CNC monosyllabic words. Northwestern University Auditory Test No. 6. Brooks Air Force Base, TX: USAF School of Aerospace Medicine Technical Report.

Tillman, T.W., & Olsen, W.O. (1973). Speech audiometry. In J. Jerger (Ed.), *Modern developments in audiology* (2nd ed.) (pp. 37–74). New York: Academic Press.

Tonndorf, J. (1968). A new concept of bone conduction. *Archives of Otolaryngology, 87*, 49–54.

Tonndorf, J. (1972). Bone conduction. In J.V. Tobias (Ed.), *Foundations of Modern auditory theory, Vol. II* (pp. 197–237). New York: Academic Press.

Tyler, R.S., Gantz, B.J., McCabe, B.F., Lowder, M.V., Otto, S.R., & Preece, J.P. (1985). Audiological results with two single channel cochlear implants. *Annals of Otology, Rhinology, and Laryngology, 94*, 133–139.

Valente, M., Valente, M., & Goebel, J. (1992). High-frequency thresholds: Circumaural earphone versus insert earphone. *Journal of the American Academy of Audiology, 3*, 410–418.

Van Camp, K.J., Margolis, R.H., Wilson, R.H., Creten, W.L., & Shanks, J.E. (1986). Principles of tympanometry. *ASHA Monograph Number 24*. Rockville, MD: American Speech-Language-Hearing Association.

Van Campen, L.E., Sammeth, C.A., & Peek, B.F. (1990). Interaural attenuation using Etymotic ER-3A insert earphones in auditory brain stem response testing. *Ear and Hearing, 11*, 66–69.

Ventry, I.M., Chaiklin, J.B., & Boyle, W.F. (1961). Collapse of the ear canal during audiometry. *Archives of Otolaryngology, 73*, 727–731.

Wegel, R.L., & Lane, G.I. (1924). The auditory masking of one pure tone by another and its probable relation to the dynamics of the inner ear. *Physics Review, 23*, 266–285.

Wiley, T.L., Oviatt, D.L., & Block, M.G. (1987). Acoustic-immittance measures in normal ears. *Journal of Speech and Hearing Research, 30*, 161–170.

Wright, D.C., & Frank, T. (1992). Attenuation values for a supra-aural earphone for children and insert earphones for children and adults. *Ear and Hearing, 13*, 454–459.

Zwislocki, J. (1953). Acoustic attenuation between the ears. *Journal of the Acoustical Society of America, 25*, 752–759.

Zwislocki, J., Kruger, B., Miller, J.D., Niemoeller, A.R., Shaw, E.A., & Studebaker, G. (1988). Earphones in audiometry. *Journal of the Acoustical Society of America, 83*, 1688–1689.

Index